Discover the Power
of Integrative Oncology

A Better Way To Treat Cancer

A Comprehensive Guide to Understanding,
Preventing, and Most Effectively Treating
Our Biggest Health Threat

Michael Karlfeldt, ND, PhD

Praise for Dr. Karlfeldt and *A Better Way To Treat Cancer*

Dr. Karlfeldt's *A Better Way To Treat Cancer* is a groundbreaking guide that mirrors my belief in the power of integrative oncology. His extensive experience and insightful exploration of cancer treatment provide not just a comprehensive guide, but a lifeline to those impacted by cancer. This book underscores the importance of a holistic approach to health and patient empowerment. I believe this is essential reading for patients, caregivers, and loved ones.

— **Dr. Paul Anderson,
author of Cancer - The Journey from Diagnosis to
Empowerment and co-author of Outside
the Box Cancer Therapies**

Dr. Karlfeldt's *A Better Way To Treat Cancer* presents a life-changing endorsement to the healing power of integrative oncology, a truly invaluable tool in the fight against cancer. Dr. Karlfeldt's decades of experience and unique perspective bring important and fresh insight into the complex landscape of cancer treatment and prevention. If there is just one book you need to read this year it is this one.

— **Ann Louise Gittleman, PhD, CNS,
multiple award-winning NY Times Best Selling Author of 35 books**

What an informative book! *A Better Way To Treat Cancer* provides a comprehensive holistic perspective on cancer and how to address it. A must-read for anyone facing cancer!

— **Dr. Isaac Eliaz, MD, MS, LAc,
author of The Survival Paradox**

In *A Better Way To Treat Cancer*, Dr. Karlfeldt masterfully outlines a comprehensive and deeply insightful approach to cancer treatment and prevention. His application of Photo Dynamic Therapy and energy healing reflects our shared vision for effective, holistic care. This book is more than a guide - it's a call to action and a beacon of hope for anyone touched by cancer. A must-read for patients, caregivers, and healthcare providers.

**— Leigh Erin Connealy, MD,
Author of the Cancer Revolution and Be Perfectly Healthy**

Having embarked on my own journey through breast cancer, I am profoundly aware of the power of comprehensive, integrative approaches to this formidable disease. Dr. Michael Karlfeldt's *A Better Way to Treat Cancer* exemplifies this approach—offering a holistic, patient-centered road map that empowers individuals to reclaim their health. As both a fellow healthcare professional and a survivor, I have experienced firsthand the potency of the strategies Dr. Karlfeldt elucidates. This book showcases his expertise, passion, and commitment to revolutionizing how we confront cancer. Whether you're seeking to prevent cancer, are currently navigating a cancer journey, or are a healthcare professional, *A Better Way to Treat Cancer* is a comprehensive resource that champions the power of integrative oncology. "

**— Dr. Veronique Desaulniers,
Chiropractor, Breast Cancer Conqueror®,
Author of Heal Breast Cancer Naturally**

As a medical oncologist with a career spanning over four decades, I've witnessed the evolution of cancer care and the urgent need for a holistic, patient-centered approach. Dr. Michael Karlfeldt's *A Better Way to Treat Cancer* delivers exactly this, presenting a comprehensive guide that is both scientifically rigorous and deeply empathetic. Our collaborative work with cancer patients over the years has revealed the necessity of such an integrative approach, and I am thrilled to see this valuable knowledge compiled in one accessible resource. I applaud Dr. Karlfeldt's work and wholeheartedly endorse *A Better Way to Treat Cancer*. It is more than a book—it's a roadmap to navigating one of life's most challenging journeys with clarity, empowerment, and hope.

— **Stephen J. Iacoboni, MD,
Oncologist, Author of The Undying Soul and TELOS**

In a world where cancer continues to affect the lives of millions, this transformative guide stands as a beacon of hope and empowerment. Dr. Karlfeldt, an esteemed expert in the field of oncology and integrative medicine, has skillfully brought together cutting-edge research, practical advice, and compassionate insights to offer a comprehensive roadmap for individuals and their loved ones navigating the challenging landscape of cancer.

What sets this book apart is Dr. Karlfeldt's unwavering empathy and dedication to providing comprehensive knowledge about this complex disease. He leaves no stone unturned in educating readers about the various risks that may cause cancer. Armed with knowledge, readers are empowered to make informed decisions and adopt preventive measures. Beyond conventional treatments, *A Better Way To Treat Cancer* explores an array of cutting-edge therapies, emerging research, and complementary approaches to cancer care, including the all-important state of mind in the battle against cancer, by offering guidance and effective self-care solutions for creating and maintaining a positive, resilient mindset.

Whether you are a patient, a caregiver, or a healthcare provider, A Better Way To Treat Cancer is an invaluable resource that will equip you with the knowledge and tools needed to face cancer with courage, resilience, and hope. I wholeheartedly endorse this book and believe it will make a meaningful difference in the lives of everyone touched by cancer.

— **Sylvie Beljanski,
Founder and Executive Vice President of The Beljanski
Foundation, and author of Winning The War On Cancer**

Having collaborated with Dr. Karlfeldt in different capacities, I can attest to his unwavering commitment to patient empowerment and his tireless pursuit of knowledge. His work as a Naturopathic Doctor and the therapies he offers are the lifeline many patients are seeking. *A Better Way To Treat Cancer* stands as an insightful, scientifically-backed resource for anyone impacted by cancer. It provides a new vision of hope and a roadmap to healing. Dr. Karlfeldt's work is a testament to his dedication to the cause, and I wholeheartedly endorse this book.

— **Jane McLelland,
author of How to Starve Cancer**

In *A Better Way to Treat Cancer*, Dr. Michael Karlfeldt expertly weaves his extensive clinical experience with the most promising advances in integrative oncology, particularly photodynamic therapy (PDT). As we've collaborated in the past, I can vouch for his commitment to patient-centered care and innovative treatment approaches. This book is an essential resource, offering hope and empowering patients and healthcare providers alike. I wholeheartedly recommend this enlightening guide.

— **Dr. Michael Weber,
Pioneer of Modern Laser Therapy, President of ISLA,
Developer of Weberneedle® Technology**

Dr. Karlfeldt's *A Better Way To Treat Cancer* is an enlightening exploration of integrative oncology, resonating deeply with my own journey from stage IV melanoma survivor to holistic health advocate. His extensive experience and genuine compassion shine through, providing not just a guide, but a lifeline to anyone facing cancer. This book is a testament to the power of the human body to heal itself when given the right tools. A must-read.

— **James Templeton,
founder of the Templeton Wellness Foundation
and author of I Used to Have Cancer**

Dr. Karfeldt has been a leader in integrative cancer care for many years, and A Better Way To Treat Cancer is a comprehensive review of the causes and treatment of cancer. It is an important contribution to the field. This wholistic approach to cancer opens up options that can improve outcomes at all stages and for all types of cancer.

— **Neil McKinney, ND,
author of Cancer Unravelled and Naturopathic Oncology -
An Encyclopaedic Guide for Patient and Physicians**

Dr. Karlfeldt offers his experienced voice to the growing number of practitioners and researchers coming forth urging the need for a more integrative approach in the care of cancer patients globally. *A Better Way To Treat Cancer* is a valuable resource for deepening our understanding of the "why" of cancer, while providing actionable ways to prevent it and to support and help someone thrive after a diagnosis.

— **Nasha Winters, ND,
FABNO, Executive Director
of the Metabolic Terrain Institute of Health**

As a MD with more than 30 years of clinical experience in the field of complementary cancer treatments and an author of a book on this topic myself, I am deeply impressed by Dr. Karlfeldt's new book. *A Better Way To Treat Cancer* leaves me in awe with its wealth of knowledge and cutting edge insights into the many causes of, and the non-toxic treatments for. cancer. It's a must read for everybody who wants to know how to manage and hopefully heal from a cancerous diagnosis. We all need *A Better Way To Treat Cancer*!

— **Henning Saupe, MD, PhD,
Founder and Medical Director of the Arcadia Clinic
in Bad Emstal, Germany**

The field of integrative oncology is rapidly becoming the future of cancer therapy. In *A Better Way to Treat Cancer*, Dr. Michael Karlfeldt gives readers *a guide to his holistic, patient-centered approach that ultimately puts the patient at the center for overcoming and defeating cancer.*

**— Dr. William Li,
President of the Angiogenesis Foundation
and New York Times bestselling author
of Eat to Beat Disease and Eat to Beat Your Diet**

As someone who chose a natural path in my own battle with cancer, I can personally attest to the significance of the approach revealed in *A Better Way to Treat Cancer*. Dr. Michael Karlfeldt speaks to the core of what many patients need—a scientific yet holistic treatment plan that not only targets the disease but also nurtures the body's innate healing powers. From his holistic perspective on prevention to his understanding of the most effective treatments, Dr. Karlfeldt guides the reader through each step, making an overwhelming journey feel navigable and hopeful. I wholeheartedly recommend this book. Dr. Karlfeldt's comprehensive guide offers a profound roadmap to navigating one of life's greatest health challenges. May it bring you the same sense of clarity, empowerment, and hope it brought me.

**— Lourdes Reynolds,
award-winning actress and filmmaker,
co-author of Our Journey to Option C
and co-host of The Lourdes and Chris Show**

Dr Karlfeldt's *A Better Way To Treat Cancer* provides hope and empowerment to cancer patients and their families, with factual, in-depth research-based solutions, including solutions to the often-overlooked emotional and spiritual aspects of healing. It's rare for a physician to convincingly combine these two modalities. You can bring this book to your oncologist and your pastor - and they would both respect and honor it. This book will be saving so many more lives.

— **Magdalena Wszelaki,
Founder and CEO Wellena and Hormones Balance**

Dr. Karlfeldt is one of the most genuine, caring, loving, and intelligent people I know. Not to mention, he's a brilliant Naturopathic Oncologist with a profound expertise in natural and integrative cancer care. His book, *A Better Way to Treat Cancer*, is a must read for anyone seeking a more holistic and effective approach to beating cancer.

— **Nathan Crane,
Certified Holistic Cancer Coach,
Award Winning Natural Health Researcher**

Legal Notice & Disclaimer

This book and the information it contains is not, nor is it claimed to be, a program to treat or diagnose cancer or any other disease, and is not intended as a substitute for medical care. Neither the author nor the publisher is engaged in rendering professional advice or services to the individual reader. If you suffer from cancer or any other disease, seek immediate medical attention, and always consult with your physician or other health care provider as appropriate before engaging in any new endeavor related to your health. The author and publisher specifically disclaim all responsibility for any liability, loss or risk, personal or otherwise, which is incurred as a consequence, directly or indirectly, of the use and application of any of the contents in this book. All matters pertaining to your personal health should be supervised by a healthcare professional.

Copyright(C) 2023 by Michael Karlfeldt, ND, PhD. All rights reserved. No part of this publication may be reproduced, stored in a retrieval system, or transmitted in any form or by any means, electronic, mechanical, photocopying, recording, or otherwise, without the prior written permission of the author and publisher. Printed in the United States of America. For information address Dr. Michael Karlfeldt c/o: The Karlfeldt Center, 3451 E Cooper Point Dr, Meridan, ID, 83642.

Cataloging-in-Publication data for this book is available from the Library of Congress.

ISBN 979-8-9890042-0-1 (hardcover)
ISBN 979-8-9890042-1-8 (trade paperback)
ISBN: 979-8-9890042-2-5 (e-book)

Book cover design and Interior formatting by 100Covers.

Dedication

This book is primarily dedicated to those, like my father, who valiantly faced the battle against cancer armed only with the standard of conventional care as their single choice of treatment. His journey illuminates the harsh reality of many who, in their fight, are unaware of the diverse therapies available, instead becoming fading echoes of themselves in the process of succumbing to the harsh effects of the therapies, the disease or a combination of the two. In honor of their struggles, this book serves as a testament to the breadth of treatment choices that exist beyond the conventional. May it illuminate your path, broaden your options, and strengthen your hope in this fight.

I also dedicate this book to my wife, Miste, an embodiment of determination and hope, who faced the daunting prospect of chemotherapy as a single mother of four young children with fierce resolve, choosing instead to explore a multitude of options. Her decision to forge her own path in battling a lethal autoimmune condition has not only gifted her with extended life beyond the prescribed expectancy but also instilled in us an irrefutable belief in the power of choice.

Lastly, I dedicate this work to my mother. Her thirst for knowledge, desire to educate, independent spirit and leadership have molded me into the person I am today.

This work stands as a testament to both my wife's and mother's journeys, their courage, and their immeasurable influence on my life and work. As I strive to shed light on the plethora of options available in the realm of cancer treatment, I endeavor to ensure that no one feels shackled by a single path. To both of them, and to all those who bravely navigate the choppy waters of life-threatening illnesses, I offer the information this book contains. May it serve you and help you to heal.

Table of Contents

Introduction: You Don't Have To Fear Cancer and I Can Prove It . . xv

Chapter 1: Cancer: An Overview 1

Chapter 2: Inflammation: The Fire Within You 45

Chapter 3: Other Significant Risk Factors For Cancer 75

Chapter 4: Cancer Stem Cells and Circulating Tumor Cells 101

Chapter 5: Know Your Risk 115

Chapter 6: The Importance of Addressing Your Spiritual Health . . . 141

Chapter 7: Optimizing Your Mindset, Beliefs, and Emotions 169

Chapter 8: Optimizing Your Gut Health With Diet and Nutrition . 203

Chapter 9: Cancer-Fighting Supplements 247

Chapter 10: The Importance of Regular Exercise 275

Chapter 11: Optimizing Immune and Mitochondrial
Function to Fight Cancer 293

Chapter 12: Why An Integrative Medicine Approach
Is Crucial For Treating Cancer 319

Chapter 13: Creating A Cancer Prevention Lifestyle 381

Chapter 14: Frequently Asked Questions 399

Resources 413

Recommended Reading 419

References 423

Acknowledgements 487

About the Author 489

Introduction

You Don't Have To Fear Cancer and I Can Prove It

Most likely, you picked up this book because either you or a loved one close to you has been diagnosed with cancer. Or, like me, perhaps someone you loved has lost their battle with cancer, and you want to do all you can to empower yourself to be able to prevent cancer from striking you and your loved ones in the first place. Whatever your reason for choosing to read this book, I applaud your decision, and I promise to provide you with hope and the knowledge you need to help create a cancer-free life.

Most likely, it is also true that when you think about cancer, you may feel a tinge or more of fear. If so, that's understandable. After all, for most people, hearing the words, "You have cancer" can be terribly frightening and cause you to experience a cascade of stressful, health-sapping emotions, leaving you filled with worries about your survival and questions about your best course of action.

This, too, is understandable, in large part because, despite the trillions of dollars that have been spent on cancer research in the U.S. since President Richard Nixon signed the National Cancer Act on December

23, 1971 to officially declare a "war on cancer," conventional cancer care, for all of the innovations and discoveries that have occurred since that time, has yet to achieve much overall progress. This despite the fact that the U.S. now spends over $200 billion each year on cancer research.

The sad, uncontestable truth, is that conventional cancer treatments—the "cut, burn, and poison" approach of, respectively, surgery, radiation, and chemotherapy drugs—still largely fail to achieve long-term remission of most types of cancer, especially when cancer has metastasized (spread) from its original location in the body to other tissues and organs. In 1971, cancer was the second leading cause of death in the U.S. The same is true today. But the statistics are now even worse. Currently, approximately 40 percent of the American population will likely develop cancer in their lifetimes, and researchers estimate that figure will soon jump to 50 percent. Clearly, the "war on cancer" has been an abject failure overall.

But, as I promised earlier, one of the purposes of this book is to provide you with hope. And there are indeed many reasons why you can be hopeful that new and better solutions are presenting themselves outside of the arena of the conventional cancer care establishment. And, as I intend to prove to you in the chapters that follow, when these innovative approaches are integrated into a cancer treatment program that also combines the best that conventional cancer medicine provides, much better outcomes for cancer patients are far more likely. As proof, I offer the following case histories from my own integrative oncology practice.

Lori G first came to my clinic in 2014, after being diagnosed with tumor in the upper region of her ascending colon. Her diagnosis was preceded by eight years of heavily stressful events for Lori, including a painful divorce, the death of both of her parents, and other family issues. Upon receiving her diagnosis, Lori says, "I knew immediately that they had found my 'emotional garbage can' where I had been stuffing everything for years." There was no history of cancer in Lori's family, so learning that she had cancer "was a shock yet it wasn't a shock. It was almost as if I had given myself cancer. For years, I was going like Mach 1 all the time, dealing with all the external issues in my life and thinking there wouldn't be any repercussions, but my body was taking the heat from all of that. I was also pretending that I was handling my mental and emotional stress. I was disconnected from myself and who I truly am."

As is common for many of my patients, cancer served as a wake-up call for Lori. She recognized that it was a message from her body and its innate intelligence that she needed to heed. She describes the ensuing decisions she needed to make to treat cancer as a "spiritual journey" that required her to rely on and deepen her connection with God. "I knew I couldn't do this on my own; I needed God's help, because when you are told you have cancer fear walks in like this huge force that is very scary. I knew I was potentially facing my death and that had to be dealt with. If you don't have God to help you through all of that, you can't get through it."

Despite her doctors insisting that she quickly have surgery, followed by chemotherapy, Lori instead "took a step back" to consciously examine her options, decided on an alternative, integrative approach, and came to see me. Once I assessed her condition, I recommended that she first debulk the tumor. She agreed and had surgery with a cancer specialist at the MD Anderson Cancer Center, who successfully removed the tumor and three involved lymph nodes. She was then urged by an MD Anderson oncologist to begin chemotherapy, and told that she would be dead within six months if she refused. The course of treatment the oncologist recommended involved two six-month stints of aggressive chemotherapy. After researching the pros and cons involved with such a course of action, Lori decided against it. "I knew that my body had what it needed to beat cancer, so long as I did all that I could to help it heal, while working on myself spiritually, mentally, and physically," she explains.

Instead of chemotherapy, Lori worked diligently at changing the inner terrain of her body. "Learning about the things cancer loves, I eliminated these types of foods and beverages, and replaced them with the foods and nutrients that cancer hates," she says. By taking complete responsibility for her health, following my recommendations, and employing the integrative treatments she received at my clinic, Lori soon began to experience greater levels of happiness in her life, fortified by the work she was doing on herself spiritually, mentally, and emotionally.

Today, eight years after originally being told she only had six months to live if she didn't undergo chemo, Lori reports that she feels "so much better and stronger" as she continues to practice her faith and receive regular supportive treatments and testing at my center. "I don't think you are ever over cancer once you're diagnosed, but cancer doesn't scare me anymore," Lori proclaims. "When you begin to enlist God's help and manage your thoughts, you discover an incredible spiritual place of strength. My journey through cancer has been a real blessing. The emotional and stressful issues that once defined so much of my life are now gone, and that's huge!"

Lori's focus on her spiritual health is something I recommend that all of my patients emphasize. You will learn why this is so important later on in this book.

This next case history illustrates how integrative therapies can support traditional cancer treatments to both minimize side effects and improve outcomes.

It concerns Artie K, a Vietnam veteran who was regularly exposed to heavy doses of agent orange while fighting in the Vietnamese jungles. "We had it dripping off of us whenever it was sprayed," Artie recounts. In 2018, Artie was diagnosed with a highly aggressive form of prostate cancer following a PSA test during his annual checkup at a VA hospital. A biopsy revealed that there was 100 percent cancer involvement throughout his prostate. His physician at the VA hospital immediately linked it back to agent orange.

Artie had surgery to remove his prostate gland, and then underwent radiation treatments. Before even beginning radiation treatments, he was told his chance of survival and becoming cancer-free was only 40 percent. "I didn't know what else to do at that time," Artie says. I told him about other treatment options that might help him, but he was highly dubious at first. After doing his own research, however, Artie says, "I decided that Michael was making more sense than any of my other doctors." As a result, he chose to be treated by me before and while he received radiation therapy.

Because of the supportive therapies Artie received at my clinic he never experienced any of the pain and fatigue that are typical of radiation treatments over time. "Most times, two-thirds of the way through radiation treatment, patients hit a wall and become weak, usually needing someone to assist them getting to and from their treatments and so forth," Artie says. "I was concerned about that, thinking, oh man, that is going to suck. But it never did suck! On the last day of my radiation treatments, when I should have been laying in bed for a week, I packed up my truck, put my motorcycle in the trailer, and drove all the way back to where I live, a distance of over 200 miles, with no pain or any other problems." Artie attributes that to the integrative treatments he received.

In all, Artie received 47 radiation treatments over a period of nine and a half weeks. Following the completion of his radiation treatments and concurrent integrative therapies, Artie reports that he felt "better than ever, even better than before he was originally diagnosed."

An avid motorcyclist, Artie was told that he likely would not be able to ride his motorcycle any more. Instead, soon after he finished receiving his last dose of radiation, he was able to take a 3700 mile long cross-country motorcycle trip with no problems on his chopper. "A chopper is not your long ride bike," Artie laughs, "and I did all that with no trouble." That spring, Artie went on more rides on his chopper, traveling a total of over 8,000 miles all told. Originally given only a 40 percent of survival, years later Artie is still going strong today.

I am very grateful to have been able to help facilitate the patient outcomes you've just read, yet my quest for learning all I can to best help cancer patients recover is never ending. Since the time that I first began treating Lori and Artie, I have learned about, and incorporated, additional tools and therapies that have further increased the likelihood of successful outcomes. To illustrate how this more comprehensive approach has aided me and my patients, consider this more recent case history.

Ron B. first came to me for treatment in 2020, after being diagnosed with aggressive prostate cancer following his first PSA test, which revealed a score of 27 ng/ml. (The normal range for men Ron's age is between 1.0 to 1.5 ng/ml.) Before seeing me, his prostate gland had been biopsied by his urologist and divided into 12 sections, all of which were shown to be between 80 to 90 percent cancerous. In addition, imaging revealed that the cancer has metastasized to the thoracic, along the intestinal wall, along with possible involvement in the pancreas. Ron also lost nearly 50 pounds in only two months, due to vomiting whenever he tried to eat solid food. Ron's urologist estimated Ron had at most another three months to live and sent him home, telling him to do whatever he had left that he desired to do before he died.

A man of deep faith, Ron surrender his situation over to God, and came to see me. Initially, Ron underwent the intensive two week treatment program that I offer all of my cancer patients. Ron's condition stabilized, he was able to again start eating and regained his lost weight within a few months. His PSA score also dropped and today, nearly two years later, Ron is still going strong. Since cancer-survivor rates are typically measured in five-year intervals, it is too early to say that Ron has achieved complete remission, he now leads a full and active life again while diligently following the daily health regimen I've prescribed for him. "I am feeling great," Ron says today, "and I'm very grateful to be able to say that, because I was not feeling great for a very long time."

These are only a few of many similar cases histories of my cancer patients that I could share with you. (I will share others throughout the rest of this book.) In reading them, you may think them remarkable, even miraculous. (Full disclosure: I believe in miracles and the power of God to heal us.) And indeed they are. Yet these and many of my other patients who have survived cancer to now lead thriving lives are living proof of what is possible once you have the knowledge and tools needed to recover from cancer and all other life threatening diseases, and to prevent them from occurring in the first place. Providing you with that knowledge and educating you about these tools, many of which are completely ignored or unknown by most oncologists and other physicians, is why I wrote this book. As the title of this Introduction says, you truly don't have to fear cancer. And in the pages that follow, you will come to understand why.

A Word About Me

My passion and desire to help people regain their health began when I was 13. It was then that I met Dr. Ingemar Wiberg, a leading Swedish naturopathic doctor (ND), in Zolikofen, Switzerland. I was fascinated by Dr. Wiberg. He took a genuine interest in me and we became fast friends. He ignited my passion for naturopathy. After I'd studied engineering for two years, Dr. Wiberg invited me to move in with his family and study full-time with him in his practice. That's when I began my seven-year apprenticeship. The training was demanding, rigorous, and carefully supervised. Being mentored by Dr. Wiberg, one of the curriculum designers for (at that time) the leading Swedish naturopathic school (Birger Ledins Naturläkarskolan), opened my eyes to a world of healing that went far beyond the drug-based, symptom management approach that conventional physicians are trained in.

I began my clinical practice in 1987. One of my specialties is integrative cancer therapy. Cancer patients fly to me from all over United States because of the unique, specialized program I've developed to assist my patients that are dealing with cancer. At my clinic, we also focus on neurological disorders, chronic infections and other diseases, and also regenerative medicine.

Since my education with Dr. Wiberg, I have continued to learn about, train in, and incorporate many other effective healing therapies in order to best serve my patients as completely as possible. Many of these therapies, such as nutritional and I.V. therapies, peptides, oxidative medicine, photodynamic therapy, anti-aging medicine, applied psychoneurobiology (APN), and more, are now included in my overall approach to treating cancer. Don't be concerned if they are unfamiliar to you. You will learn what they are and how and why they work as you read on.

As I learned from Dr. Wiberg, and have since seen proven time and time again after treating tens of thousands of patients in the more than 30 years that I've been practicing medicine, the innate intelligence and healing power of the body, properly supported spiritually, mentally, emotionally, and nutritionally, can often lead patients, including cancer patients, back to a life of good health, even in cases that oncologists and other physicians may consider hopeless. As I will continue to emphasize throughout this book:

As long as you are alive, there is always hope!

The reason I am so passionate about helping cancer patients is because of how cancer deeply affected me. I lost my father to colon cancer, making cancer very personal to me. I am committed myself to learning all I can to spare other cancer patients what my dad went through. If I known back then what I know now, perhaps I could have helped him in ways that his traditional oncologists had no clue about.

Since that time, I've recognized that when you are fighting for your life, you deserve the best and most effective medical and integrative cancer care possible, even if it doesn't fit within the scope of traditional care. That's why I've made it my mission to offer cancer patients the very best, cutting-edge, integrative oncology treatments.

I also recognize that each cancer patient is unique and that every cancer type must be treated specifically. As someone specializing in naturopathic oncology, I evaluate the individual terrain of each patient to determine what may be contributing to the cancer's growth, such as toxic emotions and belief systems, chemical exposures, chronic infections, nutritional deficiencies, lack of microbiome (gut) integrity, food and other sensitivities, and organ weaknesses. In order to triumph over cancer, patients must be supported at every level and with every method necessary to reverse cancer's multi-pronged assault on their bodies, all while maintaining each patient's maximum possible well-being. This book will teach you how to best achieve this.

What You Will Learn

This book begins by providing you with the information you need to better understand cancer, the essential keys you need to know and implement in order to most effectively prevent it, and the cutting edge cancer treatments I use to help my cancer patients, many of which most doctors don't know about.

In Chapter 1, you will learn what cancer actually is, its characteristic traits and explanations of each one, its root causes, and other risk factors to be aware of.

In Chapter 2, you will learn about chronic inflammation, which I refer to as "the insidious fire within", and how it wrecks havoc in the body, and triggers and exacerbates cancer. This chapter will also teach you about free radicals, reactive oxygen species (ROS), cellular redox, mitochondrial dysfunction, and insulin resistance and how they can also play a role in causing cancer.

Chapter 3 goes into more detail about the cancer drivers and disrupters mentioned in Chapter 1. Here you will learn about pathogens, toxins, EMF/EMR/electrosmog, trauma and unresolved/limiting mental/emotional issues and beliefs, and nutritional deficiencies, all of which need to be effectively addressed in order to optimize prevention and recovery from cancer.In Chapter 4, you will learn about cancer stem cells (CSCs) and circulating tumor cells (CTCs), both of which are far too often ignored by most oncologists. I will explain why they are both resistant to, and can become stronger as a result of, conventional cancer treatments and surgeries alone, often leading to recurrence of cancer that is more deadly than the original onset of cancer. This chapter also provides the rationale for my far more comprehensive and integrative cancer treatment approach.

Chapter 5 discusses the importance of early detection and the benefits and limitations of conventional cancer diagnostic and screening tests, as well as other recommended tests that I use and why. It also provides you with a cancer profile self-assessment questionnaire you can use to help determine your current risk for developing cancer.

Chapter 6 explains how crucial, yet often overlooked, spiritual health is when dealing with cancer, and provides you with tools you can use to deepen your connection with God or Spirit. This chapter also includes supporting research and compelling case histories of healing from cancer after patients connected to and aligned with their Divine guidance.

Chapter 7 is about how and why you need to optimize your mindset, beliefs, and emotions. This chapter augments the spiritual health component in Chapter 6, providing you with guidance and effective self-care solutions for creating and maintaining a positive, resilient mindset while addressing your fears, limited beliefs, and persistent negative emotions.

Chapter 8 instructs you in how best to optimize your diet, nutrition and gut health. It opens with a discussion of the microbiome and its importance to and connection with the brain, immune system, and other body systems, while also exploring the connection between dysbiosis, cancer, and disease in general. From there, the chapter explores the best anti-cancer dietary options and provides recommendations and guidelines for each of them.

In Chapter 9 I share the nutritional and other supplements I recommend for protecting against cancer, both preventively and therapeutically.

Chapter 10 explains the importance of regular exercise, including research documenting the role exercise can play in protecting against cancer and why it needs to be part of an overall cancer treatment program. It also includes my exercise guidelines and recommendations, including the "do's and the don'ts" and the best types of exercises to engage in. You will also learn about the importance of the "air" and "fire" elements (oxygen/carbon dioxide, healthy breathing, breathwork techniques, and the importance of daily exposure to sunlight), along with the proven health benefits of "earthing"/grounding.

Chapter 11 provides you with a deeper understanding of your immune system and its dependence on mitochondria, the "energy factories" inside your cells. In this chapter, I share effective solutions for achieving improved immune function and healthy mitochondria and overall cell health.

In Chapter 12, you will learn why an integrative oncology treatment approach is crucial for recovery from cancer. I explain the reasons for my cancer treatment approach and how and why its success rate is greater, on average, than conventional treatments alone. I also explain the pros and cons of traditional chemotherapy and radiation and their appropriate use within an integrative framework.

I then explain the various individual treatments I use and how and why each of them work, both individually and together when combined as part of a truly integrative treatment plan to target and resolve each of the causative factors and cancer drivers that you will learn about in Chapter 1 through 5.

In Chapter 13 you will learn how to create your very own cancer prevention lifestyle, with an emphasis on self-care and prevention.

Finally, in Chapter 14, I provide answers to the questions I am most frequently asked about my cancer treatment approach.

My promise to you, if you take to heart and make use of the information this book will teach you, is that you will not only have a clearer and better understanding of cancer and its causes, but, far more importantly, you will know what to do to protect yourself from cancer, and, should it strike, how to best go about treating it without fear.

Now turn the page, and let your education begin.

Chapter 1

Cancer: An Overview

In order to successfully triumph over cancer, you need to know and understand what cancer is. As the saying goes, Knowledge is power. This chapter provides you with that necessary information. In it, you will learn:

- What cancer is.
- Its characteristics.
- Its history from prehistoric times to the present.
- The three major competing theories as to how and why it develops.
- How cancer is diagnosed.
- How it progresses and can cause death.
- Its primary causes and other risk factors to consider.
- And its early warning signs.

As you read this chapter, you will also be introduced to terms and scientific concepts that may be unfamiliar to you, such as *carcinogenesis, oncogenes, suppressor genes, angiogenesis, hypoxia and the Warburg effect* and *mitochondria*. Don't worry; they will all be explained. Now let's begin by taking a look of the history of cancer down through the ages.

Ancient Illness, Modern Scourge

It may surprise you to know that the existence of cancer predates human history by millions of years. This fact was established in 2003, when scientists discovered the existence of cancer cells in fossils of dinosaurs that roamed the earth sometime between 70 and 80 million years ago.

Jumping forward in time, our human ancestors, the hominids *Homo erectus* and *Australopithecus*, who lived over 4 million years ago, during the Pleistocene era, were also susceptible to cancer. We know this thanks to the work of the famed paleoanthropologist Louis Leakey, who, in 1932, found an abnormal growth suggestive of a malignant tumor in a hominid jawbone dating back to that time period. After examining it, the growth was subsequently diagnosed as an osteosarcoma (bone cancer) by a specialist at the Royal College of Surgeons of London. Growths resembling osteosarcoma have also been found in Egyptian mummies dating back to 3,000 BCE, as have destruction of skull bones that is also suggestive of cancer.

The earliest written description of cancer, although that term was not used, also comes from Egypt and dates back to this same time period. It is known as the Edwin Smith Papyrus (named after the man who purchased it in 1862), is claimed to have been written by the Egyptian high priest Imhotep, and is part of a larger treatise on trauma surgery. In addition, it also describes eight cases of tumors in the breast being treated by cauterization.

Knowledge about the existence of cancer can also be found in historical records and writings from Babylonia, including the Code of Hammurabi (circa 1750 BCE), which established the fee that surgeons should be paid for the removal of tumors; China, as far back as 1100 BCE; in the Ramayana of India (circa 500 BCE); and in Peru, where mummies dating back to 400 BCE were found to have lesions resembling malignant melanoma.

Hippocrates (460-470 BCE), considered the "Father of Western Medicine", became the first physician to distinguish the differences between benign and malignant tumors, and coined the terms from which the word *cancer* derives—*carcinos* and *karkinoma*, both of which refer to a crab. In his view, cancer resembled a crab because of how it extends, like the claws of a crab, across cells, tissues, and organs. Centuries later, the Roman physician Celsus (25 BCE-70AD) applied these Greek terms to the Latin word *cancer*, which also means "crab".

Interestingly, it was in ancient China that the first integrative approach for treating cancer was written about, as well as the first written clinical description of breast cancer, including its progression and prognosis following its diagnosis. Both of these discussions appear in the *Nei Ching*, known in the West as The Yellow Emperor's Classic of Internal Medicine (circa 250 BCE). This classic treatise of traditional Chinese Medicine (TCM) recommends an integrative treatment approach for breast cancer, consisting of spiritual and pharmacological therapies, diet, acupuncture, and augmentative treatments for respiratory conditions.

Written records and research about cancer throughout various world cultures continued down through the ages. But it was not until the 1800s that our modern-day understanding of cancer began to take shape. During that century, discoveries by a number of noteworthy scientists provided the foundational tenets of oncology as we know it today. They include:

- Joseph Recamier, of France, who in 1829 coined the term *metastasis* to describe how cancer cells invade and spread through the bloodstream.

- Johannes Müller, of Germany, who in 1838 proved that cancer comes from cells, not lymph, as was previously considered to be the case.

- Domenico Antonio Rigoni-Stern, of Italy, who in 1842 conducted the first comprehensive study of cancer occurrence and mortality, finding that cancer cases were rising and were more common in cities than in rural areas (thus establishing an environmental link to cancer, although he may not have recognized it as such), and that the incidence of cancer increased with age.

- John Hughes Bennett, of Scotland, who in 1845 became the first physician to determine that leukemia is a condition characterized by excessive growth of blood cells.
- Hilario de Gouvea, of Brazil, who in 1886 discovered a hereditary link to cancer based upon his study of a family with an above average predisposition to develop retinoblastoma (cancer of the retina).

Three other scientists who significantly advanced our study and understanding of cancer are the physicist Wilhelm Konrad Roentgen, physician Rudolf Virchow, both of Germany, and the English surgeon, Stephen Paget.

In 1895, Roentgen discovered X-rays. As a result of his discovery, X-rays were soon used to scan for and diagnose cancer in the body. His work also led to the use of radiation therapy as a cancer treatment.

Dr. Virchow (1821-1902), a former student of Johannes Müller, pioneered and is known as the father of cellular pathology. Virchow proved that all cells, including cancer cells, are derived from other cells in the body. He established the scientific basis for the study of cancer pathology based upon his use of the modern microscope. He was also the first physician to propose that cancer was caused by chronic inflammation in the body, based on his study of wounds and wound healing. (Ironically, even today, his finding in that regard is still overlooked by many oncologists and other physicians.) Virchow also coined the term "leukemia".

Dr. Paget (1855-1926) was the first physician to determine that, although cancer cells spread to other organs via the bloodstream, they can only grow in conditions that are biochemically conducive for their growth within organs. Paget's discovery was a major contributor to our understanding of what today is known as the biological terrain theory of cancer, and also laid the groundwork for the true scientific basis and understanding of metastasis.

Current cancer researchers, oncologists and other physicians, including myself, owe these men a tremendous debt of gratitude for how their work paved the way for the numerous advances in cancer diagnostic and treatments that occurred throughout the 20th century and continue today.

Unfortunately, alongside of these advances has been a corresponding rise in the incidence of cancer. While the incidence of cancer was relatively rare for most of human history, and even in the early part of the 20th century, since that time, there has been an explosion of cancer cases throughout the Western world, to the point where today in the United States, as I pointed out in this book's Introduction, we are fast approaching a time where one of every two Americans is likely to be diagnosed with cancer in their lifetime. Cancer has truly become a major scourge of the modern era.

What is Cancer?

As Neil McKinney, ND, a leader in the field of naturopathic oncology, has stated, "Cancer is not a simple disease. It has many forms and many causes, and therefore there is no simple cure. What works for one cancer at one stage in one person will not always do the same for another person, another cancer type, or the same cancer in the same person at a later stage." This explains why there is no such thing as a "one size fits all, magic bullet" cure for cancer, and why there likely never will be. Grasping that fact is vitally important for anyone dealing with cancer.

Broadly speaking, cancer is a disease that develops when various cells cease to function properly (become cancerous) and then begin to multiply uncontrollably, while also failing to mature and die off as nature intended. This initiation and growth of cancer cells is called *carcinogenesis*. Although conventional medicine recognizes literally hundreds of different types of cancer, all of them fall into one of five major categories or classes.

Carcinomas are cancers that occur in the epithelial cells covering the surface of the skin, mouth, nose, throat, lung airways, and genitourinary and gastrointestinal tracts, and also line the breast, thyroid, and other glands. Carcinomas are the most common class of cancers. Examples of carcinomas include lung, breast, prostate, skin, stomach, and colon cancer.

Sarcomas are cancers the originate in bones and/or soft connective tissues that connect, support, and surround other body structures, such as cartilage, muscles, tendons, fat, blood vessels, and the linings of joints.

Leukemias are cancers characterized by abnormal white blood cells which originate in the blood and bone marrow and then migrate via the bloodstream to affect various organs and tissues. Unlike carinomas and sarcomas, leukemias are not solid tumors.

Lymphomas are cancers of the lymph glands. They typically are composed of abnormal white blood cells called lymphocytes that form tumors in the lymph glands. The two most common lymphomas in the United States are Hodgkin's disease and non-Hodgkin's lymphomas. A rarer form is called Burkitt's lymphoma, which is more common in parts of Africa.

Myelomas are cancers of a type of white blood cells known as plasma cells. Plasma cells produce antibodies to prevent and fight off infections. In cases of myeloma, the plasma cells over accumulate in bone marrow, crowding out other cells. In addition, the plasma cells stop producing antibodies to instead produce abnormal proteins.

In a state of health, the normal process of cell death is self-programmed in each cell by cellular DNA and is known as *apoptosis*. Cancer disrupts this process so that cancer cells do not die off as nature intended. As these "rogue" cells continue to grow, they stop working in harmony with the rest of cells, tissues, organs, and systems in the body. In addition to not dying as nature intended, cancer cells lack the specialized functions of healthy cells. Instead, they operate very much like undying parasites, sapping the body's supply of energy and nutrients as they continue to grow and eventually form into tumors capable of spreading to and invading healthy tissues. It is this invasive process that makes tumors malignant. By contrast, benign, or non-malignant tumors, are essentially harmless because they are surrounded by fiber, preventing them from spreading or creating toxic effects in the body.

The miraculous creation that is the human body is made up of trillions of cells, each of which has specific functions and a normal lifespan, and acts in tandem with all other cells to help maintain the body's overall health and equilibrium (homeostasis). What most people do not realize is that cancer cells are produced in the body every day. That's natural. In a state of health, these cells are easily identified by the body's immune system and eliminated by various immune cells, as well as pancreatin, an enyzme produced in the pancreas that is also involved in the process of digestion. What this means—though you may find it shocking—is that, in a state of good health, the formation of cancer cells in the body is a normal process that the body routinely deals with. The problem arises when various on-going factors—both internal and external—overburden the body to the point where, instead of being detected and eliminated, the cancer cells continue to grow and multiply. If this process is not corrected, eventually these rogue cells combine to form tumors. Over time, cancer cells often spread and circulate further into the bloodstream to lodge in and attack other areas of the body, causing additional tumors. This process is known as *metastasis*. The more that cancer is able to metastasize, the more difficult in becomes to treat successfully.

Genes and Cancer

Unlike healthy cells, cancer cells are abnormally shaped and contain malformed or irregular internal structures. It is widely accepted that these abnormalities are caused by biochemical insults to and mutations in cellular DNA, the genetic blueprint for all cells, tissues, and organs. Scientists have also identified a specific class of genes called *proto-oncogenes* which are responsible for helping to regulate normal cell division. But when the proto-oncogenes are mutated, or expressed at greater than normal levels, they transform into *oncogenes*, which can trigger normal, healthy cells to turn into cancer cells. According to the National Human Genome Research Institute, "Some oncogenes work like an accelerator pedal in a car, pushing a cell to divide again and again. Others work like a faulty brake in a car parked on a hill, also causing the cell to divide unchecked."

Another class of genes that impact the likelihood of whether or not a person will develop cancer is tumor suppressor genes, sometimes also referred to as *anti-oncogenes*. Tumor suppressor genes produce proteins that regulate cell growth. There are three different types of tumor suppressor genes, each with a specific function. One type signals cells to stop dividing, a second type repairs cellular DNA that can be damaged by cell division, and the third type triggers apoptosis in aged and damaged cells. Like oncogenes, tumor suppressor genes are also susceptible to damage and mutation, both of which can cause tumor suppressor genes to malfunction or become inactivated.

Typically, for the cancer process to begin, mutations or damage to both proto-oncogenes and tumor suppressor genes must first occur. For this reason, cancer is commonly considered to be a genetic disease, which how it is defined by the National Cancer Institute (NCI). However, there is more to cancer than genes alone, and an increasing number of cancer researchers and physicians now regard cancer to be a metabolic disease, as well. This is discussed later in this chapter.

The chief traits that differentiate cancer cells from normal cells are the following:

- Cancer cells grow without receiving growth signals, whereas normal cells do not grow in the absence of growth signals.

- Cancer cells ignore the apoptosis signals that cause normal cells to die at the end of their normal life cycle.

- Cancer cells migrate to and invade various areas of the body. By contrast, normal cells typically don't move around the body. They also stop growing when they come in contact with other cells, whereas cancer cells do not.

- Cancer cells evade detection by the immune system, which is designed to rid the body of aged and/or damaged cells. Unlike normal cells, certain cancer cells also have the ability to cause various immune cells to actually protect, rather than attack, them.

- Cancer cells can also produce changes to their chromosomes, including duplicating or deleting various chromosome elements. In some cases, these changes can result in certain cancer cells having twice as many chromosomes than normal cells have.

- Cancer cells also feed on different kinds of nutrients than normal cells do, and in some cases can also produce energy in an abnormal fashion, enabling them to more rapidly increase their growth and spread.

In order to support themselves and their growth, cancer cells can also form their own network of blood vessels to divert the nutrients they need to stay alive away from the rest of the body's cells, tissues, and organs, all of which are "fed" by the body's blood supply. The end result is that the cancer cells grow stronger while the rest of the body, sapped of its normal supply of energy because of nutrient loss, becomes increasingly weaker and unable to mount an effective response to cancer. Matters are made worse by the toxic waste products cancer cells give off, which act like poison to nearby healthy cells, tissues, and organs.

The creation of the blood vessel networks that support the growth and spread of, and feed, cancer cells and tumors is called *angiogenesis*. More broadly, angiogenesis is defined as the formation of new blood vessels to support the growth of tissues of any kind. It plays a crucial role in the development of babies and children, and is also important for tissue repair in the body, such as for the healing of wounds or when the lining of the uterus is shed each month during menstruation. Under such circumstances, angiogenesis is obviously good, and when the tissue repair is complete, body signals "switch off" angiogenesis. In the case of cancer, however, angiogenesis typically does not "switch off" without medical intervention, enabling cancerous tumors to grow and metastasize.

Were cancer cells not able to initiate angiogenesis, cancerous tumors would be unable to grow beyond a few millimeters in size, which would make them far less of a health threat and much easier to treat. This is why halting angiogenesis in cancer patients is vitally important as part of an overall comprehensive treatment approach (as well as in cases of various autoimmune diseases and other conditions in which angiogenesis is also involved). Once the angiogenesis process is arrested, cancer cells and tumors are cut off from their "food supply" and begin to starve and weaken, making it easier for the full battery of integrative therapies to target and destroy them. Please note, however, that arresting angiogenesis alone is not enough to reverse cancer. That can only be achieved by also addressing cancer's root causes.

Cancer As A Metabolic Disease

Although the National Cancer Institute, as well as many oncologists and cancer researchers, still continue to regard cancer as a genetic disease, an increasing body of evidence indicates that it is not. In fact, researchers now estimate that no more than 15 percent of all cancer cases are primarily due to inherited genetic predispositions. This is a significant finding and should go a long way to alleviate the fears people may experience when told they have cancer genes passed down to them by their parents.

According to Dr. McKinney, the cancer as a genetic disease theory falls short in part because, "Cancer cells grow too fast. This is because they have too many growth-promoting programs in their genes turned on, while growth-controlling genetic programs are turned down or off. Very seldom is it a single or simple set of genes that is mutated. There is exactly one kind of cancer that involves a single gene mutation. Most cancers have 40 to 80 distinct mutations in the parental, nuclear DNA by the time they are well established. What is driving cancer cell growth is a primitive program called the *fetal growth cassette*, making masses of new cells that are not specialized or differentiated. They are genes that are focused on growth of crude biomass. This is not at all some sort of random mutation event. This is a cluster-fuss with a purpose."

What matters is not so much the genes themselves, but whether or not they are activated ("switched on"). And as it happens, we all have a great deal of control over the factors that can cause that activation in the form of our daily dietary and other lifestyle choices, and how we manage stress, our thoughts, and our emotions. You will learn much more about how you can harness that control as you continue to read this book.

So, if genes are not the primary cause of cancer, what is?

It turns out that the answer to that question first began to be formulated in the early 20th century by the German scientist Dr. Otto Warburg. Beginning in the early 1920s, Warburg began studying cellular respiration, especially the respiration of cancer cells and its relationship to the metabolism of cancer tumors. During that decade, among his discoveries were "the nature and mode of action of the respiratory enzyme" for which he was awarded the Nobel Prize In Physiology or Medicine in 1931 (he was previously nominated for the award 46 times, beginning in 1923), and the fact that cancer tumors in animals produce large amounts of lactic acid. He also found that cancer tumors are highly acidic and prone to cause fermentation. Of his work, the Nobel Committee wrote, "This discovery has opened up new ways in the fields of cellular metabolism and cellular respiration. He [Warburg] has shown, among other things, that cancerous cells can live and develop, even in the absence of oxygen."

Based on these and other discoveries, Warburg theorized that cancer growth is caused by tumors producing energy by breaking down (metabolizing) glucose (sugar) within a low oxygen state known as anaerobic respiration or, more simply, fermentation. By contrast, healthy cells produce energy by using oxygen to metabolize pyruvate, an end product of glycolysis that is oxidized within the mitochondria of the cells. (Warburg termed mitochondria *grana*.) As a result of his findings, Warburg proposed that cancer is a disease caused by metabolic mitochondrial dysfunction, stating, "Cancer, above all other diseases, has countless secondary causes.

But, even for cancer, there is only one prime cause. Summarized in a few words, the prime cause of cancer is the replacement of the respiration of oxygen in normal body cells by a fermentation of sugar. All normal body cells meet their energy needs by respiration of oxygen, whereas cancer cells meet their energy needs in great part by fermentation...Oxygen gas, the donor of energy in plants and animals, is dethroned in the cancer cells and replaced by an energy yielding reaction of the lowest living forms, namely a fermentation of glucose."

We now know that this statement is somewhat of an oversimplification, yet there still is much truth to it.

Dr. McKinney summarizes the Warburg Theory of Cancer as follows:

1. Cancer arises from damage to cellular respiration (burning fuel with oxygen).
2. Energy production by fermentation (metabolizing without oxygen) gradually compensates for insufficient respiration.
3. Cancer cells continue to ferment lactate in the presence of oxygen = Warburg Effect.
4. Enhanced fermentation is the signature malady of all cancer cells.

Despite his stature as a Nobel laureate, Warburg's discoveries were, until recently, mostly overlooked by the cancer establishment in favor of other theories, especially since the 1970s, following the discovery of oncogenes and the subsequent emphasis on cancer as a genetic disease caused by damaged or mutated cellular DNA. But Warburg's work has more recently begun to be revisited in a more favorable light, in part because of ongoing research into mitochondria and mitochondrial metabolism and dysfunction.

In simple terms, mitochondria are the "energy factories" within all of trillions of cells in your body (except blood cells). They produce approximately 95 percent of all the energy your body uses on a daily basis. These microscopic powerhouses accomplish this by taking in the nutrients delivered to the cells from the bloodstream. They then break the nutrients down (metabolize them) and combine them with oxygen to produce *adenosine triphosphate* (ATP), the main fuel supply for your body's energy needs. This is the process known as cellular respiration. Mitochondria are the only components of the cell where food molecules and oxygen can be combined.

Not only are mitochondria essential for supplying your body with adequate energy, they also play important roles in protecting against disease and helping you to live longer. In addition, they are involved in cell growth and division, cell signaling, and normal cell death (apoptosis). They also regulate cell metabolism and cellular and genetic repair, and help to control the function of immune cells. Research confirms that mitochondria are essential for establishing and maintaining both the innate adaptive responses of immune cell responses. Damaged or dysfunctional mitochondria can weaken the body's immune response, promote genetic mutations, activate oncogenes, and deactivate suppressor genes.

A remarkable characteristic of mitochondria that is unique among all other cellular components is that they possess their own DNA, which is distinct from the DNA found in the nucleus of the cells. This means that mitochondria have the ability to increase their number inside each cell. This fact has important implications, as scientists now believe that overall health and longevity in humans depends in large part on the amount of mitochondria within human cells, and on how well the mitochondria function.

Unfortunately, their very function—metabolizing nutrients with oxygen to generate ATP for energy—make mitochondria highly susceptible to impaired functioning and premature death due to accelerated degradation and destruction of their DNA. Because of the large amount of oxidative activity that mitochondria require to produce ATP, they are constantly exposed to large amounts of free radicals, one of the primary causes of aging and disease. Cellular DNA is defended from free radicals by the cells' double-membrane structure that shields it from the rest of the cell, along with a plentiful supply of protective proteins. The DNA of mitochondria lacks such protections and therefore has few defenses against free radical damage. As a result, as we age mitochondria function tends to decline.

In recent decades, a growing body of research has found that the decline of mitochondria in the body and impaired mitochondrial functioning are primary causes of many disease conditions today, including cancer, confirming Warburg's findings.

One of the leaders in this field of research is Thomas N. Seyfried, PhD. As he wrote in a scientific paper published in the medical journal *Frontiers in Cell and Developmental Biology* in 2015, "Cancer is widely considered a genetic disease involving nuclear mutations in oncogenes and tumor suppressor genes. This view persists despite the numerous inconsistencies associated with the somatic [genetic] mutation theory. In contrast to the somatic mutation theory, emerging evidence suggests that cancer is a mitochondrial metabolic disease, according to the original theory of Otto Warburg. The findings are reviewed from nuclear cytoplasm transfer experiments that relate to the origin of cancer. The evidence from these experiments is difficult to reconcile with the somatic mutation theory, but is consistent with the notion that cancer is primarily a mitochondrial metabolic disease."

Dr. Seyfried and other researchers point out that scientific evidence continues to add weight to Warburg's original theory that cancer is the result of damaged mitochondrial respiration. While there is no question that genetic mutations play a role in cancer, they only do so when there is damage to cellular metabolism. Regardless of whether the damage is caused by viral, bacterial, fungal, or various environmental factors, it inevitably directly or indirectly causes insufficient respiration in the mitochondria. It is this dysfunction within the mitochondria that causes cancer cells to depend on glucose, as well as glutamine, a non-essential amino acid, in order to produce the energy they need. Without these fuel sources, cancer cells cannot survive, whereas healthy cells can generate energy and keep themselves alive by using many substances besides glucose. A primary fuel source for healthy cells is fat, which is one of the reasons why the ketogenic diet, which I will explain later in this book, can be an effective strategy for many cancer patients. Such a diet is rich in healthy fats and low in glucose and other sugars found in carbohydrate-rich foods such as grains, legumes, potatoes, and breads, as well as many types of fruits. The reliance of cancer cells on glucose and glutamine also explains why cancer thrives in a low-oxygen, fermentation state.

Questions about the genetic basis for cancer intensified in 2015, the year when The Cancer Genome Atlas (TCGA) officially came to an end. This project successfully sequenced 10,000 tumors, uncovering nearly 10 million genetic mutations in the tumors. However, the project failed to discover any genetic patterns that might lead for a cure for cancer, leading some researchers to call for a shift away from an emphasis on gene sequencing.

Meanwhile, other research gave further support to the metabolic theory of cancer over the belief that cancer is primarily a genetic disease. For example, the emerging science of epigenetics has shown researchers that a wide range of factors influence genes and overall cellular expression. An example of this is Asian women and their risk of breast cancer. From a genetic standpoint, Asian women living in their native lands and following a traditional diet and lifestyle have a lower risk of breast cancer compared to Western women. However, studies show that when Asian woman migrate to the U.S. and adopt a Western lifestyle, including the standard American diet, their risk of breast cancer increases by 60 percent. This is a clear case of epigenetic influences, rather than their genes, being responsible for their increased breast cancer risk.

Studies in which genes from mutated cancer cells are transplanted into healthy cells also support the metabolic theory of cancer. Were cancer truly first and foremost a genetic disease, then it follows that transplanting genes from cancer cells into normal cells should be all that is necessary to turn normal cells cancerous. But multiple animal studies have found that transplanting a cancer cell nucleus (site of the cell's damaged DNA and mutated genes) into the body (cytoplasm) of a normal cell, in fact, does not cause the normal cell to become malignant.

Summing up the results of these experiments, Dr. Seyfield states, "Normal cells beget normal cells. Tumor cells beget tumor cells. Transfer of a tumor cell nucleus into a normal cytoplasm begets normal cells, despite the presence of the tumor-associated genomic abnormalities. Transfer of a normal cell nucleus into a tumor cell cytoplasm begets dead cells or tumor cells, but not normal cells. The results suggest that nuclear genomic defects alone cannot account for the origin of tumors and that normal mitochondria can suppress tumorigenesis [production of malignant tumors]."

He adds, "The genomic damage in tumor cells follows, rather than precedes, the disturbances in cellular respiration... I attribute the slow progress in the 'War on Cancer' to the persistent embrace of the somatic mutation theory, and to the failure in recognizing mitochondrial dysfunction as a credible alternative explanation for the origin of the disease."

However, there may be even more to this story of what cancer is.

Cancer As A Survival Mechanism

Over the last two decades, a new theory has emerged about why cancer develops in the body. Rather than dismissing the genetic and metabolic theories of cancer, this theory adds a new twist to them. Namely that cancer, instead of being a disease that attacks the body, is actually a survival mechanism that the body triggers as a last resort attempt to cope with an ongoing onslaught of toxins, nutritional deficiencies, stress and various other factors so common to our modern world.

Proponents of the theory of cancer as a survival mechanism hold that cancer is not a chance occurrence caused by damaged DNA and mutated cells, recognizing—as do proponents of the metabolic theory of cancer—that more than 100 oncogenes have thus far been discovered within the human genome. Obviously, they are there for a reason, not as a freak fluke of Nature.

Just as significantly, the nature of cancer cells and the way that they proliferate has now come to be recognized by some researchers as a "default state" common to all cells that dates back to the origin of life, at a time when organisms were unicellular (single-celled). One of these researchers is Dr. Barnali Majumdar of the Department of Surgical Oncology at Dharamshila Narayana Superspeciality Hospital, in New Delhi, India. In a research paper she published in 2021, she explained, "In the Pre-Cambrian era before the evolution of complex organisms, the early life-forms existed as unicellular, asexual, immortal, non-specialized (not differentiated) [organisms], exhibited genomic instability and executed simple fermentation (aerobic glycolysis or Warburg effect) for sustenance. They survived in an environment compris[ed] of high radiation, free radicals, low oxygen and, low pH. Eons later, as the environment underwent conducive transitions, it instigated evolutionary changes in the early life-forms to explore the new oxygen-rich atmosphere. It is enthralling to note that in the present environment when a cell is exposed to direct and indirect carcinogens (similar to primitive extreme conditions), the cells attempt to revert back to early-life survival strategies which we term as 'malignant transformation'. The primitive cells that endured and sustained in a nutrient-deprived and extreme environment display striking similarities with the hallmark characteristics of a malignant cell. It appears as if 'cancer' is nature's ancient encrypted code embedded in every cell as a life-boat, ensuring the survival of the cell when challenged with hostile conditions."

Dr. Majumdar's statement is supported by various studies which confirm that key biological cell traits were established as unicellular organisms evolved into multicellular life-forms, such as limited cell proliferation, programmed cell death, cell differentiation, and specific cell functions, all of which are characteristic traits of healthy human cells, but not found in cancer cells. For this reason, some cancer researchers hypothesize that healthy, differentiated cells evolved by suppressing the genetic programming that enabled unicellular life forms to survive, and that this pre-historic programming is reactivated as a last resort by the body when it becomes overwhelmed by cancer drivers. For example, in a research paper published in 2018 in the *British Journal of Cancer*, the authors wrote, "Neoplastic [cancer] growth and many of the hallmark properties of cancer are driven by the disruption of molecular networks established during the emergence of multicellularity. Regulatory pathways and molecules that evolved to impose regulatory constraints upon networks established in earlier unicellular organisms enabled greater communication and coordination between the diverse cell types required for multicellularity, but also created liabilities in the form of points of vulnerability in the network that when mutated or dysregulated facilitate the development of cancer. These factors are usually overlooked in genomic analyses of cancer, but understanding where vulnerabilities to cancer lie in the networks of multicellular species would provide important new insights into how core molecular processes and gene regulation change during tumourigenesis [sic]... Mounting molecular evidence suggests altered interactions at the interface between unicellular and multicellular genes play key roles in the initiation and progression of cancer."

Another researcher, Dr. Mark D. Vincent, of the Department of Oncology at the University of Western Ontario in Canada, agrees with this assessment. In one of his many published research papers on cancer, he wrote, "The genes of cellular cooperation that evolved with multicellularity about a billion years ago are the same genes that malfunction to cause cancer." He defines cancer as "an atavistic [reverting to an ancestral] condition that occurs when genetic or epigenetic malfunction unlocks an ancient 'toolkit' of pre-existing adaptations, re-establishing the dominance of an earlier layer of genes that controlled loose-knit colonies of only partially differentiated cells, similar to tumors."

In another published paper, Dr. Vincent and his co-authors point out that "Current therapeutic treatments attack the strengths of cancer: they predominantly target what cancer cells, and all cells, have deeply embedded in their genomes–strategies for cellular proliferation. It may seem rational to treat a proliferative disease with anti-proliferative drugs. However, after 4 billion years of evolution (the first 3 billion of which were characterized by the largely unregulated proliferation of unicellular organisms) cellular proliferation is probably the most protected, least vulnerable, most redundant and most entrenched capability that any cell has. The redundant and robust supports for cellular proliferation are 2 billion years older than the many layers of recent differentiation and regulation that evolved with multicellular eukaryotes [cells with a clearly defined nucleus]. Thus proliferation, not differentiation, is the ancestral and default state of cells." This statement goes a long way towards explaining why conventional cancer therapies so often fail.

Another researcher who gives credence to the theory of cancer as a survival mechanism is Sayer Ji, founder of the health information website GreenMedInfo. Addressing this theory, he notes that, "Cancer cells are, in fact, surprisingly well-coordinated for cells that are supposed to be the result of strictly random mutation...What if cancer was the unmasking of a more ancient survival program within the cell, activated as a last ditch effort to survive an increasingly hostile bodily environment, saturated through with carcinogenic and immunotoxic agents?...In other words, cancer is not some predestined gene-time bomb setting itself off within us; rather, it is the logical result of decades' worth of cell shock/damage/adaptation to environmental poisoning, nutrient deprivation and psycho-spiritual and/ or emotional stress. These cells have learned to survive the constant abuse, and have flipped into survival mode, which is self-centered, hyper-proliferative (constant self-repair/replication) and aggressive (metastatic).

"Instead of a monolithic 'disease,' it makes more sense to view cancer as a *symptom* of a bodily milieu gone awry; in other words, the environment of the cell has become inhospitable to normal cell function, and *in order to survive*, the cell undergoes profound genetic changes associated with the cancerous personality (phenotype). This ecological view puts the center of focus back on the preventable and treatable causes of the disease, rather [than] on some vague and out-dated concept of 'defective genes' beyond our ability to influence directly. It also explains how the disease process may conceal an inherent logic, if not also healing impulse, insofar as it is an attempt of the body to find balance and survive in inherently unbalanced and dangerous conditions."

In my own clinical practice, I have found that there is a lot of truth to this theory, while also recognizing the causative roles that both genetic and mitochondrial metabolic dysfunctions play in the onset and progression of cancer. What is most important to me is not theory, however, but practical solutions that offer my cancer patients the best hope for remission and long-term survival. I have no doubt that as our understanding of cancer continues to evolve, so too will the theories that underpin how and why cancer is treated. Keeping an open mind and having a willingness to try new options is vitally important on the part of both physicians and cancer patients alike.

Causes Of Cancer Deaths You May Not Know About

A surprising fact about cancer is that it is often not cancer itself that can prove fatal, but its side effects. Many cancer deaths are actually due to infections by bacteria, viruses, and fungi and other harmful pathogens that normally would be eliminated by the body's immune system. Cancer interferes with immunity by suppressing the immune system, as do surgery, chemotherapy and radiation. This explains why many cancer patients die from pneumonia, for example.

Organ dysfunction is another common cause of death in cancer patients because of how tumors can impinge upon, and even in some cases, strangle, organs as tumors grow. In addition, tumors divert nutrients from organs via angiogenesis and can also produce toxins that infiltrate organs to further weaken and damage them.

Another important issue cancer patients need to be aware of is a condition known as *cachexia*. It is caused by angiogenesis and results in severe malnutrition and starvation at the cellular level, and can be compounded by the loss of appetite many cancer patients experience as cancer progresses. Signs of cachexia are edema and ascites, a condition in which fluid collects within the spaces of tissues in the abdominal cavity. Both conditions result from lack of amino acids and minerals in the bloodstream, causing fluid to leak into tissues.

Finally, some cancer patients hemorrhage to death. This is most common among leukemia patients, but can also occur in other cancer patients because of how tumors can interfere with the body's ability to form blood clots, especially if a tumor invades and starts to grow within blood vessels. Tumors can also cause excessive blood clotting, resulting in the blood supply being cut off from organs.

Cancer Grading, Staging, and Tumor Markers

When determining the best course of action for treating cancer, two factors known as grading and staging come into play, both of which are based upon cancer diagnostic tests and imagery from X-rays, PET, CT and/or MRI scans. These tests, scans, and methods of grading and staging determine whether or not the cancer is localized, meaning not spreading beyond the tissue or organ in which it was discovered, or if it has metastasized to other parts of the body.

Grading and staging also determine whether the cancer is aggressive or not. Aggressive cancers metastasize rapidly and are more malignant than cancers that progress slowly. Aggressive cancer cells are also typically less differentiated from localized cancer cells. Differentiation in this context refers to how physically defined, or shaped, cancer cells are, as well as to what degree they possess or lack the elements of normal cells.

Cell differentiation also refers to the process by which cells mature and undergo changes in their gene expressions to become specialized in order to perform their specific tasks. The human body's trillions of cells are differentiated into hundreds of different types of cells. Cancer cells that bear little resemblance to the normal cells are termed "poorly differentiated", and are known to be the most destructive and difficult to treat.

Aggressive, poorly differentiated cancers are also known to double within 60 days or less, further complicating their treatment. The more undifferentiated cancer cells appear, the higher their grade.

Cancer Grading: Although some cancers have their own grading system, most cancers are graded on a scale of 1 to 4 based on their appearance. Grade 1, or low grade, cancer cells and tissues are well-differentiated and most resemble healthy cells. Grade 2 cancer cells and tissues, while more abnormal in appearance, are still moderately differentiated, and are called intermediate cancers. Grade 3 and grade 4 cancer cells and tissues are the least differentiated and most abnormal in appearance, and are both considered high grade, with grade 4 cancers being the most aggressive.

Cancer Staging: Cancer staging is based on the size of the primary tumor and how much the cancer has metastasized to other areas of the body. The most common staging system ranks cancer on a scale of 0 to 4.

Stage 0 is the category given to cells that appear abnormal but have not spread or turned cancerous, although there is the risk of them doing so over time. This stage is also known as "carcinoma in situ".

Stages 1, 2, and Stage 3 are used to describe cancers that are either localized or have only spread to nearby tissues. The higher the stage number, the larger the tumor size is, and the more the cancer has spread.

Stage 4 refers to cancers that have metastasized to distant areas of the body.

Tumor Markers: Oncologists and other physicians also employ blood (and in some cases urine or bone marrow) tests to both detect cancer and monitor cancer patients' progress as they undergo treatment. These tests measure the levels of various proteins and other substances that cancer cells produce, all of which are known as tumor markers. In some cases, the tests analyze tumors directly. The following are among the most common tumor markers, the cancers they screen for, and how they are used, according to the National Cancer Institute (NCI):

ALK gene rearrangements and over-expression
Cancer types or cancer-like conditions: Non-small cell lung cancer, anaplastic large cell lymphoma, histiocytoses
What's analyzed: Tumor
How used: To help determine treatment and prognosis

Alpha-fetoprotein (AFP)
Cancer types: Liver cancer and germ cell tumors
What's analyzed: Blood
How used: To help diagnose liver cancer and follow response to treatment; to assess stage, prognosis, and response to treatment of germ cell tumors

B-cell immunoglobulin gene rearrangement
Cancer type: B-cell lymphoma
What's analyzed: Blood, bone marrow, or tumor tissue
How used: To help in diagnosis, to evaluate effectiveness of treatment, and to check for recurrence

BCL2 gene rearrangement
Cancer types: Lymphomas, leukemias
What's analyzed: Blood, bone marrow, or tumor tissue
How used: For diagnosis and planning therapy

Beta-2-microglobulin (B2M)
Cancer types: Multiple myeloma, chronic lymphocytic leukemia, and some lymphomas
What's analyzed: Blood, urine, or cerebrospinal fluid
How used: To determine prognosis and follow response to treatment

Beta-human chorionic gonadotropin (Beta-hCG)
Cancer types: Choriocarcinoma and germ cell tumors
What's analyzed: Urine or blood
How used: To assess stage, prognosis, and response to treatment

Bladder Tumor Antigen (BTA)
Cancer types: Bladder cancer and cancer of the kidney or ureter
What's analyzed: Urine
How used: As surveillance with cytology and cystoscopy of patients already known to have bladder cancer

BRCA1 and BRCA2 gene mutations
Cancer types: Ovarian and breast cancers
What's analyzed: Blood and/or tumor
How used: To help determine treatment

BCR-ABL fusion gene
Cancer types: Chronic myeloid leukemia, acute lymphoblastic leukemia, and acute myelogenous leukemia
What's analyzed: Blood or bone marrow
How used: To confirm diagnosis, predict response to targeted therapy, help determine treatment, and monitor disease status

BRAF V600 mutations
Cancer types or cancer-like conditions: Cutaneous melanoma, Erdheim-Chester disease, Langerhans cell histiocytosis, colorectal cancer, and non-small cell lung cancer
What's analyzed: Tumor
How used: To help determine treatment

C-kit/CD117
Cancer types: Gastrointestinal stromal tumor, mucosal melanoma, acute myeloid leukemia, and mast cell disease
What's analyzed: Tumor, blood, or bone marrow
How used: To help in diagnosis and to help determine treatment

CA15-3/CA27.29
Cancer type: Breast cancer
What's analyzed: Blood
How used: To assess whether treatment is working or if the cancer has recurred

CA19-9
Cancer types: Pancreatic, gallbladder, bile duct, and gastric cancers
What's analyzed: Blood
How used: To assess whether treatment is working

CA-125
Cancer type: Ovarian cancer
What's analyzed: Blood
How used: To help in diagnosis, assessment of response to treatment, and evaluation of recurrence

CA 27.29
Cancer type: Breast cancer
What's analyzed: Blood
How used: To detect metastasis or recurrence

Calcitonin
Cancer type: Medullary thyroid cancer
What's analyzed: Blood
How used: To aid in diagnosis, check whether treatment is working, and assess recurrence

Carcinoembryonic antigen (CEA)
Cancer types: Colorectal cancer and some other cancers
What's analyzed: Blood
How used: To keep track of how well cancer treatments are working and check if cancer has come back or spread

CD19
Cancer types: B-cell lymphomas and leukemias
What's analyzed: Blood and bone marrow
How used: To help in diagnosis and to help determine treatment

CD20
Cancer type: Non-Hodgkin lymphoma
What's analyzed: Blood
How used: To help determine treatment

CD22
Cancer types: B-cell lymphomas and leukemias
What's analyzed: Blood and bone marrow
How used: To help in diagnosis and to help determine treatment

CD25
Cancer type: Non-Hodgkin (T-cell) lymphoma
What's analyzed: Blood
How used: To help determine treatment

CD30
Cancer types: Classic Hodgkin lymphoma, B-cell and T-cell lymphomas
What's analyzed: Tumor
How used: To help determine treatment

CD33
Cancer type: Acute myeloid leukemia
What's analyzed: Blood
How used: To help determine treatment

Chromogranin A (CgA)
Cancer type: Neuroendocrine tumors
What's analyzed: Blood
How used: To help in diagnosis, assessment of treatment response, and evaluation of recurrence

Chromosome 17p deletion
Cancer type: Chronic lymphocytic leukemia
What's analyzed: Blood
How used: To help determine treatment

Chromosomes 3, 7, 17, and 9p21
Cancer type: Bladder cancer
What's analyzed: Urine
How used: To help in monitoring for tumor recurrence

Circulating tumor cells of epithelial origin (CELLSEARCH)
Cancer types: Metastatic breast, prostate, and colorectal cancers
What's analyzed: Blood
How used: To inform clinical decision making, and to assess prognosis

Cytokeratin fragment 21-1
Cancer type: Lung cancer
What's analyzed: Blood
How used: To help in monitoring for recurrence

Cyclin D1 (CCND1) gene rearrangement or expression
Cancer types: Lymphoma, myeloma
What's analyzed: Tumor
How used: To help in diagnosis

Des-gamma-carboxy prothrombin (DCP)
Cancer type: Hepatocellular carcinoma
What's analyzed: Blood
How used: To monitor the effectiveness of treatment and to detect recurrence

DPD gene mutation
Cancer types: Breast, colorectal, gastric, and pancreatic cancers
What's analyzed: Blood
How used: To predict the risk of a toxic reaction to 5-fluorouracil therapy

EGFR gene mutation
Cancer type: Non-small cell lung cancer
What's analyzed: Tumor
How used: To help determine treatment and prognosis

Estrogen receptor (ER)/progesterone receptor (PR)
Cancer type: Breast cancer
What's analyzed: Tumor
How used: To help determine treatment

FGFR2 and FGFR3 gene mutations
Cancer type: Bladder cancer
What's analyzed: Tumor
How used: To help determine treatment

Fibrin/fibrinogen
Cancer type: Bladder cancer
What's analyzed: Urine
How used: To monitor progression and response to treatment

FLT3 gene mutations
Cancer type: Acute myeloid leukemia
What's analyzed: Blood
How used: To help determine treatment

Gastrin
Cancer type: Gastrin-producing tumor (gastrinoma)
What's analyzed: Blood
How used: To help in diagnosis, to monitor the effectiveness of treatment, and to detect recurrence

HE4
Cancer type: Ovarian cancer
What's analyzed: Blood
How used: To plan cancer treatment, assess disease progression, and monitor for recurrence

HER2/neu gene amplification or protein overexpression
Cancer types: Breast, ovarian, bladder, pancreatic, and stomach cancers
What's analyzed: Tumor
How used: To help determine treatment

5-HIAA
Cancer type: Carcinoid tumors
What's analyzed: Urine
How used: To help in diagnosis and to monitor disease

IDH1 and IDH2 gene mutations
Cancer type: Acute myeloid leukemia
What's analyzed: Bone marrow and blood
How used: To help determine treatment

Immunoglobulins
Cancer types: Multiple myeloma and Waldenström macroglobulinemia
What's analyzed: Blood and urine
How used: To help diagnose disease, assess response to treatment, and look for recurrence

IRF4 gene rearrangement
Cancer types: Lymphoma
What's analyzed: Tumor
How used: To help in diagnosis

JAK2 gene mutation
Cancer type: Certain types of leukemia
What's analyzed: Blood and bone marrow
How used: To help in diagnosis

KRAS gene mutation
Cancer types: Colorectal cancer and non-small cell lung cancer
What's analyzed: Tumor
How used: To help determine treatment

Lactate dehydrogenase
Cancer types: Germ cell tumors, lymphoma, leukemia, melanoma, and neuroblastoma
What's analyzed: Blood
How used: To assess stage, prognosis, and response to treatment

Microsatellite instability (MSI) and/or mismatch repair deficient (dMMR)
Cancer types: Colorectal cancer and other solid tumors
What's analyzed: Tumor
How used: To guide treatment and to identify those at high risk of certain cancer-predisposing syndromes

MYC gene expression
Cancer types: Lymphomas, leukemias
What's analyzed: Tumor
How used: To help in diagnosis and to help determine treatment

MYD88 gene mutation
Cancer types: Lymphoma, Waldenström macroglobulinemia
What's analyzed: Tumor
How used: To help in diagnosis and to help determine treatment

Myeloperoxidase (MPO)
Cancer type: Leukemia
What's analyzed: Blood
How used: To help in diagnosis

Neuron-specific enolase (NSE)
Cancer types: Small cell lung cancer and neuroblastoma
What's analyzed: Blood
How used: To help in diagnosis and to assess response to treatment

NTRK gene fusion
Cancer type: Any solid tumor
What's analyzed: Tumor
How used: To help determine treatment

Nuclear matrix protein 22
Cancer type: Bladder cancer
What's analyzed: Urine
How used: To monitor response to treatment

PCA3 mRNA
Cancer type: Prostate cancer
What's analyzed: Urine (collected after digital rectal exam)
How used: To determine need for repeat biopsy after negative biopsy

PML/RARα fusion gene
Cancer type: Acute promyelocytic leukemia (APL)
What's analyzed: Blood and bone marrow
How used: To diagnose APL, to predict response to all-trans-retinoic acid or arsenic trioxide therapy, to assess effectiveness of therapy, to monitor minimal residual disease, and to predict early relapse

Prostatic Acid Phosphatase (PAP)
Cancer type: Metastatic prostate cancer
What's analyzed: Blood
How used: To help in diagnosing poorly differentiated carcinomas

Programmed death ligand 1 (PD-L1)
Cancer types: Non-small cell lung cancer, liver cancer, stomach cancer, gastroesophageal junction cancer, classical Hodgkin lymphoma, and other aggressive lymphoma subtypes
What's analyzed: Tumor
How used: To help determine treatment

Prostate-specific antigen (PSA)
Cancer type: Prostate cancer
What's analyzed: Blood
How used: To help in diagnosis, to assess response to treatment, and to look for recurrence

ROS1 gene rearrangement
Cancer type: Non-small cell lung cancer
What's analyzed: Tumor
How used: To help determine treatment

Soluble mesothelin-related peptides (SMRP)
Cancer type: Mesothelioma
What's analyzed: Blood
How used: To monitor progression or recurrence

Somatostatin receptor
Cancer type: Neuroendocrine tumors affecting the pancreas or gastrointestinal tract (GEP-NETs)
What's analyzed: Tumor (by diagnostic imaging)
How used: To help determine treatment

T-cell receptor gene rearrangement
Cancer type: T-cell lymphoma
What's analyzed: Bone marrow, tissue, body fluid, blood
How used: To help in diagnosis; sometimes to detect and evaluate residual disease

Terminal transferase (TdT)
Cancer types: Leukemia, lymphoma
What's analyzed: Tumor, blood
How used: To help in diagnosis

Thiopurine S-methyltransferase (TPMT) enzyme activity or TPMT genetic test
Cancer type: Acute lymphoblastic leukemia
What's analyzed: Blood and buccal (cheek) swab
How used: To predict the risk of severe bone marrow toxicity (myelosuppression) with thiopurine treatment

Thyroglobulin
Cancer type: Thyroid cancer
What's analyzed: Blood
How used: To evaluate response to treatment and to look for recurrence

UGT1A1*28 variant homozygosity
Cancer type: Colorectal cancer
What's analyzed: Blood and buccal (cheek) swab
How used: To predict toxicity from irinotecan therapy

Urine catecholamines: VMA and HVA
Cancer type: Neuroblastoma
What's analyzed: Urine
How used: To help in diagnosis

Urokinase plasminogen activator (uPA) and plasminogen activator inhibitor (PAI-1)
Cancer type: Breast cancer
What's analyzed: Tumor
How used: To determine aggressiveness of cancer and guide treatment

FoundationOne CDx (F1CDx) genomic test
Cancer type: Any solid tumor
What's analyzed: Tumor, blood
How used: As a companion diagnostic test to determine treatment

Guardant360 CDx genomic test
Cancer type: Any solid tumor
What's analyzed: Blood
How used: As a companion diagnostic test to determine treatment and for general tumor mutation profiling

5-Protein signature (OVA1)
Cancer type: Ovarian cancer
What's analyzed: Blood
How used: To pre-operatively assess pelvic mass for suspected ovarian cancer

17-Gene signature (Oncotype DX GPS test)
Cancer type: Prostate cancer
What's analyzed: Tumor
How used: To predict the aggressiveness of prostate cancer and to help manage treatment

21-Gene signature (Oncotype DX)
Cancer type: Breast cancer
What's analyzed: Tumor
How used: To evaluate risk of distant recurrence and to help plan treatment

46-Gene signature (Prolaris)
Cancer type: Prostate cancer
What's analyzed: Tumor
How used: To predict the aggressiveness of prostate cancer and to help manage treatment

70-Gene signature (Mammaprint)
Cancer type: Breast cancer
What's analyzed: Tumor
How used: To evaluate risk of recurrence

While tumor marker tests can be very helpful in helping to detect cancer and monitor treatment progress, they do have their limitations, and by themselves should not be relied upon to diagnose cancer. Rather, they serve as indications that other more conclusive tests are warranted, both to confirm the existence of cancer and to detect a possible cancer recurrence.

Tumor marker tests can also sometimes result in a "false positive" reading, indicating cancer is present when in actuality it is not. That's because, in some cases, people without cancer can still exhibit high tumor marker levels. Additionally, the existence of other health conditions can sometimes raise tumor marker levels.

Tumor marker levels are also sometimes not consistent, meaning the tests results may not always be the same despite being given successively within a short time frame. In some cases, tumor markers may stay the same even as cancer progresses. Finally, for some types of cancer no known tumor markers have been found. Despite these shortcomings, I still recommend tumor marker tests, with the caveat that they are not perfect.

In Chapter 5, you will learn more about the benefits and limitations of conventional cancer screening tests, and I will also introduce you to other tests that I recommend that many oncologists and other physicians may not use or are not aware of.

Missing The Forest For the Trees

Based on my clinical experience and many years of working with cancer, I have come to recognize that one of the primary reasons why conventional oncology so often fails cancer patients is because of its myopic focus on tumors, without regard to the underlying systemic causes that initiated the cancer process in the first place. Addressing tumors is certainly important, especially in cases where tumors have grown so large that they are impinging upon organs and interfering with organ function. In such cases, debulking via surgery is almost always a wise course of action. But even when surgery is warranted, cancer patients need to recognize that when their doctors tell them, "We got it all," it does not mean that they are cancer-free. In point of fact, surgery by itself is almost always incapable of "getting it all", because during the surgical procedures, invariably microscopic pieces of the tumor, known as circulating tumor cells (CTCs), break off from the tumor as it is being removed to enter into the bloodstream and migrate to other parts of the body undetected, where they can then begin to form other tumors. In addition, the radiation and/or chemotherapy treatments that usually follow tumor removal often cause cancer stem cells (CSCs) to become stronger and more resistant to such treatments over time, also setting the stage for cancer recurrence later on. Usually, when cancer recurs, it is more malignant and widespread than it was originally. (You will learn more about CTCs and CSCs in Chapter 4.)

The focus on surgical tumor removal originated with Dr. William S Halstead (1852-1922), a surgeon at Johns Hopkins Hospital in Baltimore, Maryland. In 1894, Dr. Halstead developed and named the surgical procedure known as radical mastectomy to treat breast cancer. This highly invasive surgery involves removing breast tissues (usually the complete breast), chest muscles, and lymph nodes in the armpit in order to remove breast cancer tumors. Radical mastectomy remained the standard treatment for breast cancer until the 1970s, and is still performed today in some cases due to the conventional model of cancer theory, which emphasizes the tumor over the cancer patient.

Fortunately, in recent decades, this emphasis has begun to be challenged by a growing number of cancer researchers, such as Gershom Zajicek, MD, of the Department of Developmental Biology and Cancer Research at Hebrew University in Jerusalem, Israel. As early as the 1990s, Dr. Gershom pointed out that from 1930 to 1990 the age-adjusted mortality rate for breast cancer patients had basically remained unchanged, indicating that the tumor treatment model of cancer had failed. Dr. Zajicek maintains that it failed because it is "based on false premises." In a paper he published in 1996, he wrote, "This hypothesis implies that tumor removal should cure the patient, yet 60 years of intensive effort to remove the tumor did not change the biological outcome of the disease. Obviously, the hypothesis is wrong and should be modified." It also bears mentioning that Dr. Zajicek views cancer as both a metabolic disease and a survival mechanism, and that tumors are formed by the body as a self-protective mechanism.

I agree with Dr. Zajicek's views, which is why I have chosen the naturopathic oncology model over the conventional oncology model. A key component that we need to recognize is that cancer is not an isolated event. It's a systemic experience caused by multiple factors, all of which must be properly addressed. In addition, in line with the idea that cancer is a survival mechanism, I've come to view cancer as the body's way of walling off toxins and infections to protect the rest of the body, just as we build prisons to protect society from the effect of harmful individuals. Thus, the solution is not to destroy the tumor, letting the toxic debris loose in the body. It is to clean up the environment so that the toxic debris in the cancer can be handled as the tumor is diminishing.

If you just focus on cancer by removing tumors and then using radiation or chemotherapy, you are overlooking or ignoring the environment that the cancer developed within. We call this environment the biological terrain. Naturopathic oncology focuses on that terrain in order to best determine the factors that that led to the development of cancer. This enables physicians and cancer patients alike to know what needs to change in order to be able help ensure that cancer can no longer thrive in that environment.

The analogy I sometimes use to explain the difference between conventional oncology and naturopathic oncology is that of rats in an infested area. You can kill the rats, but if you don't also clean up the area, then the infestation is likely to reoccur, and more rats will keep coming back again and again. It's the same thing with cancer. Conventional cancer therapy, even though it can be very powerful at times, and start to produce immediate results in the form of a reduction in tumor size and so forth, ultimately will still fail if the patient still has the same terrain and continues to be affected by the cancer drivers that caused the cancer in the first place.

Moreover, it's a well-known fact that surgery, radiation, and chemotherapy all leave cancer patients weaker, further suppressing immune function and making the terrain even worse, thus increasing the likelihood that cancer will eventually come back, which is an all-too common scenario.

In order to have the best chance of preventing recurrence and achieving long-term remission, it is vital to create a cancer treatment plan that is individualized to most effectively address all of the factors—nutritional, environmental, mental/emotional, and spiritual— that caused the patient's cancer in the first place. Because it addresses each of these factors while also improving the overall terrain, naturopathic oncology is a "whole person" treatment approach that results in a more balanced state of overall health. To return to my analogy, not only are the rats dealt with, but the environment is also cleaned up and transformed into one that is no longer conducive for attracting other rats.

To conclude this chapter, let's take a brief look at the most common drivers that can cause and exacerbate cancer, followed by early warning signs that you need to be aware of.

The Multiple Factors That Drive Cancer

As I hope you now understand, after reading this far, cancer is not some random occurrence that happens "out of the blue". Rather, it results from a chronic mix of factors known as cancer drivers, all of which I discuss in more detail later on in this book, beginning in Chapter 2. Here, I will simply list each of the most common drivers so that you can be aware of them and start to recognize those that may currently be present in your own life.

- Chronic stress (physical, mental/emotional, spiritual)
- Chronic inflammation and related factors (free radicals, reactive oxygen species, cellular redox, insulin resistance)
- Trauma (physical and psychological)
- Life shocks, e.g. death of a loved one, divorce, job loss, "crisis of faith", etc.

- Unresolved or repressed emotions
- Poor diet and low quality foods (processed foods, "junk foods", GMOs, farm-raised fish, non-grass fed/grass finished meats and poultry, etc)
- Nutritional imbalances (both deficiencies and excesses)
- Unhealthy microbiome (gut) and related gastrointestinal disorders
- Poor lifestyle choices, e.g. lack of exercise/sedentary lifestyle
- Excessive alcohol consumption
- Smoking and exposure to secondhand smoke
- Being overweight/obesity/high body mass index (BMI)
- Heavy metals and other environmental toxins, including asbestos, chemicals in household and cosmetic products, fluoridated water
- Pathogenic infections (bacterial, viral, fungal, parasitic)
- Electrosmog (EMFs, EMRs, dirty electricity, cell phones, cell phone towers, smart meters, etc)
- Ultraviolet (UV) radiation
- Frequent X-rays, CT scans
- Unhealthy home or work environments (sick building syndrome, geopathic stress)
- Poor sleep/unhealthy sleep habits
- Endocrine (hormone) imbalances
- Unsafe sex/promiscuity
- Occupational risks/exposures.

As you review the list above, you will come to realize that you have a great deal of control over many of these risk factors based upon the choices you make and how committed you are to becoming and staying healthy. This fact has been confirmed by numerous studies, including a 2022 study published in *The Lancet* which found that nearly half of all annual cases of cancer around the globe are caused and driven by unhealthy lifestyle choices, and thus are highly preventable. Throughout the rest of this book, I will show you how to address and protect yourself from these cancer drivers.

Be Aware Of Cancer's Early Warning Signs

Recognizing the early warning signs of cancer can help to ensure an early diagnosis. This makes it potentially easier to treat cancer before it spreads to other areas of the body. Cancer that is detected early typically has not yet had the opportunity to deplete the body of its disease-fighting resources, and therefore cancer is far more likely to respond to treatment that results in remission.

What follow are the most common early warning signs, or initial symptoms, of cancer. If you experience any of them, seek immediate medical attention so that you can be properly screened for cancer.

Lumps of Thickening in Breast or Testicle Tissues: Since breast and testicular cancer have increasingly shown signs of developing earlier, all men and women above the age of 25 should regularly (at least once a month) examine themselves for telltale signs of cancer of the breasts and testicles. By gently yet firmly pressing into the breasts, women are often able to detect lumps or thickening breast tissue that can be a sign of breast cancer. In a similar fashion, men can massage their testicles, being on the lookout for any noticeable changes in the way they feel.

Changes in Warts or Moles: Warts or moles that begin to change appearance can be a sign of various types of skin cancer, such as melanoma or squamous carcinoma. One indication that skin cancer might be developing is bleeding that occurs in warts and moles. A change in wart or mole size is another common indicator. In addition, the appearance of chronic pimples or patches of dry, scaly skin are other warning signs, as is skin that becomes inflamed or ulcerated. Sores that are slow to heal are another indicator, as are chronic sores in the mouth.

Persistent Sore Throat: A chronic sore throat can be a potential indicator that cancer is developing in an area of the throat (esophagus, larynx, or pharynx). Other early warning signs of throat cancer include persistent hoarseness, lumps in the throat, and difficulty swallowing.

Changes in Bowel and Bladder Habits: Any noticeable and persistent change in your bowel movements or in the way you urinate can be an indication of cancer in the genitourinary tract (bladder, prostate, and testicular cancer), or in the gastrointestinal tract (colon or stomach cancer). Such changes include unexplained constipation or diarrhea, blood in the urine or stool, pain during urination and elimination, difficulty urinating or passing stool, abdominal pain, and stools that are dark and resemble tar.

Coughing Blood/Persistent Coughing: Persistent coughing and coughing up of blood can be signs of lung cancer, as well as other types of cancer, especially in people who smoke, although in recent years the incidence of lung cancer in nonsmokers has also begun to rise.

Chronic Digestion Problems: The following digestive symptoms can all be indications of cancer: abdominal pain, bloating of the stomach or abdomen, chronic heartburn or indigestion, nausea, and loss of appetite. Chronic flatulence is another potential early warning sign, as is a persistent "growling" or a "rumbling" stomach.

Unexplained Weight Loss: Any sudden and unexplained loss of weight should immediately be brought to the attention of your doctor.

Persistent Fatigue and Feelings of Exhaustion: Ongoing loss of energy or chronic fatigue are other possible indications that cancer is present and beginning to spread.

Abnormal Vaginal Discharges and/or Bleeding: These signs can be indications of cervical, ovarian, or vaginal cancer.

In addition to the general early warning symptoms mentioned above, specific types of cancers usually result in specific symptoms. What follows is a list of some of the most common cancers and the symptoms that most commonly accompany them.

Bladder Cancer Symptoms: blood in the urine, rust-colored urine, pain and/or burning sensations during urination, frequent need to urinate, difficulty urinating, pus-filled urine.

Bone Cancer (Sarcoma) Symptoms: unexplained weakness in areas of the musculo-skeletal system, unexplained pains in and around areas of the bones, increased susceptibility to fractures.

Breast Cancer Symptoms: lumps in the breast and/or thickening breast tissue, nipple discharge, retraction of the nipple, dimpling of breast tissue, reddened breast skin tissue, swollen breasts, sensation of heat in the breasts, swelling in the lymph nodes beneath the armpits.

Colon and Rectal Cancer Symptoms: blood in the stools, bleeding from the rectum, dark and tarry stools, abdominal pains and cramping, unexplained constipation or diarrhea, alternating constipation and diarrhea, unexplained weight loss, loss of appetite, unexplained fatigue, poor skin pallor.

Kidney Cancer Symptoms: Blood in the urine, dull aches or pains in the lower back or on the sides of the abdomen, lumps or swelling in the kidney area of the abdomen or lower back, unexplained elevations in blood pressure levels, unexplained abnormalities in red blood cell count.

Leukemia Symptoms: Unexplained weakness or fatigue, pale skin, unexplained fever, flu-like symptoms, prolonged bleeding, unexplained bruising, enlarged lymph nodes, swollen spleen and/or liver, frequent infections, unexplained bone or joint pain, unexplained weight loss, night sweats.

Lung Cancer Symptoms: persistent coughing or wheezing, persistent chest pain, persistent lung congestion, swollen lymph nodes in the neck, blood produced upon coughing.

Melanoma (Skin Cancer) Symptoms: changes in skin tone and texture; changes in the size, shape, and/or color of moles; unexplained bleeding from the skin.

Non-Hodgkin's Lymphoma Symptoms: Swelling (without pain) of the lymph nodes in the neck, armpits, and/or groin; persistent fever; persistent fatigue; unexplained weight loss; unexplained skin rashes and/or itching; small lumps in the skin; bone pain; swelling in the liver, spleen, and/or areas of the abdomen.

Oral (Lip, Mouth, or Throat) Cancer Symptoms: Lumps or sore spots in the mouth, pain while eating or drinking, persistent ulcers on the lip, tongue or inside the mouth, difficulty swallowing, oral pain, loosening teeth, bleeding in the mouth, blood produced by coughing, persistent bad breath.

Ovarian Cancer Symptoms: Abdominal swelling, unexplained vaginal bleeding or discharge, persistent and unexplained digestive problems.

Pancreatic Cancer Symptoms: Persistent pain in the upper abdomen, unexplained weight loss, persistent pain in the mid-back and center of the back, loss of appetite, sudden inability to properly digest/tolerate fatty foods, yellow skin tone (jaundice), abdominal swelling, swelling of the liver and spleen.

Prostate Cancer Symptoms: Difficulty urinating, pain or burning sensations upon urination, frequent need to urinate, incomplete urination, blood in the urine, pain in the area of the bladder, dull, persistent aching in the area of the pelvis and lower back.

Uterine Cancer Symptoms: (Approximately 70 to 75 percent of all cases of uterine cancer occur after menopause.) Vaginal bleeding or discharge after menopause, painful urination, collection of fluids in the uterus, pain during intercourse, persistent pains in the area of the pelvis.

Note: Relying on self-care screening methods alone is not enough to detect cancer. People 40 years and older, as well as anyone with a family history of cancer, should consider receiving professional cancer screening tests on an annual basis.

Now that you have a deeper understanding of what cancer is, let's examine one of its primary underlying causes, chronic inflammation. That is the topic of Chapter 2.

Chapter 2

Inflammation: The Fire Within You

John had a history of stage-2 non-Hodgkin's follicular lymphoma, which he thought was under control. The CAT scans he had received every six months to monitor his health showed that the cluster behind his left kidney was stabilizing and starting to shrink. But then his next scan revealed his spleen had enlarged and the lymphoma had expanded across his entire chest area. Follow-up lab tests shows that he had cancer in 50 percent of his bone marrow, and his diagnosis was changed from follicular lymphoma to chronic lymphocytic leukemia CLL.

Lisa is a health practitioner who ate a healthy diet and supported herself with nutritional supplements. So she was shocked to find out she'd developed stage 4 triple negative breast cancer that had metastasized to her bones and lungs. Soon thereafter, she ended up in a wheel chair with five compression fractures along her spine.

Susie had been diagnosed with ductal carcinoma in the situ (DCIS) when she was 49 and living in Seattle. DCIS is a condition characterized by the presence of abnormal cells inside a milk duct in the breast. It is considered the earliest form of breast cancer, but is noninvasive, meaning it hasn't spread out of the milk duct and has a low risk of becoming invasive. Nonetheless, Susie elected to have a lumpectomy to remove it. Four months later, following a routine mammogram, she was diagnosed with microinvasive lobular carcinoma, a rare form of breast cancer, in her right breast.

In addition to cancer, what John, Lisa, and Susie had in common was a high degree of inflammation and infection.

In John's case, an inflammation marker revealed that the level of inflammation in his body was ten times higher than a normal, healthy reading. Lisa's onset of cancer and rapid decline followed an examination by her biological dentist who discovered that she had hidden dental infections so severe that he did not dare to touch them. The infections were due to bad root canal procedure from a prior dentist, who subsequently removed them, leaving her with a lot of cavitations that had not been treated. This enabled colonies of infection to accumulate in the cavitation sites and then spread further into her body, causing systemic inflammation.

In Lisa's case, lab tests revealed she had a wide range of serious infections, including high levels of *Streptococcus mutans*, *Helicobacter pylori*, *Blastocystis hominis*, *Aspergillus*, cytomegalovirus, human herpes virus-6, and *Borrelia burgdorferi*, all of which kept her body in a chronic inflammatory state.

Unfortunately, the above case histories are far from rare. Both chronic inflammation and infection are very common among cancer patients. This chapter explains why.

Inflammation—Both Good and Bad

The word "inflammation" is derived from the Latin words *inflammatio*, which means "to set on fire", and *inflammatus*, which means "inflamed". And just like fire itself, inflammation can be both protective and destructive. When left unchecked, it is a major driver of cancer and many other disease conditions, including autoimmune disease. The names of all conditions that end in *itis* are also inflammatory diseases. If you suffering from any type of persistent health challenge, there is a good chance that your body is in a state of low-grade, chronic inflammation.

There are two types of inflammation responses: Acute and chronic. Acute responses are short-lived and serve as an important component of the immune system's response to infections. Acute inflammation is also crucial for healing wounds, burns, and other injuries. Once these conditions are dealt with and healed, this type of inflammation response soon ends, as nature intended.

Chronic inflammation, on the other hand, is a persistent, uncontrolled response. It is caused when the body is unable to heal infections or injuries, but can also occur in their absence. In either case, chronic inflammation can often go undetected because its symptoms differ from those of acute inflammation. The longer that chronic inflammation is not addressed, the greater its harmful effects can become, to the point where they can even be life-threatening. In 2011, the Centers for Disease Control and Prevention (CDC) noted chronic, low-level inflammation contributes to the onset and progression of cancer, as well as Alzheimer's disease, chronic lower respiratory disease, diabetes, heart disease, stroke, and kidney disease. Since then, the range of disease conditions linked to chronic inflammation has continued to expand. In order to reverse cancer and these other diseases, chronic inflammation must be properly dealt with and eliminated.

Common Causes of Chronic Inflammation: Besides lingering injuries and infections, chronic inflammation is often caused by other factors. One of the most common is an unhealthy diet, especially one consisting of processed foods, hydrogenated and other unhealthy fats/oils (canola, corn, safflower, soybean, sunflower, etc), sugars and simple ("white") carbohydrates. These pro-inflammatory foods, as well as foods that are baked, fried, smoked, or otherwise heated or grilled at high temperatures, increase the production of substances called glycotoxins, also known as advanced glycation end products (AGEs). AGEs, once they enter the body, stick to tissues and oxidize them, triggering and sustaining chronic inflammation, which is why AGEs are now recognized as a primary risk factor for premature aging and chronic illness, including cancer.

Eliminating AGEs from your diet can go a long way towards improving your health, as was shown in a published study conducted by researchers at Mount Sinai School of Medicine. In the study, participants were randomly assigned into two groups. The first group consumed a typical Western diet that was rich in AGEs. The participants in the second group avoided eating grilled, fried, or baked foods, instead eating foods that were poached, steamed, or stewed. This reduced their intake of AGEs to about half of the AGEs the first group consumed. The amount of calories and nutrient content in both groups were the same and did not change during the course of the study. At the end of four months, researchers found that the participants in the AGE-reduced diet group achieved as much as a 60 percent reduction in their blood AGE levels, lipid peroxides (markers of oxidative stress), inflammatory markers, and biomarkers of vascular function.

"What is noteworthy about our findings is that reduced AGE consumption proved to be effective in all study participants, including healthy persons and persons who have a chronic condition such as kidney disease," said the study's lead author Helen Vlassara, MD, Professor and Director of the Division of Experimental Diabetes and Aging at Mount Sinai School of Medicine. "This suggests that oxidants may play a more active role than genetics in overwhelming our body's defenses, which we need to fight off disease. It has been said that nature holds the power, but the environment pulls the trigger. The good news is that unlike genetics, we can control oxidant levels, which may not be an accompaniment to disease and aging, but instead due to the cumulative toxic influence of AGEs."

Other causes of chronic inflammation include excessive alcohol intake, smoking and/or regular exposure to secondhand smoke, exposure to heavy metals and other environmental toxins, and regular exposure to ultraviolet (UV) radiation. Chronic stress and poor sleep are other common risk factors, as is the regular use of certain pharmaceutical drugs, which can cause vasculitis (inflammation of blood vessels) and inflammation in the gastrointestinal tract, including inflammatory bowel disease (IBD). People who are overweight or obese also have a higher risk of chronic inflammation, and therefore cancer and other serious illnesses.

Poor circulation is another significant, yet often overlooked, risk factor. Poor, or sluggish, circulation causes blood to become too thick and "sticky", a condition known as hyperviscosity. How much energy the body needs, as well as how efficiently it produces energy, depends on the availability of oxygen and various nutrients in the blood, as well as the heart's ability to continually circulate blood. Thick, sticky blood impairs blood circulation, placing a strain on the heart. The combination of hyperviscosity and chronic inflammation impairs the functioning of every system in the body, including the immune system.

Another overlooked risk factor for chronic inflammation is excess iron buildup (also known as iron overload) in the body. While iron plays many important roles in the body, including forming hemoglobin, regulating cell growth, and helping to maintain brain function, metabolism, endocrine function, and immune function, too much iron can cause oxidative stress and can be toxic. Multiple studies link excess iron to many degenerative diseases, including cancer. Iron overload is very common in most adult Americans today, especially as they age. This is not surprising, since iron, unlike other minerals such as magnesium, accumulates in the body. Iron is now found in many iron-enriched food products and supplement formulas. Since the 1940s, it has also been commonly added to crop soil, where it is absorbed by food grown in that soil. The link between iron overload and cancer is discussed further later in this chapter.

It is also well-established that excess visceral (belly) fat is another significant risk factor for chronic inflammation, and that chronic inflammation is a contributor to visceral fat and obesity. Combined, both also increase the risk of metabolic syndrome (prediabetes). Elevated levels of the hormone cortisol, which is released during times of stress, can also cause visceral fat to produce even more inflammation.

All of these risk factors trigger the release of pro-inflammatory proteins that contribute to cancer.

Inflammation and Cancer

As mentioned above, inflammation is a normal and vital response when the body is wounded or otherwise injured. Without such a response, injured tissues would not be able to heal. The inflammatory process starts when chemicals within the injured tissues get released. When this occurs, white blood cells respond by producing various substances that promote the growth of new blood vessels and cause cells to divide and grow, healing and rebuilding tissue in the process.

Interestingly, the same mechanisms of action—new blood vessel growth, cell division, etc—involved in wound healing are very similar to those involved in the development and progression of cancer. Moreover, various genes that play key roles in wound healing can also be activated by cancerous tumors, making the tumors more likely to spread. This fact was confirmed by researchers at Stanford University School of Medicine. "The molecular features that define this wound-like phenotype are evident at an early clinical stage, persist during treatment, and predict increased risk of metastasis and death in breast, lung, and gastric carcinomas," the researchers reported. (A phenotype is the set of observable and biochemical traits based on genetic and/or environmental influences.) "Wound healing is a process that allows cells to break normal constraints on their growth and cross boundaries," Howard Chang, MD, PhD, lead author of that study, explained. "If a cell can access that program, that's a good environment for cancer."

The findings of Dr. Chang and his research team built upon research dating back to the mid-1980s. By then, microscopic tissue analysis by other researchers had already revealed a similarity between the microenvironment of cancer tumors to that of a healing wound. One of these researchers was pathologist Harold F. Dvorak, MD, founding Director of the Center for Vascular Biology Research at the Beth Israel Deaconess Medical Center and the Mallinckrodt Distinguished Professor of Pathology at Harvard Medical School. In a research paper he published in 1986 in the *New England Journal of Medicine (NEJM)*, Dvorak dubbed tumors "wounds that do not heal".

As you will recall from reading Chapter 1, however, modern day researchers were not the first to link inflammation to tumors. That honor belongs to the father of cellular pathology, Rudolph Virchow. In 1858, Virchow, based on his observations that cancerous skin lesions often developed at skin sites that were chronically irritated, proposed his irritation theory for cancer. According to Virchow, irritations of any type were key components contributing to the spread of cancerous tissues. Continuing his research by examining cells and tissues under a microscope, he observed that areas of skin irritation were also always associated with inflammation cells, leading him to later state that there is a direct link between inflammation and cancer.

In a research paper published in *The Lancet* that supported Virchow's theory and further addressed the link between inflammation and cancer, researchers Frances Balkwill, PhD and Alberto Mantovani, MD wrote, "If genetic damage is the 'match that lights the fire' of cancer, some types of inflammation may provide the 'fuel that feeds the flames'."

In another research paper published in 2021, its authors wrote, "Recent reports showed that there is a direct causal link between inflammation and cancer development, as several cancers were found to be associated with chronic inflammatory conditions. In patients with cancer, healthy endothelial cells [cells that line the interior surface of blood vessels, and lymphatic vessels] regulate vascular homeostasis [the state of equilibrium in the body maintained by its self-regulating processes], and it is believed that they can limit tumor growth, invasiveness, and metastasis. Conversely, dysfunctional endothelial cells that have been exposed to the inflammatory tumor microenvironment can support cancer progression and metastasis."

How Inflammation Triggers Cancer

To understand how inflammation triggers cancer and enables it to grow and spread, we first need to understand what happens when the body's inflammation response is initiated.

At the onset of the inflammation response, neutrophils, the most abundant type of white blood cells and part of the body's immune system, are activated and travel to where the body is injured or has been invaded by infectious microorganisms. There, they are soon joined by other inflammatory cells, such as leukocytes, lymphocytes, macrophages, and mast cells.

The activation of these inflammatory cells is initiated and regulated by a cell signaling network consisting of various growth factors (either proteins or steroid hormones), along with cytokines and chemokines. Growth factors stimulate cell proliferation, wound healing, and, to a lesser extent, cell differentiation. Cytokines belong to a class of proteins known as peptides. They play an important role in cell signaling and stimulate normal cell growth in order to repair and replace aged or damaged tissues. Chemokines are a subclass of cytokines that guide the migration of cells, including inflammatory cells that they recruit to areas in the body of injury and infection.

All inflammatory cells work together to repair damaged tissues and to fight infections. Typically, though, neutrophils are more actively involved in cases of acute inflammation, while other inflammatory cells play a more active role in chronic inflammation.

Once the inflammatory cells have performed their tasks, they need to be rapidly cleared. This programmed clearance is regulated by other cells that induce apoptosis (programmed cell death) and promote phagocytosis, a process in which other cells engulf and "eat" the inflammatory cells. Phagocytosis of inflammatory cells that undergo apoptosis also initiates various other anti-inflammatory responses by our bodies.

If the inflammation response is not controlled and resolved, inflammatory cells continue to operate beyond their original task, and chronic inflammation ensues. When this occurs, various inflammatory cells, such as lymphocytes, and macrophages, start generating increased amounts of growth factors, cytokines, and reactive oxygen and nitrogen species, all of which can cause DNA damage in cells, tissues, and organs. This creates an ideal microenvironment for chronic inflammation to cause cancer.

A growing body of research confirms that chronic inflammation can both trigger and increase the risk of cancer and also cause it to worsen. For example, studies show that chronic prostatitis (inflammation of the prostate gland) increases the risk of prostate cancer. Other studies have found that chronic inflammatory conditions of the gastrointestinal tract, such as Crohn's disease and ulcerative colitis, can increase the risk of colorectal cancer by as much as 1,000 percent. Research has also demonstrated that the use of anti-inflammatory drugs to manage colitis symptoms reduces the risk of developing colon cancer.

In addition, studies have also linked *Helicobacter pylori* (*H. pylori*), an infectious bacteria linked to peptic ulcers and other ulcers of the stomach and small intestine, as the primary risk factor for non-cardia gastric cancer (cancer of the stomach that occur one inch or more below the esophagus; stomach cancer that occurs in the top inch of the stomach is known as cardia gastric cancer) and of gastric mucosa-associated lymphoid tissue (MALT) lymphoma.

Gastric cancer is the second most common cause of cancer-related deaths in the world, according to the National Cancer Institute (NCI). The increased risk H. pylori poses appears to be restricted to non-cardia gastric cancer. A 2001 analysis of 12 studies of *H. pylori* and gastric cancer estimated that the risk of non-cardia gastric cancer was nearly six times higher for *H. pylori*-infected people than for uninfected people. Another study comparing people with non-cardia gastric cancer with cancer-free control subjects revealed that people with *H. pylori*-infections individuals had a nearly 800 percent increased risk for non-cardia gastric cancer.

Gastric MALT lymphoma is a rare type of non-Hodgkin lymphoma that is characterized by the slow multiplication of B lymphocytes, a type of immune cell, in the stomach lining. According to the NCI, "nearly all patients with gastric MALT lymphoma show signs of *H. pylori* infection, and the risk of developing this tumor is more than six times higher in infected people than in uninfected people."

H. pylori is also known to increase the risk of gastric adenocarcinoma. Adenocarcinoma is a type of cancer that affects glands and glandular tissues. Other studies have found a possible association between *H. pylori* infection and pancreatic cancer, but the evidence is not conclusive.

Research has also found an increased risk for bile duct cancer (cholangiocarcinoma) resulting from inflammation caused by a liver fluke called *Clonorchis sinensis*. Similarly, hepatitis B and C infections and the resultant inflammation they cause are known to increase the risk for liver cancer.

In addition, just as chronic prostatitis increases the risk for prostate cancer, and inflammatory conditions of the GI tract increase the risk for colorectal cancer, inflammatory diseases such as esophagitis and chronic pancreatitis increase the risk of esophageal and pancreatic cancers, as well as gallbladder cancer. And, of course, a variety of environmental factors known to cause inflammation, such as asbestos, heavy metals, pesticides, herbicides, and other toxins, are also well-known carcinogens.

Although there is no question that chronic inflammation is a primary cause of cancer, it is important to point out that researchers are still exploring the question of whether or not it is able to trigger cancer without at least one carcinogen also being present. Given the vast and growing number of known carcinogens, however, and how prevalent chronic inflammation is among the populace today, the answer to that question may prove to be a moot point.

Inflammation, Cancer, and Mitochondria

At the cellular level, a number of factors contribute to both inflammation and cancer. Perhaps the most significant of these is dysfunction of the mitochondria. Recapping what you learned in Chapter 1, through the process of cellular respiration, mitochondria produce nearly all of the energy our bodies need by metabolizing nutrients and combining them with oxygen to produce ATP, the main cellular "fuel". In addition, mitochondria play essential roles in cell growth and division, cell signaling, and normal cell death (apoptosis), while also regulating cell metabolism, and cellular and genetic repair. They are also critical for maintaining the health of immune cells, including T cells, and activating the body's immune response to infectious disease. As the authors of one research study wrote, "Mitochondrial ROS (mtROS) [mitochondrial reactive oxygen species] production, mitochondrial DNA (mtDNA) release, [and] mitochondrial antiviral signaling protein (MAVS) are key triggers in the activation of innate immune response following variety of stress signals that include infection, tissue damage and metabolic dysregulation." Healthy immune function is essential for protecting our bodies against cancer.

However, as you also learned in Chapter 1, the very process by which mitochondria metabolize nutrient food molecules with oxygen to produce energy can impair their ability to function and even cause them to die prematurely because this process is highly oxidative and therefore constantly exposes mitochondria to large amounts of inflammation-causing free radicals. Over time, this exposure, along with other factors, can cause mitochondrial damage and dysfunction. Damaged mitochondria weaken the body's immune response, promote genetic mutations, activate oncogenes, and deactivate suppressor genes. Numerous studies have established a link between mutations in mitochondrial DNA and various cancers, including bladder, brain, breast, colon, gastric, head and neck, kidney, liver, lung, ovarian, and thyroid cancers, as well as leukemia.

Lipid peroxides play a central role in this oxidative process. They are produced in the presence of a free radical by the oxidation of unsaturated fatty acids in the cell in the presence of molecular oxygen. The formation of lipid peroxides results in the destruction of the original lipid, leading to damaged cell membranes, as well as a variety of other toxic effects. However, lipid peroxides also stimulate oxygen metabolism to improve mitochondrial efficiency.

There are two aspects to oxygen metabolism when it comes to health. One aspect is getting oxygen into the body. The other aspect is how well the body is able to use oxygen. Oxygen goes to every cell to create energy to the level that the cells can use the oxygen. The problem for many of us is that we can have decent levels of oxygen in our bodies, but we are using it poorly. The inability to process oxygen properly is a major factor of aging and age-related diseases. Almost half of the cells consist of mitochondria. The rest of the cell, the part that uses the energy produced by mitochondria, pretty much stay intact until about age 90 if no genetic disorders are present. Metabolism of oxygen becomes impaired and inefficient with age. We become like a flashlight with a battery that is fading. The oxygen that is not processed in the mitochondria results in free radical production (oxidative stress). The more we age, the less efficient the mitochondria work, leading to less energy production and more oxidative stress within the cells.

Mitochondria and Reactive Oxygen Species (ROS): Reactive oxygen species are highly reactive chemicals formed from oxygen. They are primarily produced at the cellular level by mitochondria, but can also form as a result of other metabolic processes in the body. ROS are byproducts of oxygen reacting with electrons, which is what happens when oxygen and electrons meet within what is known the electron transport chain (ETC). The ETC is a cluster of proteins that transfer electrons through a membrane within mitochondria during the process that creates ATP.

Scientists have long known that ROS at proper levels play various important roles in the body's overall health, including being involved in immune function, destruction of harmful bacteria and fungi, control of the body's inflammation response, and aiding the production of thyroid hormone. But excessive amounts of ROS can damage cells, proteins, lipids (fats), carbohydrates, and DNA, RNA, and other nucleic acids, leading to cancer, heart disease, and various neurodegenerative conditions. Insufficient levels of ROS, though less common, is also a detriment to health and has been linked to certain autoimmune diseases and recurrent infections, including pneumonia.

mtDNA mutations and dysfunctions within the mitochondrial respiratory chain (MRC), have been linked to both inflammation and cancer. Damaged respiratory chain proteins and mitochondrial genes increase the production of mitochondrial ROS. The more that mitochondria malfunction, the more that ROS levels increase, creating a vicious cycle. In addition, tumor cells typically exhibit higher ROS production compared to ROS production in normal cells.

ROS have also been linked to hypoxia-inducible factors (HIFs). HIFs are protein complexes that get activated in response to low concentrations of oxygen levels in the body (hypoxia), thereby helping to protect against cancer by limiting cancer cell metabolism and metastasis. (Recall, as you learned in Chapter 1, that cancer cells cannot thrive in an oxygen-rich environment, a discovery first made by the Nobel laureate Otto Warburg.) ROS have been shown to limit the activation of HIFs even under conditions of normal oxygen levels, thus potentially promoting the formation and spread of cancerous tumors.

ROS, as well as mtDNA damaged by ROS, have also been found to activate multiprotein molecules called *inflammasomes*, causing them to become dysregulated. Inflammasomes are a part of the body's innate immune system and are responsible for activating its inflammatory responses to injuries and infections. The most studied inflammasome is called NLRP3, which research confirms can be activated by damaged mtDNA, triggering the release of pro-inflammatory cytokines, such as interleukin (IL)-1β and IL-18, at excessively high levels. These cytokines, when overactive, suppress the immune system's ability to detect and eliminate cancer cells, thus enabling tumors to continue to grow.

You may recall the term "cytokine storm", which was commonly talked about during the height of the COVID-19 outbreak, and which was responsible for much of the serious illness and death caused by the SARS-

Co-V2 virus. This same type of cytokine storm has also been implicated in cancer, neurodegenerative diseases, and other conditions.

Once again, a vicious cycle is at play since ROS, by damaging mtDNA and by other means, can unleash harmful cytokines, and the cytokines, once unleashed, can trigger further production of ROS in certain types of immune cells.

Not only do excessively produced ROS increase the risk of cancer because of how they activate proliferation pathways via the innate immune system, as well as their inactivation of the immune surveillance system, they also cause a sustained innate immune response, furthering the damage caused by chronic inflammation. The end result is a dangerous cycle of mtDNA mutations caused by ROS, leading to impaired production of proteins of the mitochondrial respiratory chain, thus triggering the production of more ROS.

Nuclear Factor-kappaB (NF-κB)

Another key player in both inflammation and the initiation and spread of cancer is nuclear factor-kappaB (NF-κB), also known as nuclear factor kappa-light-chain-enhancer of activated B cells. This protein complex regulates other proteins in the body and plays key roles in cellular transformation, proliferation, and apoptosis, as well as in coordinating the innate and adaptive immune system responses to stress, free radicals, heavy metals, ultraviolet (UV) irradiation, oxidized LDL cholesterol, and bacterial and viral infections. It also controls cytokine production and cell survival. When NF-κB is activated, it moves to the cell nucleus, where it regulates the expression of over 200 immune, growth, and inflammation genes.

NF-kappaB signaling also plays a critical role in the development and progression of cancer. As biochemist and cancer researcher Bharat B. Aggarwal, PhD, of MD Anderson Cancer Center in Houston, Texas, explains, "The activation of NF-κB is a double-edged sword. While needed for proper immune system function, inappropriate NF-κB activation can mediate inflammation and tumorigenesis. That duality is especially striking in relation to cancer." During the inflammatory process, activated NF-kB can trigger the expression of oncogenes involved in cancer cell proliferation, carcinogenesis, and blockage of apoptosis, as well as the production of additional pro-inflammatory cytokines to increase the potency of this response. This process also links back to ROS levels.

"Most inflammatory agents mediate their effects through the activation of NF-κB, and the latter is suppressed by anti-inflammatory agents." Aggarwal explains. "Similarly, most carcinogens and tumor promoters activate NF-κB, whereas chemopreventive agents suppress it, suggesting a strong linkage with cancer. Paradoxically, most agents, including cytokines, chemotherapeutic agents, and radiation, that induce apoptosis also activate NF-κB."

This fact indicates that "NF-κB is a part of the cells' autodefense mechanism," Aggarwal says, which may explain why, when it is activated in cancer cells, NF-κB aids cancer cells and tumors to resist chemotherapy, radiation, and other cancer treatments.

Research has found that NF-κB is active in most tumor cell lines derived from both solid and blood cell tumors, and that it is rarely active in most normal cells. Active NF-κB has also been found in tumor tissues taken from patients with multiple myeloma, various leukemias, and prostate and breast cancers. "Suppression of NF-κB in these tumor samples inhibits proliferation, causes cell cycle arrest, and leads to apoptosis, indicating the crucial role of NF-κB in cell proliferation and survival," according to Aggarwal.

Since activation and inactivation of NF-κB have both positive and negative effects when it comes to cancer, Aggarwal cautions that drug treatments intended to inhibit NF-κB should be tested and used with caution. I agree, and I also agree with his suggestion that nontoxic blockers of NF-κB, such as plant foods rich in compounds known as polyphenols may be a more beneficial option. (You will learn much more about such foods and why they are useful for both preventing and treating cancer in Chapter 8.)

Other Pro-Inflammatory Molecular Compounds Linked To Cancer

What follow are brief overviews of molecular compounds that are also involved in the body's inflammation responses and which can cause the development and spread of cancer.

Cytokines: Cytokines are chemical signals that trigger normal cells to grow in order to repair and replace aged and damaged tissues. They also play key roles in regulating the activation, growth, and differentiation of immune cells. Examples of cytokines are interleukin-6 (IL6), elevated levels of which have been linked to colon cancer; vascular endothelial growth factor (VEGF), which stimulates blood vessel formation, and is up-regulated in many tumors and supports tumor angiogenesis; and tumor necrosis factor (TNF), which plays important roles in normal cell survival, proliferation, differentiation, and apoptosis, yet can also damage DNA and inhibit DNA repair, and aid the growth, proliferation, angiogenesis, and metastasis of cancer cells and tumors.

Chemokines: Chemokines regulate the movement of leukocytes, the white blood cells of the immune system that capture and digest bacteria and fungi, to inflamed areas of the body. Chemokines can trigger cancer formation by influencing precancerous cells to transform into cancerous cells. Research has also shown that chemokines help facilitate tumor metastasis by regulating the migration of tumor cells to other areas of the body in much the same way that they regulate the movement of leukocytes.

Inducible Nitric Oxide Synthase (iNOS): iNOS is an enzyme that catalyzes nitric oxide (NO) production in the body, resulting in increased NO levels. NO helps regulate the body's inflammation response. Excessive, or over-expressed, levels of NO are known to play a role in chronic inflammatory diseases and in the development of cancer. In such cases, this is due in part to DNA damage and impaired DNA repair caused by excess nitric oxide. Research shows that iNOS is influenced by pro-inflammatory cytokines, such as tumor necrosis factor, as well as by NF-κB. For example, in an experimental model of colitis, TNF caused inflammation by triggering the expression of iNOS. Research has also shown that, once tumors are formed, iNOS may be continuously stimulated by cytokines and NF-κB located within the tumor's inflammatory microenvironment.

Cyclooxygenase-2 (COX-2) and **Prostaglandins:** Cyclooxygenase (COX) is an enzyme in the body that occurs in two forms, COX-1 and COX-2. COX-1 is expressed in most tissues, whereas COX-2 usually is absent until it is produced by the body as part of an inflammatory response. When this happens, COX-2 produces inflammatory messengers called prostaglandins. Pro-inflammatory cytokines and other stimuli are known to trigger COX-2 expression. Conversely, the synthesis of prostaglandin E2 (PGE2) by COX-2 triggers the production of more inflammatory cytokines, setting up a vicious cycle.

Studies have linked COX-2 to various types of cancer, and show that when it is over-expressed it plays a role in cancer cell proliferation and angiogenesis, interferes with the process of apoptosis, and increases the risk of metastasis. Research also shows that it is highly expressed in nearly all tumors, and has also found a correlation between COX-2's level of expression and tumor size and the likelihood of tumors to invade other tissues. Additional research shows that prostaglandins also possess the same cancer-inducing mechanisms of action as those of COX-2.

Aspirin and nonsteroidal anti-inflammatory drugs (NSAIDs) act as COX-2 inhibitors, and epidemiological studies have shown a 40 to 50 percent reduction in deaths caused by colorectal cancer in people who use NSAIDs drugs on a regular basis compared with people not taking such drugs. Similar studies have found that NSAIDs can reduce the risk of other cancers, as well. The regular use of NSAIDs can cause serious side effects, however, including heart attack, high blood pressure, kidney damage and sudden kidney failure, stroke, stomach bleeding.

Fortunately, there are a variety of safer natural substances and herbs that also act as COX-2 inhibitors. Zinc, for example, has been shown to regulate COX-2 expression in cancer better than the NSAID drugs Celecoxib or Indomethacin. I cover these natural COX-2 inhibitors in more detail in Chapter 8.

Hypoxia-Inducible Factor-1α (HIF-1): HIF-1 helps to ensure that the delivery of oxygen to cells is greater than, or at least equal to, the oxygen demand of the cells. In response to low oxygen levels in the body (hypoxia), HIF-1 activates various molecules, including iNOS and VEGF. Since hypoxia often occurs at inflammation sites due to metabolic shifts during the body's inflammation response, it's likely that HIF-1 is involved in the inflammation response and capable of driving its progression. Research also indicates that HIF-1 may contribute to chronic inflammation by preventing the normal cell death (apoptosis) of the white blood cells neutrophils and T lymphocytes. In cancer cells, HIF-1 is activated by various proinflammatory cytokines. It also plays a role in tumor development because it facilitates the expression of cancer cell DNA, enhances glycolysis activity, and increases VEGF levels, all of which are necessary for tumor growth and metastasis.

Galectin-3

Another significant risk factor for chronic inflammation and cancer, as well as other diseases, is galectin-3.

Galectins are a specific class of proteins that act like glue because of how they bind various molecules with different types of sugar in the body. There are many subclasses of galectins in the body that perform this glue-like function, with galectin-3 being of most concern among doctors and scientists dealing with inflammation and cancer. Normally, galectin-3 is mostly present in small amounts within the body's various cells. It is primarily produced by macrophages. Chronic inflammation can cause galectin-3 to trigger injured organs in the body to form scar tissue.

Scar tissue formation triggered by galectin-3 is well-known to occur when the liver becomes subject to chronic inflammation. Over time, the scar tissue can impair liver function and cause liver fibrosis, cirrhosis, and other liver problems.

Increased levels of galectin-3 are present in many solid cancer tumors. Studies indicate that the higher the levels of galectin-3 are, the more aggressive the cancer is likely to be. Galectin-3 has been shown to enhance the ability of cancer cells to invade other tissues, thus aiding metastasis. Moreover, tumors in areas of the body where metastases occur usually have higher galectin-3 levels than the original tumor. Galectin-3 also promotes angiogenesis that support tumor growth, while simultaneously impairing immune function, making it more difficult for the immune system to detect and kill cancer cells and tumors. It produces these effects by encouraging cancer cells to clump together and bind to surrounding tissues, further triggering chronic inflammation and cancer growth.

According to Isaac Eliaz, MD, a leading expert on galectin-3 and its harmful effects, galectin-3 acts as a "survival protein" because of how it is activated in response to injury, infection, and other health threats. But when the body's acute inflammation turns chronic, galectin-3 continues to be produced, sending out inflammatory survival signals "like an alarm that won't turn off."

"Thousands of studies show how this harmful galectin-3 activity leads to chronic inflammation, fibrosis (uncontrolled scar tissue build-up) of organs and tissues, tumor formation and metastasis, immune imbalances, and much more," Eliaz says. "Galectin-3 has even been called, 'The Guardian of the Tumor Microenvironment' because it helps cancer grow while shielding it from your immune system."

Recent research that examined a type of immune cells known as tumor-associated macrophages, or TAMS, revealed how TAMS and hypoxia (low oxygen environment) combines with galectin-3 to increase the risk of death by breast cancer. High levels of TAMS are typically located near tumors, especially tumors where surrounding cells and tissues lack enough oxygen. The study revealed for the first time that TAMS in a hypoxic environment increases the production and secretion of galectin-3. The study also found that "hypoxia-induced galectin-3 expression and secretion from TAMs promotes tumor growth and metastasis."

According to Eliaz, modified citrus pectin is the only natural ingredient known to block and reverse the harmful effects of galectin-3. It has also been shown to be effective in halting and even reversing heart disease, kidney disease, and various other conditions, as well as gently removing stored toxins stored in the body's tissues and organs.

You will learn much more about modified citrus pectin and the research that confirms its anticancer and other health benefits in Chapter 8.

Iron Overload and Cancer

Although iron is an important trace mineral that is necessary for good health, when iron excessively builds up in the body, the body is unable to excrete it. This causes excess iron to be stored in various organs, including the heart and liver, where, over time, it can damage them. Excess iron also contributes to inflammation, can impair mitochondrial function, and is a significant risk factor for cancer. As the authors of a research paper on iron and cancer, wrote, "Most experimental and human data support the hypothesis that iron overload is a risk factor for cancer in general and liver cancer in particular. This oncogenic effect could be explained by an overproduction of reactive oxygen species and free radicals."

These same researchers also noted that even mild excess levels of iron have been found to be present in over 50 percent of cases of hepatocellular carcinoma, the most common type of liver cancer. They also note that iron overload is likely to be an equally important risk factor in liver cancer as alcohol, smoking, and viral hepatitis.

Other studies have found that even mild elevations of iron in the body increase the risk of cancer in general and death by cancer. Research has also established that iron overload, in addition to contributing to excess production of ROS and other free radicals, can also cause cancer by activating pro-inflammatory cytokines and triggering hypoxia in cells and tissues. Excess iron also initiates tumor growth and then acts as a tumor growth factor, furthering the likelihood of metastasis, while also enhancing the survivability of cancer cells.

A class of proteins called transferrins (TF) bind iron and transport it throughout body via the bloodstream. When iron levels are low, the body manufactures more transferrins. Conversely, transferrin levels decrease as iron levels become excessive. However, higher levels of transferrin saturation in the body has also been shown to be a risk factor for cancer because of the iron that is bound to TF. It is also well known that people born with or develop hemochromatosis, a hereditary genetic condition of iron overload, have an elevated risk for cancer, especially liver cancer, but also breast, colorectal, prostate, and other cancers. Other studies have found that donating blood, which reduces iron levels in the body, reduces the risk of cancer, whereas blood transfusion can increase cancer risk because of the iron levels the transfused blood contains.

Transferrin is often used as a marker to determine if patients are anemic, but it is also a useful marker for determining if iron overload is present, although other factors must first be ruled out, as I discuss later in this chapter.

Regularly consuming iron-enriched foods, such as breads, cereals, and pasta, is a common dietary contributor to excess iron buildup in the body. Avoiding such foods is therefore recommended.

Iron is also often found in tap water. Common signs of iron in tap water include yellowish stains in sinks, ring stains in toilets, and constantly clogging pipes. Avoid drinking tap water, and using a shower filter (iron in tap water is absorbed through the skin during bathing and showering) are therefore also advisable.

Older homes are other common source of iron exposure. Typically, such homes have iron piping that connects municipal water supplies to them. If possible, replacing iron piping with copper pipes can reduce iron exposures.

Getting in the habit of regularly donating blood every three to six months can significantly reduce iron levels in your body. In addition to potentially saving lives by donating blood, you will also be reducing your risk of both inflammation and cancer, as well as gaining other health benefits.

Insulin Resistance

Insulin resistance is a blood sugar disorder that occurs when the body fails to properly regulate the amount of insulin in the blood. This makes it more difficult for the body to use sugar (glucose) for energy, thus interfering with mitochondrial function.

Insulin is a hormone produced in the pancreas. When you eat, as foods get digested and metabolized, the glucose foods contain enters the bloodstream, triggering the pancreas to release insulin. Insulin then helps usher glucose into cells, where mitochondria use it to produce energy. Insulin also moves excess glucose that is not needed by the cells into the liver, where it is stored for later use. Insulin also plays an important role in helping your body metabolize and use fats.

Insulin levels in the body fluctuate depending on how much glucose is in the bloodstream. When glucose enters your cells and the levels in your bloodstream decrease, it signals your pancreas to stop producing insulin. But several factors can make cells resistant to insulin, causing insulin levels to be chronically elevated, a condition known as hyperinsulinemia. Chief risk factors for insulin resistance and hyperinsulinemia are a diet high in processed foods, sugars and other simple carbohydrates, and unhealthy fats; being overweight or obese; excess body fat, especially belly fat; and lack of exercise. Hormonal imbalances and certain medications, such as high blood pressure drugs and steroids, can also cause insulin resistance.

When insulin resistance persists, blood glucose levels become elevated, causing hyperglycemia (high blood sugar), which in turn can cause metabolic syndrome and type-2 diabetes. Insulin resistance is also a known risk factor for cancer, as well as heart disease, kidney and liver conditions, and other diseases.

Insulin resistance typically results in the body creating more fat cells and also interferes with the body's ability to break fat cells down. This leads to weight gain, while also causing chronic inflammation, as well as various disruptions in overall hormone function.

In addition, insulin resistance impairs apoptosis, increasing the risk of healthy cells becoming cancerous. Changes in insulin production can also stimulate the body to increase pro-inflammatory prostaglandins that also increase the risk of cancer. Moreover, because insulin resistance is a leading cause of hyperglycemia, it also helps to "feed" cancer cells and tumors that thrive on the excess sugar that is produced because of insulin resistance.

Insulin resistance is a key component of type-2 diabetes, and chronic insulin resistance is almost always present prior to people developing type-2 diabetes. This is troublesome, since a growing body of research indicates that people with diabetes have an increased risk for cancer, and that cancer is now the leading cause of death of diabetic patients. Studies show that chronic low-grade inflammation is often a co-factor with insulin resistance in cases of obesity and type-2 diabetes, further linking these metabolic conditions and cancer.

Cytokines, prostaglandins, and other pro-inflammatory agents inflammatory that initiate cancer and promote cancer progression can cause the effects of insulin resistance to become more severe. For example, research indicates that the cytokine tumor necrosis factor alpha (TNF-α) may trigger and enhance insulin resistance by inhibiting the insulin receptor (INSR) signaling pathway that regulates metabolic responses to insulin in insulin target cells and tissues. In addition, elevated levels of circulating TNF-α have been found in insulin-resistant, overweight patients with cancer. Insulin resistance can also cause an overproduction of reactive oxygen species, further increasing the risk of cancer. The large number of inflammatory cells in adipose (fat) tissues produced by insulin resistance also increases the likelihood of systemic inflammation, further creating a pro-cancerous environment.

For all of these reasons, you can see why preventing and reversing insulin resistance and maintaining a healthy weight are important measures for reducing cancer risk.

Measuring Your Body's Inflammation Levels

These are the markers I most commonly use to gauge my patients' levels of inflammation. You should be able to obtain them from your doctor, although you may have to request them, since not all physicians pay attention to all of them.

C-reactive Protein (CRP) and Fibrinogen: These inexpensive tests measure the amount of the pro-inflammatory markers C-reactive protein and fibrinogen in the bloodstream. They can both be used to detect chronic inflammation and to monitor your progress as you work to reduce inflammation levels in your body. The CRP test can also be used to determine your risk of heart disease and stroke.

Any CRP reading above 3.0 mg/L is an indication of chronic inflammation. The higher the reading, the more likely it is that systemic chronic inflammation is present. The optimal CRP level for men is anything under 1 mg/L, while for women it should be under 1.5 mg/L.

Fibrinogen is a protein that acts as a blood clotting agent. Like CRP, it is also a useful marker for determining the presence of chronic inflammation. In both men and women, the optimal fibrinogen level is between 295 - 370 mg/dL.

Eosinophil Count (EOS Blood Test): This test measures eosinophils in levels. Eosinophils are a class of white blood cells that are crucial players in the body's inflammation response to infectious and other disease conditions. Prolonged elevated eosinophil levels can cause chronic inflammation and tissue damage.

Under normal conditions, eosinophils only comprise about five percent of your body's total white blood cell count. Normal eosinophil counts can range from zero to 500 cells per microliters (UL) of blood, with the average being between 30 and 350 cells per UL. Elevated eosinophil cell levels fall into three categories: mild (500 to 1,500 cells per UL), moderate (1,500 to 5,000 cells per UL), and severe (5,000 or more eosinophil cells per UL). All higher than normal counts are categorized as cases of eosinophilia, and are signs of chronic inflammation and infection, and can be indications of various disease conditions, including leukemia.

Ferritin Test: This test measures iron storage in the body and screens for iron overload and unbound iron in the blood. It is also used to screen for possible inborn genetic errors of metabolism, such as hereditary hemochromatosis.

While a ferritin range between 200 and 300 ng/mL is considered normal for both women and men, an ideal range is between 30 and 80 ng/mL for men and non-menstruating women. (Menstruating women are more likely to suffer from iron deficiency than iron overload.)

LDH Test: LDH stands for lactate dehydrogenase, an enzyme in the body that plays an important role in cellular respiration (the process by which glucose from food is transformed into energy by mitochondria). LDH is found in nearly all body tissues, as well as in the blood. In the presence of various infections, or when tissues are damaged, more LDH is produced and enters the bloodstream. For these reasons, the LDH test can be useful for detecting and monitoring tissue damage and infections. It is also helpful for determining the severity of cancer, as well as the effectiveness of chemotherapy and other cancer treatments.

In men, the normal range for LDH is 135 – 225 U/L (units per liter of blood). In women, the normal range is 135-214 U/L.

Sed Rate Test: A sed rate test, also known as a erythrocyte sedimentation rate or ESR test, is a common test used to detect inflammation and to monitor the progression of inflammatory diseases. Sedimentation rate is the rate that red blood cells, also known as erythrocytes, fall when a blood sample is placed in a vertical test tube. In cases of inflammation, red blood cells clump together, making them fall more quickly than single red blood cells. The sed rate measures how far red blood cells fall in an hour after blood is placed in the test tube. The greater the distance they fall, the higher the degree of inflammation in the body. In men, the normal sed rate ranges between a distance of zero to 22 millimeters per hour (mm/hr). In women, the normal rate is zero to 29 mm/hr.

Transferrin: Normal transferrin levels range from 200 to 370 mg/dL. Readings above those levels are an indication of iron deficiency and anemia, while lower levels indicate iron overload and inflammation, and can also be indicators of hereditary conditions such as hemochromatosis, thalassemia, or sickle cell anemia. Nutritional deficiencies, as well as kidney and liver disorders, can also result in lower than normal transferrin levels. All of these factors need to be taken into consideration before making a definitive diagnosis of iron overload based on transferrin readings.

I also recommend two immune system marker tests: neutrophil-to-lymphocyte ratio, and lymphoctye-to-monocyte ratio. Neutrophils, lymphocytes, and monoctyes are types of white blood cells that play important roles in the body's inflammatory response, in particular in fighting infection. Neutrophils, under normal conditions, comprise between 55 to 70 percent of all white blood cells, while lymphocytes and monocytes comprise 20 to 40 percent and zero to eight percent, respectively. Percentages, and therefore ratios, of all classes of white blood cells can be measured using a white blood cell (WBC) differential test.

The **neutrophil-to-lymphocyte ratio (NLR)** is now recognized as a useful marker for evaluating immune system function. Research shows that it also correlates well with mortality related to cancer and various other diseases, including pneumonia, sepsis, and Covid-19. (During the Covid-19 pandemic, NLR was often used to determine whether Covid patients required hospitalization and as a marker to determine how well they were recovering.) Both a lower than normal neutrophil count (a condition known as neutropenia), and a higher than normal lymphocyte count (lymphocytosis) can be indicators of infection, especially viral infection, and also indications of lymphomas, leukemias, or certain autoimmune diseases.

Conversely, a high NLR reading (high neutrophil and low lymphocyte levels), can also indicate the presence, and be a measure of the severity, of cancer, cardiovascular disease, and many infectious disease conditions. A normal NLR is between 1 and 4. NLR above 6 is a good indicator of inflammation and possible disease. In cancer and other serious condition, NLR can go as high as 100.

The **lymphocyte-to-monocyte ratio (LMR)** is often used to predict the severity of cardiovascular conditions, including stroke, with low LMR found to be associated with severe stroke and poorer outcomes, whereas the opposite (high LMR) is associated with greater recovery and survival rates.

LMR can also be used to help determine both the progression of cancer and the likelihood of survival of cancer patients. As in cases of cardiovascular disease, high LMR is associated with a greater likelihood of recovery and patient survival. Studies confirm this is true for cases of colorectal, urological, and various other cancers. Research has also found that LMR is a better predictor of the likelihood of survival of patients with colorectal cancer who undergo colon resection surgery compared to more established biomarkers.

LMR below 4.25 is a good indicator of inflammation and possible disease. In cancer and other serious conditions, LMR can go as low as below 1. Studies indicate LMR above 3 is associated with better overall survival of cancer patients. There are some fluctuations depending on type of cancer, age and sex.

Action Steps For Preventing and Reversing Chronic Inflammation

Taming inflammation is one of the most important steps you can take to minimize your risk of cancer, as well as helping to reverse it if you to develop it. Fortunately, there are a number of self-care measures you can employ to help you achieve this goal, starting with your diet. This means eliminating, or at least minimizing your intake of alcohol, processed foods, fried foods, iron-enriched foods, hydrogenated and other unhealthy fats/oils (canola, corn, safflower, soybean, sunflower, etc), sugars and simple ("white") carbohydrates from your diet.

Also avoid baking and cooking foods at high temperatures to avoid advanced glycation end products (AGEs). Increasing your intake of nuts, seeds, and wild caught fish, such as haddock, halibut, herring, mackerel, sardines, and salmon, is also advisable, since all of these foods are rich food sources of omega-3 essential fatty acids, which are known to protect against inflammation. If you enjoy meat, lamb, and poultry, focus on grass-fed and grass-finished meats and free-range poultry.

If possible, also eat only organic foods free of harmful pesticides or herbicides, which are known carcinogens, and make organic, non-starchy vegetables a regular part of your meals throughout each week.

Garnishing your meals various spices, such as black and red pepper, cinnamon, cumin, garlic, ginger, rosemary, and turmeric, can also help since they all have proven anti-inflammatory properties. Regularly drinking green tea can also be very helpful.

You can further support your diet and overall nutritional status with various supplements that also protect against inflammation. These include boswellia, ginger, curcumin, vitamin A (as opposed to beta-carotene), B-vitamins (especially B3 and B6), food-based vitamin C, vitamin E, green tea extract, quercetin, magnesium, modified citrus pectin, resveratrol, and zinc.

Molecular hydrogen tablets added to pure, filtered water can also be very helpful. According to Jim Wilson, Director of Hydrogen Technologies in Australia, molecular hydrogen supplementation acts against inflammation in two ways. "First," he notes, "it suppresses the oxidative stress signal and, in turn, reduces the risk of unnecessarily triggering or over sustaining an inflammatory response. Second, it also dampens the NF-kB pathway, directly avoiding a highly detrimental runaway inflammatory response."

More detailed information about diet and nutrition is provided in Chapters 3 and 8.

Other important self-care steps you can take include not smoking and avoiding secondhand cigarette smoke, minimizing your exposure to heavy metals and other environmental toxins, avoiding regular exposure to ultraviolet (UV) radiation (discussed further in Chapter 3), getting at least 30 minutes of exercise or other physical activity every day (see Chapter 11), and losing weight if necessary. Regularly donating blood is also recommended.

Finally, improve your sleep and learn how to most effectively manage stress (see Chapters 6 and 7), both of which can cause and worsen chronic inflammation.

In the next chapter, we will explore other common risk factors for cancer.

Chapter 3

Other Significant Risk Factors For Cancer

In addition to chronic inflammation and related infections, which we discussed in Chapter 2, there are other significant cancer risk factors you need to be aware of and address. This chapter provides overviews of the most common of them.

Chronic Stress

It's estimated that stress in a primary causative factor in at least 95 percent of all cases of disease in the United States. And certainly it plays a significant role in cancer, as I can attest based on my many years of helping cancer patients deal with and heal their stressors. Unfortunately, despite the compelling scientific evidence linking stress to cancer, little attention to managing stress is usually given by oncologists and other doctors when they consult with their patients.

I take a much more proactive approach, taking time to learn what types of stress my patients may be dealing with, as well as the fears they typically experience after being diagnosed with cancer. Helping my patients to become aware of and acknowledge their stress, and teaching them self-care techniques they can use to release their fears and become better able to resiliently cope with stress can go a long way in preparing them for their journey through cancer, as well as improving their prospects for remission and long-term survival.

When it comes to cancer, oncologists and other health care practitioners correctly focus on the immune system. But there is another system that is equally as important as the immune system, and which has a direct bearing on how well the immune system functions. It's called the hypothalamus-pituitary-adrenal axis, or HPA axis for short.

The purpose of the HPA axis is to spring into action at the first sign of stress and any threats—both real and perceived—that we may face. When there aren't any threats, the HPA axis is in "idle mode." But when we are stressed or the hypothalamus center in the brain perceives an outside threat, it signals the HPA axis to "roll out" and do its job. This is known as the "freeze, flight, or fight" response.

As soon as this signal is given, your body's adrenal glands increase the production of cortisol and other stress hormones, releasing them into the blood stream. Once this happens, blood vessels that supply oxygen and nutrients to your body's cells and organs are constricted so that more blood can be made available to nourish the tissues of your body's arms and legs, since it is primarily these extremities that the body uses to fend off external attacks and get out of harm's way. Prior to this response, the blood in the body is concentrated in what are known as the visceral organs. These are the organs responsible for digestion and absorption of food and nutrients, excretion, and various other functions that provide for proper cell growth and production of cellular energy. As blood is rushed to the tissues of the arms and legs, the visceral organs, such as the stomach, kidneys, and liver, cannot function at 100 percent. This inhibits all growth-related activities in the body. If this process continues for sustained periods of time, overall body functioning suffers.

This situation is further compounded by the impact sustained "freeze, flight, or fight" responses have on the immune system. During these responses, the HPA axis causes the adrenal glands to suppress immune function in order to conserve the body's energy reserves via the adrenals' increased production of stress hormones. Stress hormones are so effective at suppressing immune function that they are administered to patients receiving organ transplants to prevent their bodies' immune systems from rejecting the organs.

To recap, what is important for you to understand is that chronic stress causes the HPA-axis to release stress hormones that suppress immune function, impairing the ability of immune cells to detect and eliminate cancer cells. This cascade of events both helps set the stage for cancer to occur, and to impair the body's ability to recover from cancer once it develops.

There are different categories of stress. They include mental and emotional stress, physical and environmental stress, stress caused by trauma (both physical and psychological), and life shock events, such as the death of a loved one, divorce, job loss, and the loss of friendships (as, sadly happened with friends and family members during the Covid crisis based on each other's stances regarding masking, vaccines, and so forth). Spiritual stress, such as a "crisis of faith," is another common factor among cancer patients. Recognizing and dealing with stress in all categories is essential for good health and for recovery from cancer and all other illnesses.

Limited Beliefs and Unresolved Or Repressed Emotions

This category of risk factors is closely interrelated with chronic stress and must also be properly addressed.

As I will repeatedly emphasize throughout this book, cancer is not something to fear, yet very often, and quite understandably, fear is often the emotion that most takes hold of people upon learning that they have cancer. Intertwined with fear, in most cases, are various unhealthy, limited beliefs, starting with the belief that "cancer is a death sentence". That simply isn't true, but as long as such beliefs are held onto, the likelihood of recovery is lessened. For example, many people, upon being diagnosed with cancer, automatically assume the worst, even when there is no reason to do so. As a result, they can unconsciously sabotage their ability to recover even when they receive the most appropriate and effective types of cancer treatment.

This goes back to the "freeze, flight, or fight response". Decades ago, researchers in the field of psychoneuroimmunology (PNI, more commonly known as mind/body medicine) discovered that actual physical danger is not necessary to trigger this response. It can also be triggered by our thoughts and beliefs. Simply put, if you habitually focus on thoughts and beliefs of a limiting or negative nature, you are causing your body to act as if it is in danger. Though the adrenaline rush that occurs in the face of an actual physical threat usually doesn't result, a stress response still takes place, often for long periods of time as the limited beliefs are held onto. This results in chronic production of stress hormones, resulting in chronic suppression of immune function.

Chronic, unresolved emotions have also been shown to significantly affect the immune system by lowering the immune response. In fact, PNI research shows that many people who die of cancer (as well as heart disease) suffer from chronic, serious depression, anger or a combination of both emotions.

A prevalent emotion associated with cancer is depression and often depression is suppressing a deeper underlying chronic state of anger. Other common emotional characteristics of cancer patients are anxiety, fear, grief, hopelessness, indecisiveness, and loneliness. (Some cancer patients live isolated lives and lack meaningful personal relationships.) Other emotional issues include hostility, resentment, and selfishness.

It is vitally important that all of us, whether or not we have cancer, learn how to properly manage and express our emotions, resolve limited beliefs, and do all that is necessary to heal and recover from any unexpected life shocks or traumas we may have sustained. In Chapters 6 and 7, I provide you with proven self-care methods and other techniques for doing so.

Poor Diet and Nutritional Imbalances

Next to smoking, unhealthy eating is the second most preventable cause of cancer. It is also the factor you have the most control over. The food choices you make either support or harm your health. Healthy eating means eliminating all low quality foods from your diet, including processed and "junk foods", genetically modified foods (GMOs), refined grain products, and sugar and sweets. You should also avoid farm-raised fish, non-free range poultry, and non-grass-fed, grass-finished meats. Excessive alcohol consumption should also be avoided, as should sodas and commercial fruit juices and artificial energy booster drinks.

Poor eating habits also increase your risk for cancer because of the nutritional imbalances they create. While nutritional deficiencies seem most common, nutritional excesses, such as too much iron, discussed in Chapter 2, and excess intake of pro-inflammatory omega-6 fatty acids, also affect many people. Omega-6 fatty acids are found in most vegetable and seed oils, such as canola, corn, cottonseed, safflower, soybean, and sunflower oils, all of which are rich in lineolic acid, which accounts for approximately 90 percent of omega-6 fatty acids in the standard American diet. Lineolic acid triggers free radicals, impairs mitochondrial function, and creates inflammation. In order to not be harmful, omega-6 fatty acids must be balanced with omega-3 fatty acids, ideally in a one to one ratio, but the standard American diet typically contains up to 16 times or more omega-6 than omega-3 fatty acids.

In addition, a regular diet of unhealthy, low-quality foods creates unhealthy gut health and related gastrointestinal disorders, further increasing cancer risk, as does overcooking foods because of the advanced glycation end products (AGEs) this creates (see Chapter 2).

In Chapter 8, you'll learn how you can create the best anti-cancer diet for yourself, and how to improve your body's overall nutritional status and gut health.

Smoking and Regular Exposure To Cigarette Smoke

Smoking is the number one cause of cancer around the world. Despite all that is known about the dangers of smoking, over one billion people worldwide, mostly men, still smoke on a daily basis. Globally, cigarette smoking is directly responsible over a third of all cases of cancer in men, and more than ten percent of cases in women.

Although lung cancer is most thought of as being caused by smoking, at least 19 other types of cancers can also be caused by smoking. Types of cancer deaths in both men and women directly attributable to smoking are bronchial and tracheal cancer, which, combined with lung cancer, account for nearly 40 percent of cancer deaths, followed by colon and rectal cancer, esophageal cancer, stomach cancer in men, and cervical cancer, colon and rectal cancer, and breast cancer in women.

Although most incidences of smoking related cancers are due to cigarette smoking, cigar and pipe smoking can also cause cancer, especially cancers of the lung and upper digestive tract, including the oral cavity, esophagus, larynx, and pharynx. E-cigarette smoking (vaping) is no safer than normal cigarette smoking.

Regular exposure to secondhand smoke from people who smoke is also well-established as a risk factor for cancer, most especially lung cancer. Smokers and nonsmokers alike increase their risk of cancer by regularly associating with other smokers. And recent U.S. government-funded research *in vivo* and with humans found that even exposure to third-hand cigarette smoke is a cancer risk. Third-hand smoke is defined as handling smokers' hair and clothing, which typically contain embedded particles of carcinogenic chemicals contained in cigarettes, as do furniture and carpets, rugs, and drapes in smokers' homes and places of business.

In one study, three volunteers were asked to wear clothing of heavy cigarette smokers for only three hours. At the end of that time, urinalysis of the volunteers found concentrations of two carcinogenic compounds that were 86 times higher than their urine samples taken before the experiment began. In a related study, researchers exposed human lung tissue to the same two toxins and found that the toxins caused DNA damage associated with cancer.

If you are a nonsmoker, don't smoke, and do your best to avoid smokers and their environments. If you do smoke, seek help so that you can stop. I had a patient in her sixties, a doting grandmother who struggled with her smoking habit. Her difficulty breathing wasn't enough to deter her. When she uncharacteristically missed an appointment one day, we reached out, only to discover she'd tragically passed away. Her death highlights the serious risks associated with smoking.

Lack Of Exercise/Sedentary Lifestyle

Lack of exercise and an overall sedentary lifestyle is another significant cancer risk factor, especially lack of exercises and other activities that increase aerobic capacity, such as walking, jogging, bicycling, hiking, and swimming, and sports such as tennis, basketball, and so forth.

Research has found that a physically inactive lifestyle is responsible for 1.5 percent of all cancers in men and 4.4 percent of cancers in women, with similar percentages for cancer deaths for men and women, respectively. This increased risk was especially true for colon cancer in both sexes, as well as breast and endometrial cancer in women. Additional evidence indicates lack of physical activity plays a role in the development of many other types of cancers, as well.

See Chapter 9 to learn the most effective exercise strategies for safeguarding your health, and how you can easily begin to incorporate exercise and physical activities into your daily lifestyle.

Being Overweight/Obesity/High Body Mass Index (BMI)

It's no secret that being overweight, and especially obese, is not healthy. What is less known is that people who are overweight or obese have a greater risk of developing cancer.

According to the CDC's National Center for Health Statistics, over 73 percent of all adult Americans age 20 and older are overweight, with nearly 42 percent of them being obese. America is not the only nation facing this problem. According to the World Cancer Research Foundation International, approximately two billion adults worldwide are overweight, with 800 million of them obese. Sadly, this trend in the US and abroad is also increasingly prevalent among children and teens.

Overweight means having a body mass index (BMI) between 25 and 29.9. Obese means having a BMI of 30 or greater. The normal BMI range is 18.5 to 24.9. To calculate your BMI, visit www.calculator.net/bmi-calculator.html.

According to both the National Cancer Institute (NCI) and the American Cancer Society (ACS), being overweight or obese is directly linked to various types of cancer. They include breast cancer in women post menopause, colon and rectal cancer, endometrial cancer (more than half of all cancers in this category are among overweight women), esophageal cancer, gallbladder cancer, kidney cancer, liver cancer, ovarian cancer, pancreatic cancer, stomach cancer, and thyroid cancer, as well as multiple myeloma and meningioma (cancer in the lining of the brain and spinal cord). According to the NCI, the risk for developing these cancers is between two to seven times higher for men and women who are overweight or obese, depending on the cancer and how severely overweight they are.

There is also evidence suggesting that being overweight or obese may raise the risk of breast cancer in men, non-Hodgkin's lymphoma, aggressive prostate cancer, and cancers of the mouth, throat, and voice box.

Possible ways in which excess body weight can increase cancer risk include triggering and maintaining chronic inflammation, negatively impacting cell and blood vessel growth, interfering with apoptosis (normal cell death), and aiding metastasis. Being overweight or obese can also cause excess levels of various hormones that have been linked to cancer, especially estrogen, insulin, and insulin-like growth factor-1 (IGF-1).

Given these risks, if you are dealing with unhealthy weight gain, I strongly encourage you to do all you can to lose your excess weight, starting with healthy eating and regular exercise. (See Chapters 8 and 10.)

Infections

In the early 20th century, researchers began to discover that infectious microorganisms were a cause of cancer in animals. Since then, harmful bacteria, fungi, parasites, and viruses have been shown to also be risk factors for various types of cancers in humans. Worldwide, it's estimated that infections play a role in 15 to 20 percent of all cancer cases, with higher percentages in third-world countries, and lesser percentages in the U.S. and other developed countries due to better sanitation, cleaner water, and safer food production methods, but also because of a greater incidence of more prevalent risk factors, such as obesity, sedentary lifestyles, and other causes discussed in this chapter.

Research shows that infections can cause or worsen cancer by weakening the immune system, making it less able to detect and eliminate cancer before it takes hold in the body, and also by triggering inflammation that becomes persistent. In addition, viruses, because they directly affect growth-regulating genes inside cells by inserting their own genes into them, can disrupt normal cell function, causing uncontrolled cell growth and interfering with apoptosis.

Bacteria: Bacteria linked to cancer include *H. Pylori* (discussed in Chapter 2) and *Chlamydia trachomatis*, which can be transmitted during sex and may interact with human papillomavirus (HPV) to increase the risk of cervical cancer.

Parasites: Certain types of parasites can also be risk factors for cancer. Two of the most common are *Opisthorchis viverrini* and *Clonorchis sinensis* both of which are flatworms called liver flukes. They have been shown to increase the risk for bile duct cancer. (Bile ducts are tubes connecting the liver and intestines.)

Viruses: Viruses that can cause cancer include cytomegalovirus (CMV), Epstein-Barr virus (EBV), hepatitis B virus and hepatitis C virus (HBV and HCV), human immunodeficiency virus (HIV), human papillomaviruses (HPVs), human T-cell leukemia/lymphoma virus Type 1 (HTLV-1), Kaposi sarcoma-associated herpesvirus (KSHV), and Merkel cell polyomavirus (MCPyV).

CMV is a type of herpes virus. Estimates of its infection rate around the world range from 50 to 100 percent. Typically, CMV infection persists throughout a person's life. Although most people with CMV never experience any symptoms, the virus can cause serious health problems, and even be fatal, for people with seriously compromised immune systems. CMV has also long been linked to many chronic disease conditions, as well as to cancer. Moreover, research has established an association between CMV and cancer mortality, with the risk being higher in patients with CMV. However, this risk also depends on the patients' socioeconomic status and other risk factors they may be affected by.

A number of researchers have reported the presence of CMV antigens in specimens derived from patients with glioblastoma, a deadly form of brain cancer. Antigens are produced by the immune system in response to infections. The presence of CMV antigens indicates that CMV may play a role in glioblastoma. CMV has also been shown to advance the progression of glioma tumors in a mouse genetic model. Various CMV proteins have also been found to promote cancer traits in *in vitro* studies. These findings have led to antiviral drugs and immunotherapies sometimes being used as part of overall treatments for glioblastoma.

EBV, another type of herpes virus, infects over 90 percent of the world's population during their lifetime. In some people, it can cause mononucleosis, and it has also been linked to certain types of lymphoma, nose, and throat cancers. Fortunately, most people with EBV never develop any symptoms.

Chronic HBV or HCV infections can cause liver cancer. Both viruses can be transmitted by sharing needles, through blood transfusions, and via sexual contact. They can also be passed on from mothers to babies at birth in cases of drug use, needle sharing, and unprotected sex.

HIV is considered to be a cause of AIDS. It does not cause cancer directly, but because it can weaken immunity it can increase cancer risk. According to the NCI, people infected with HIV have increased risks of a number of cancers, especially Kaposi sarcoma, lymphomas (including both non-Hodgkin lymphoma and Hodgkin disease), and cancers of the cervix, anus, lung, liver, and throat.

According to the NCI, infection with high-risk types of HPVs have been linked to most types of cervical cancer, as well as most anal cancers and many oropharyngeal, vaginal, vulvar, and penile cancers. HPVs spread easily through direct sexual contact, including oral sex.

HTLV-1 is a significant risk factor for adult T-cell leukemia/lymphoma (ATLL), an aggressive type of non-Hodgkin's lymphoma. Like HBV and HCV, HTLV-1 can be transmitted by sharing needles, blood transfusions, sexual contact, and from mother to child in the womb or via breastfeeding. HTLV-1 infections are more common in Japan, Africa, the Caribbean, and South America than they are in the United States. In addition, like EBV, most people with HTLV-1 infection never experience symptoms or develop disease.

Kaposi sarcoma-associated herpesvirus (KSHV), also called human herpesvirus-8 (HHV-8), can cause Kaposi sarcoma, a cancer characterized by the formation of masses in the skin, lymph nodes, mouth, or in other organs. KSHV is also the main cause of primary effusion lymphoma, a rare and aggressive cancer. KSHV most commonly spreads through saliva. KSHV infection in the U.S. most commonly affects gay men who have sex with each other.

MCPyV is a primary cause of Merkel cell carcinoma, a rare type of skin cancer. According to the NCI, most adults have MCPyV infections that usually do not cause any symptoms. However, the risk of Merkel cell carcinoma is greatly increased in elderly people with MCPyV, as well as in other adults with who are infected with HIV or are immunosuppressed for other reasons.

Fungi: Recently, the link between cancer and fungal infections has gained renewed interest among cancer researchers. In part, this is because in 2022 researchers at the Weizmann Institute of Science in Israel discovered that certain cancers can be detected by blood tests that identify the DNA of various fungi that grow within tumors because fungal DNA is shed in blood.

The cancer-fungus connection has been known for decades. What makes the findings of the Weizmann group noteworthy is how common this connection is. "We were surprised to find that it's actually more common to find tumors with fungi than without," the Institute's Dr. Ilana Livtatan stated, discussing the discovery.

Assisted by US and other Israeli scientists, Livyatan and her team "studied the relationship between the fungi population and tumors, which were samples of 17,400 cancer patients, all of whom were part of four cohorts. The presence of specific fungal DNA in the blood samples of each patient was correlated with one of the 35 cancer types studied, creating an 'atlas' that mapped the fungus with the tumor type." Over 20 different types of fungus, including *Candida albicans*, were found in tumors of all 35 cancer types.

Also of great interest to the researchers is the fact that the biomes of the fungi, instead of competing with the biome of the tumors, co-existed with each other in a mutually "permissive" state to create "cancer-type-specific mycobiomes". This led the researchers to conclude that fungal DNA screening tests may lead to "powerful" new methods of cancer screening.

Though the cancer-fungus connection and their co-existing microbiomes have not been widely researched, because of this discovery scientists speculate that fungal infections may be a significant factor in the development and growth of tumors. It may also mean that inexpensive yet effective anti-fungal medications may be effective for preventing and treating certain cancers. Although this remains to be proven, as Livyatan states,"[B]eyond diagnostics, this could really shake things up in tumor research. This is one of these eye-opening moments that makes us revisit our assumptions about cancer, as fungi now represent a whole new consideration in analyzing tumors."

Though there is still much to learn about the cancer-fungus connection, being screened for fungal infections, and being treated for them if they are present, is another important way of potentially reducing your cancer risk. Be aware, however, that many doctors don't consider fungal infections when treating patients, so you may have to request to be screened for them.

Environmental Toxins

Heavy metals and other toxins, including asbestos, chemicals in household and cosmetic products, fluoridated water, pesticides, and herbicides, continue to contaminate our environment and impair our health. In May 2009, the President's Cancer Panel, a bipartisan committee responsible for monitoring the development and execution of the activities of the federal government's National Cancer Program, issued a report based on findings compiled during the course of a two-year investigation. The report confirmed that environmental toxins from a variety of sources play a significant, yet still largely unrecognized, role in the development of cancer, causing "grievous harm" to a large segment of the American population each year.

The report also further substantiated studies that found that children in America today are born "pre-polluted" due to environmental toxins that are passed on to them from their mothers' bodies while they are still in the womb. One such study, commissioned by the Environmental Working Group, found the presence of over 200 environmental toxins in the umbilical cord blood of newborns, including industrial chemicals, pesticides, and other contaminants, all of which have been shown to be carcinogenic in previous studies.

According to the Panel, the primary means of exposure to environmental toxins for the majority of Americans are:

- Contaminants from industrial and manufacturing sources
- Contaminants from agricultural sources (antibiotics, food additives, food colorings and dyes, pesticides, preservatives, etc)
- Contaminants related to our modern lifestyle (cell phones, computers, etc)
- Hazards from medical sources (x-rays, CT scans, nuclear medical tests, various pharmaceutical drugs, etc)
- Hazards from natural sources (toxins in our nations, air, land, and water supply).

Prefacing their report, the Panel wrote, "With nearly 80,000 chemicals on the market in the United States, many of which…are un- or understudied and largely unregulated, exposure to potential environmental carcinogens is widespread…All levels of government, from federal to local, must work to protect every American from needless disease through rigorous regulation of environmental pollutants…The Panel urges you [then President Obama] most strongly to use the power of your office to remove the carcinogens and other toxins from our food, water, and air that needlessly increase health care costs, cripple our Nation's productivity, and devastate American lives."

Unfortunately, to this day, neither the White House nor Congress has shown much willingness to tackle the serious problems the Panel identified. Therefore, it is up to each of us to do what we can to minimize our exposure to environmental toxins in order to reduce our risk of developing cancer and other serious diseases. Fortunately, there is much that we can do on our own, starting with the following recommendations.

Get Tested: Although the human body has its own system of detoxification, if it is continually exposed to toxins eventually it is overwhelmed, allowing a buildup and storage of toxins in the body, especially in fat cells and tissues, where they start to wreck havoc on the body's immune system. For this reason, consider working with a health practitioner who specializes in the prevention and treatment of environmental toxicity. Such doctors can screen you for toxins and create a program of detoxification specific to your needs. You can find a list of these doctors by contacting the American Academy of Environmental Medicine (AAEM) at www.aaemonline.org.

Filter Your Tap Water: Most sources of tap water in the US contain carcinogens such as arsenic, chromium, and other chemicals. To avoid this problem, more and more people have chosen to drink bottled water. However, research shows that most types of bottled water are no healthier than tap water, and in some cases actually unhealthier. Moreover, the plastic used to manufacture drinking water bottles often contain toxins that leech into the water during storage. Additionally, the proliferation of plastic water bottles has led to a serious environmental problem due to the fact that many bottles are never properly recycled. Instead, they wind up in landfills, and even in water supplies, where the chemicals they contain leech into the soil and water to further pollute the earth.

A much better solution than drinking bottled water is to invest in a home water filter. (To find out how your town or city's tap water ranks in terms of cleanliness, visit www.ewg.org/tap-water/home.)

Eat Organic Food: Nonorganic fruits and vegetables tend to be higher in pesticides and a host of other potentially dangerous chemicals, while commercially harvested fish, meats, and poultry are rife with unhealthy toxins ranging from antibiotics, growth hormones, dyes, and chemicals such as arsenic (found in nonorganic poultry). To avoid such toxins, choose organically grown fruits and vegetables (ideally grown within 100 miles of where you live) as well as free-range, grass-fed meats and poultry, and wild-caught, as opposed to farm-raised, fish. Also avoid eating canned foods, which often contain bisphenol A and lack the nutrient value of fresh, whole foods. And beware of aflatoxins, which are associated with an increased risk of liver cancer. Aflatoxins are produced by fungi found on agricultural crops such as corn, peanuts, cottonseed, and tree nuts.

Avoid Stain- and Grease-Proofing Chemicals: Such chemicals, known as *fluorochemicals*, are commonly used as optional stain repellants on carpets and couches, and as greaseproof coatings for packaged and fast foods. You can avoid them by simply not choosing stain treatments for carpets and furniture, and by not eating packaged foods. Also consider replacing commercial home cleansing products with safer, more natural brands.

Beware of Commercial Cosmetic Products: Such products often contain chemicals that are carcinogenic, and which are easily absorbed into the skin and then into the body's tissues.

Read Product Labels: A growing number of products sold in the US today list warnings of cancer risks. Be sure to read product labels and warnings of all products before you buy them.

While the above recommendations alone are not enough to clean up the toxins that pollute our planet, by following them, you can significantly reduce your risk of exposure.**Consider the Health Risks of Pharmaceutical Drugs:** The list of potential side effects of pharmaceutical drugs, including those that interfere with the body's immune functions, continues to grow. Therefore, it is important that you discuss the "risk to benefit" ratio of such drugs with your doctor.

EMFs

One of the most overlooked health threats today is the rapidly increasing spread of radiation from harmful, human-made electromagnetic fields (EMFs). EMFS are emitted by cell phones, WIFI, Bluetooth, laptops and tablets, so-called "smart" meters and appliances, cell phone towers, and many other sources. Even new cars emit EMFs due to the now standard features of satellite tracking and Bluetooth they include.

Most people are unaware of the ways EMFs can negatively impact their health. And in many cases, even if they are aware, they regard EMFs as an acceptable trade-off because of the many advantages which EMF-based technologies provide. There is no question these advantages exist and we all enjoy our cell phones, surfing the Internet, sending emails and texts, being aided by GPS as we travel, and so forth. Still, it is important to cautiously make use of these still developing technologies due to the fact that EMF toxicity continues to be found in studies of animals and humans alike. Ongoing research shows EMF exposures can, over time, contribute to the onset of a range of illnesses, including cancer. For example, in 2011, the World Health Organization (WHO) and the International Agency for Research on Cancer (IARC) jointly classified EMF radiation from wireless phones as a carcinogen "based on an increased risk of glioma, a malignant type of brain cancer, associated with wireless phone use".

One of the leading researchers investigating the effects that EMF exposures have on humans is Martin Pall PhD. Based on his extensive review of the scientific literature, along with his own research and published studies, he reports that there are eight primary ways that EMFs impact us:

1. Attack the nervous system, including the brain, resulting in a wide range of neurological and neuropsychiatric disorders.
2. Negatively impact the body's endocrine (hormonal) system.
3. Cause oxidative stress and free radical damage, both of which are causative risk factors for virtually all chronic diseases.
4. Attack and damage DNA, causing both single strand and double strand breaks in cellular DNA, as well as oxidation of DNA.
5. Cause higher than normal levels of apoptosis, increasing the risk for both neurodegenerative diseases and infertility.
6. Lower male and female fertility and libido, reduce sex hormones, attack DNA in sperm cells, and increase the risk of miscarriage.
7. Produce excessive intracellular calcium and excessive calcium signaling.
8. And directly attack the cells of the body to cause cancer. According to Dr. Pall, "Such attacks are thought to act via 15 different mechanisms during cancer causation."

(Dr. Pall's full assessment of these dangers are outlined in the book-length report he wrote and compiled, entitled *5G Risk: The Scientific Perspective— Compelling Evidence for Eight Distinct Types of Great Harm Caused by Elec-*

tromagnetic Field (EMF) Exposures and the Mechanism that Causes Them. You can obtain a free PDF copy at www.radiationresearch.org/wp-content/uploads/2018/06/EU-EMF2018-6-11US3.pdf.)

Given how prevalent EMFs are, as well as our reliance on EMF-based devices, completely avoiding EMF exposure is both impractical and virtually impossible. Still, there are steps you can take to reduce your exposures. They include limiting your cell phone use and choosing to text instead of talking on cell phones, as texting keeps your phone away from your head and brain. You can also keep your phone in airplane mode when it's not in use, and shut it off completely and keep it out of your bedroom when you go to bed. Turning off your WiFi is also recommended when you do not need it, especially during bedtime.

To learn more about EMFs and more solutions for protecting yourself from EMF exposures, I recommend the resources provided by the Environmental Health Trust, which is led by Devra Davis, PhD, MPH, another leading researcher and educator in this field. For more information, visit www.ehtrust.org.

Ionizing Radiation

Like EMFs, ionizing radiation can damage DNA and therefore cause cancer. Common sources of ionizing radiation are x-rays, CT scans, and PET scans. Although these medical imaging tools play important roles in detecting and monitoring disease, they have also been linked to cancer when used repeatedly on patients. Radiation therapy can also increase cancer risk.

As the 2009 President's Cancer Panel reported, "It is becoming increasingly clear that some of these same technologies…[that] have contributed so greatly to health status and longevity also carry risks." The report pointed out that Americans "now receive nearly half of their total radiation exposure from medical imaging and other medical sources, compared with only 15 percent in the early 1980s…Computed tomography (CT) [scans] and nuclear medicine tests alone now contribute 36 percent of the total radiation exposure" that Americans receive each year. For these reasons, I recommend you avoid such tests unless they are absolutely necessary. In many cases, diagnostic ultrasound can be just as useful as x-rays, CT and PET scans and carry no ionized radiation risks.

Radon, a radioactive gas that is released from the normal decay of the elements uranium, thorium, and radium in rocks and soil. is another type of ionizing radiation that increases cancer risk, especially lung cancer. Both invisible and odorless, it seeps up through the ground and diffuses into the air. Though radon gas usually exists at very low levels outdoors, it can enter homes through cracks in floors, walls, or foundations to accumulate at dangerous levels. The highest levels in homes are usually in basements and first floors.

Radon can also be released from building materials and sometimes be found in well water. Radon levels may be higher in well-insulated, tightly sealed homes, and/or homes built on soil rich in the elements that release radon as they decay.

Effective and inexpensive home tests can reveal whether or not radon is a problem in your home. They are available at most hardware stores. You may also wish to install a home radon detector unit.

If your home tests positive for radon, you will want to seal cracks in floors and walls with plaster, caulk, or other sealants and increase the air flow by opening windows. Ideally, though, you should also contact your state radon office to locate a trained and qualified professional to fully safeguard your home.

Poor Sleep and Sleep Disorders

Increasing evidence demonstrates that poor sleep and sleep disorders impair overall health, both physically and mentally/emotionally. Research also shows that lack of deep, restorative sleep and conditions such as insomnia and sleep apnea can increase the risk of cancer and cause elevated levels of stress hormones and inflammation.

It is when we sleep that our bodies conduct most of their repair processes, including producing various extra protein molecules that help to repair cells and counteract damage caused by stress, inflammation, infection, toxins, and free radical damage. A good night's sleep for at least seven hours also releases substances that strengthen immunity. In addition, deep sleep releases a significant amount of growth hormone, further boosting immunity and aiding in the growth and repair of the body. Conversely, poor sleep can impair proper immune function, increasing susceptibility to infection, cancer, and other diseases. The majority of the body's detoxification processes also take place while we sleep, which is another reason why deep, restorative sleep is so necessary for preventing and reversing the buildup of toxins that can cause cancer.

One of the lesser known benefits of sleep is that it helps to maintain healthy weight by regulating the hormones that control appetite. Poor sleep interrupts this normal hormone balance, and can increase food cravings, especially for foods high in calories, such as fats and carbohydrates, including sweets.

Here are some guidelines I recommend for improving your sleep:

- Keep your bedroom clean and free of dust. An unclean bedroom not only interferes with restful sleep, it also makes you more susceptible to infectious microorganisms. To prevent dust build up, consider using an air purifier in your home, and also be sure that the filters on your heat ducts are professionally examined at least once a year and replaced as necessary.

- Maintain a flow of fresh air throughout your bedroom as you sleep. You can do this easily by keeping at least one window of your bedroom slightly open.

- Sleep on a comfortable mattress. Despite the investment a new mattress may mean, if your current mattress is uncomfortable you will find the cost of a new mattress that fosters better sleep well worth it.

- Be aware that you might be sensitive to the materials in your pillow, blankets, and sheets. As a general rule, cotton or wool blankets and sheets and feather pillows are healthier choices than the same items made from synthetic materials.

- Keep the temperature in your bedroom a comfortable level. Temperatures that are too hot or cold can significantly interfere with your ability to get a good night's sleep.

- If you have a TV in your bedroom, consider moving it to another room in your home. Watching TV in bed keeps your brain in active mode, making sleep more difficult to come by. Also keep it free of other electrical devices, such as stereos, cell phones, computers, radios, etc. Such devices can interfere with healthy, restorative sleep because of the EMFs they emit, even when they are not in use.

- Sleep in complete darkness. This will help your body to produce the hormone melatonin, which is essential for healthy sleep, as well as many other functions in your body.

If you suffer from chronic sleep problems, consult with a sleep specialist or other integrative health practitioner.

Unhealthy Home and Work Environments

Healthy home and work environments are essential for good health, while unhealthy home and work environments can harm your health over time, increasing your susceptibility for cancer and other illnesses. EMFs, radon, the quality of the indoor air you breathe, and other environmental toxins in your home or work place all need to be addressed and rectified.

Two other significant factors, both of which are usually overlooked, are sick building syndrome and geopathic stress.

Sick building syndrome (SBS) refers to home and indoor work places with toxic environmental conditions within them that often go unnoticed, and which can cause a wide range of symptoms that increase susceptibility to a wide range of diseases, including cancer.

SBS is typically caused by problems with a building's engineering, construction, or ventilation system, but can also be caused by volatile organic compounds released by particleboard desks, furniture, carpets, glues, paints, office machine toners, and perfumes. Other indoor air pollutants, such as asbestos, cigarette smoke, radon, and formaldehyde, all of which are known cancer risk factors, can also contribute to SBS.

If you suspect you are affected by SBS, consult with your doctor and consider contacting a building inspector trained in remediation measures for SBS. You can also contact your local regional office of the Environmental Protection Agency (EPA) at www.epa.gov/indoor-air-quality-iaq/epa-regional-office-and-state-indoor-air-quality-information.

Geopathic stress refers to magnetic radiation from the Earth that usually combines with underground geological fractures and water veins. Though it has long been linked to an increased risk of cancer, most American physicians are unaware of geopathic stress, whereas it is more commonly considered as a health factor in Europe.

The causes of geopathic stress are most often due to sudden or unusual changes or anomalies in localized magnetic fields beneath the ground. In 1971, the concept of geopathic stress was confirmed by research that showed that water flowing underground, especially subterranean streams that crossed one another, produces measurable increases in magnetic abnormalities, and can also increase electrical conductivity in soil and the air above it. Even when these changes are minor, they can still increase the risk of illness, including cancer. One large-scale study by the U.S. government conducted in 1979 reported that geopathic stress is a possible factor in between 40 and 50 percent of all human cancers, and that it accounts for between 60 and 90 percent of all cancers attributed to environmental radiation.

Hormone Imbalances

Hormone imbalances, especially imbalanced estrogen hormones, are known human carcinogens. Although estrogens, when balanced, are essential to good health in both women and men, they can increase the risk of certain cancers, particularly breast cancer.

This risk is increased by the use of synthetic estrogen therapies (hormone replacement therapy, or HRT), as well as oral contraceptives. These therapies increase the levels of estrogen relative to progesterone (another hormone) in women and can be dangerous. This is particularly true of prolonged use of oral contraceptives or HRT by postmenopausal women, which studies show cause an increased risk of breast and endometrial cancers.

Researchers have known about the cancer risk of oral contraceptives for decades. For example, one study published in 1991 found that women who use birth control pills for more than four years were twice as likely to develop breast cancer by age 50 than women who did not use oral contraceptives. Other research confirms that HRT therapy using synthetic estrogen combined with progestin, a synthetic version of progesterone, also increases the risk of breast cancer, while menopausal synthetic HRT with estrogen alone increases the risk of endometrial cancer. Bioidentical hormone therapy, on the other hand, decreases the risk of cancer in women as they move through menopause. The impact synthetic hormones have on the body compared to bioidentical hormones is quite significant. Bioidentical hormones fit easily as a key in the locks of the body, as it were, whereas synthetic hormones act as a key that must be forced into the locks, often with harmful results. Bioindentical testosterone therapy also helps protect men against prostate cancer.

Studies have also shown that a woman's risk of breast cancer depends on the level of estrogen and progesterone produce by her ovaries. Prolonged high levels of these hormones produced naturally by the body have been linked to increased breast cancer risk. Increases in these naturally produced (endogenous) hormones can be triggered by starting menstruation early, starting menopause late, first become pregnant at a later age, and never having given birth. Conversely, giving birth is a protective factor for breast cancer.

Unsafe Sex/Promiscuity

As noted earlier in this chapter, many of the viruses that can trigger cancer are often transmitted sexually during unprotected sex. In addition, researchers have found that people who have more sex partners often also have a higher risk of developing cancer over the course of their lives. In one study, for example, 2537 men and 3185 women 50 or older participated in a longitudinal study of aging. The average age of the participants was 64 and approximately 75 percent of them were married. The study found that men who had sex with 10 or more people over the course of their lives had a nearly 70 percent higher likelihood of developing cancer, compared to men who were either celibate or who had a single lifetime sex partner. Men who had two to four sex partners had a nearly 60 percent greater likelihood. The risk for cancer among women who'd had sex with 10 or more people was 91 percent higher than for women who'd never had sex or had a single sex partner. The increased likelihood of cancer in the men and women who had multiple sex partners was in part attributed to a corresponding higher risk of contracting sexually transmitted infections (STIs). That risk is obviously higher during unprotected sex.

By no means does this mean that sex itself is a cancer risk factor. It isn't. What this and related research underscores is the importance of practicing safe sex to avoid contracting STIs.

Occupational Risks/Exposures

Certain occupations can also increase cancer risk due to various carcinogens that workers are exposed to in such jobs. Worldwide, it is estimated that between three to six percent of all cancer cases are caused by carcinogenic exposures in the workplace, with the incidence being higher in low- to middle-income countries. The degree of risk depends on both the duration and intensity of the exposures.

Among the most common exposures are asbestos, arsenic and inorganic arsenic compounds, benzene, chromium compounds, coal tar pitch, formaldehyde, plutonium, soot, and wood dust, as well as gamma-ray, x-ray, and ultraviolet radiation exposures. If you work in any industry in which such exposures are likely, take all appropriate precautions to protect yourself.

Keys To Remember

You can help reduce your cancer risk by doing the following:

1. Learn how to better manage and alleviate stress, exploring and improving your mindset, and getting help to heal your emotions are vitally important.
2. Commit to eating healthy and improving your body's nutritional status.
3. Avoid second- and third-hand smoke. If you smoke, seek help so you can quit.
4. Commit to regularly exercising or engaging in other physical activities.
5. Maintain a healthy weight. If you are overweight, work with your health practitioner to help your lose excess weight.
6. Beware of infections and do all you can to avoid them and boost your immunity.
7. Become aware of environmental toxins in your home and workplace and do your best to minimize your exposures to them, creating healthier home and workplace environments.
8. Minimize your exposures to EMFs, especially during bedtime.
9. Avoid exposures to ionizing radiation and test your home for radon.

10. Get at least seven hours of restorative sleep each night, and work with your doctor or a sleep specialist if you suffer from sleep problems.

11. Maintain healthy hormone balance by working with your doctor or another hormone specialist to test your hormone levels and keep them optimal.

12. Practice safe sex and avoid being promiscuous.

Prevalent as the categories of cancer risk factors discussed in this chapter may be, the one important element that most of them have in common is that they greatly depend on your lifestyle choices. The more wisely you choose, the greater the likelihood that your risk of cancer will be lessened. Knowing these risk factors and acting to reduce them can go a long way toward helping you remain cancer-free.

Chapter 4

Cancer Stem Cells and Circulating Tumor Cells

In this chapter you will learn about two of the most significant internal drivers of cancer—cancer stem cells (CSCs) and circulating tumor cells (CTCs)—and how and why, unless they are properly screened for and dealt with, they can cause a recurrence of cancer that is often more deadly and more difficult to treat than the original cancer may have been. You will also learn why conventional cancer treatments and surgeries alone often fail to address CSCs and CTCs, and can actually make them stronger and more resistant to conventional care.

Cancer Stem Cells

Stem cells are the basic building blocks from which your body and all of its organs were formed. They are different from other cells because they are unspecialized, meaning they have no specific function. Rather, they act as the raw material from which the body, in its inherent wisdom, creates the many types of specialized cells that make up other cells, tissues, and organs. Unlike other body cells, stem cells are capable of transforming themselves into any type of cell that the body needs to regenerate itself and its component parts. For example, they can mature into heart cells, pancreatic cells producing insulin, brain cells, liver cells, and so forth. All other cells are specialized cells and incapable of doing this.

In addition, unlike other cells, which under healthy conditions undergo programmed cell death (apoptosis) over time, stem cells can renew themselves indefinitely through the process of cell division. In that respect, stem cells act very much like cancer cells, which also evade apoptosis. Tumors also contain stem cells, and it is these cancer stem cells (CSCs) that enable tumors to grow, regenerate, and spread beyond their original locations. Although CSCs comprise only a small number of total cancer cells in tumors, they are the only type of cancer cells that are tumorigenic, meaning able to create cancer tumors. CSCs ability to renew themselves and to change into other types of cells—in this case, other cancer cells—is one of the primary reasons tumors can resist treatment. For this reason, a growing number of cancer researchers now consider CSCs to be the primary driver of tumor growth and metastasis. This hypothesis has not been universally accepted, however.

The idea that CSCs play pivotal roles in the onset and spread of cancer is not new. Though the discovery of stem cells, let along cancer stem cells, did not occur until much later, the concept of such cells dates back to the 1800s, and was first postulated by researchers such as Rudolf Virchow and Stephen Paget, both of whom you were introduced to in Chapter 1. In 1889, Paget first wrote of his "seed and soil" theory of cancer, suggesting that cancer cells within tumors are capable of "seeding" the spread of cancer to other areas of the body with favorable conditions (the "soil") for additional tumors to take hold, and that these tumors were not necessarily of the same type as the original tumor. Paget's theory, beginning in the 1960s, led researchers to consider the possibility that cancer cells existed within a hierarchical order, with the principal cancer cells driving cancer situated at the top. (However, the first evidence for CSCs was documented in research conducted in 1937, when researchers discovered that even a single cell from mice with leukemia could cause a new tumor to grow when it was transplanted into a healthy mouse.) In 1994, cancer stem cells were finally discovered and isolated, initially within leukemia. This discovery confirmed that CSCs sit atop the hierarchy of cancer cells. However, it was not until the early 21st century that researchers were able to isolate cancer stem cells in solid cancers, such as brain and breast cancers, and melanoma.

Research has since confirmed that CSCs give rise to many types of cells that make up tumors, and that, in many cases, they are directly responsible for tumor formation. Therefore, addressing CSCs is essential for successfully treating cancer. As researchers of one study wrote, "With the growing evidence that cancer stem cells exist in a wide array of tumors, it is becoming increasingly important to understand the molecular mechanisms that regulate self-renewal and differentiation because corruption of genes involved in these pathways likely participates in tumor growth."

Both normal stem cells and cancer stem cells are able to renew themselves and differentiate through what are known as stemness pathways. In normal stem cells, these pathways are highly regulated, but CSC stemness pathways are not. This is a primary reason why CSCs are able to differentiate into the various components involved in tumor formation and tumor growth and spread.

Cancer tumors cause inflammation and acidification as they develop and grow, both of which are necessary for tumor survival. In an effort to deal with these acidification and inflammatory processes, one of the body's responses is to call on normal stem cells derived from bone marrow and the mesenchyme, a meshwork of connective tissues of undifferentiated cells. But research indicates that these mesenchymal and bone marrow-derived stem cells also aid in the development of cancer stem cells.

Once formed, CSCs are able to activate oncogenes and also gain the ability to essentially replicate themselves for an unlimited number of times. Moreover, they also produce various chemicals that help maintain tumor survival. In addition, CSCs are able to fuse with other types of cancer cells, creating hybrid cancerous cells capable of growing more uncontrollably and creating more tumor cells and additional tumors.

Now that researchers know of the existence of CSCs, they also recognize that CSCs are not only the primary driving force behind tumor growth and metastasis, but also are the sole factor that give rise to all other cancer cells, none of which are capable of "seeding" and maintaining cancer. What this means is that in order for any cancer treatment approach to be able truly cure cancer, it has to be capable of eliminating or silencing *all* CSCs, not just some of them. Unfortunately, this is not what conventional cancer treatments—chemotherapy, radiation, surgery, and even conventional gene and immunotherapies—do. As cancer researcher John A. Pachter, PhD, noted in 2012 in an article published in the *Journal of the National Cancer Institute*, "Most anticancer compounds have brought only incremental benefit. What we need is a focus on attacking the cancer cells that are most resistant to current therapies and most aggressive in forming secondary tumors in vital organs."

Echoing that thought in the same article was Daniel Hayes, MD, clinical director of the breast oncology program at the University of Michigan, who pointed out that conventional treatment options might relieve symptoms and shrink tumors, but ultimately cannot cure cancer. "The CSC concept would suggest that what we're treating are the terminally differentiated cells but that the CSCs remain untouched," he said.

Compounding this problem is the fact that chemotherapy can cause "hyper proliferation" in CSCs, potentially resulting in cancer recurrence. This was confirmed in 2014 by animal studies conducted by a team of researchers from the University of Massachusetts Amherst and Harvard Medical School. One of the researchers, molecular biologist Michele Markstein, stated, "We discovered that several chemotherapeutics that stop fast growing tumors have the opposite effect on stem cells in the same animal, causing them to divide too rapidly. This was a surprise, because it showed that the same drug could have opposite actions on cells in the same animal: Suppressing tumor growth on one cell population while initiating growth in another... Indeed, the side effect that we observed is caused by damage [from] the chemotherapy drugs to cells in the stem cell microenvironment. The stem cells respond to this damage by hyper proliferating."

Studies indicate that radiation therapy can also induce other types of cancer cells to turn into cancer stem cells. This has been demonstrated in studies of human breast cancer cells.

As with other forms of solid cancer, breast cancer stem cells sit atop a hierarchal pyramid of cancer cells, with only breast cancer stem cells (BCSCs) being tumorigenic and thus capable of triggering the re-growth of breast cancer tumors. In one study, samples of differentiated non-tumorigenic cancer cells transformed into BCSCs after they were exposed to radiation. According to the researchers, it was the radiation that "reprogrammed differentiated breast cancer cells into induced BCSCs". Additional research found that BCSCs "increase in numbers after short courses of fractionated irradiation".

In another study, researchers found that when breast cancer stem cells were irradiated, they "survived and retained their self-renewal capacity for at least four generations". In addition, this study revealed that radiation not only spared the BCSCs, but also shifted them from a dormant, inactive cell cycle into active cycling cells, "while the surviving non-tumorigenic cells were driven into senescence [meaning they were weakened and died; to learn more about immunosenescence, see Chapter 3]".

Research has also found that, compared to other cancer cells, cancer stem cells are more resistant to both chemotherapy and radiation therapy. Moreover, these therapies can cause CSCs to become even more resistant to chemo and radiation depending on how often they are used to treat cancer patients. This buildup of resistance is similar to how bacteria become resistant to antibiotics the more that they are exposed to such drugs.

Another problem posed by CSCs is the fact that they are slow cycling, meaning that they do not grow rapidly, as other cancer cells do. Conventional cancer treatments typically target fast growing cancer cells in order to slow tumor growth. While this is an admirable goal, it leaves CSCs untouched, and may also be one reason why CSCs are able to develop resistance to chemotherapy and radiation.

As cancer researchers Erina Vlashi and Frank Pajonk of the Department of Radiation Oncology, David Geffen School of Medicine at UCLA, Los Angeles, California noted in one of their published studies about CSCs, "Experimental and clinical data provide a growing body of evidence supporting the hierarchical organization of cancers with a small number of CSCs able to self-renew, repopulate a tumor after treatment and initiate metastatic growth." As they point out, the ability of CSCs to resist chemotherapy, as well as, in many cases, radiation therapy, explains why how well the primary tumor responds to treatment is not enough to accurately predict whether or not cancer patients will achieve lasting remission. "Yet," they continue, "most established chemotherapies, including targeted therapies, have been and continue to be developed based on their effects on bulk tumor cell populations despite the knowledge that responses of the bulk tumor cell populations are unable to predict effects on the CSC population."

Vlashi and Pajonk also noted that aging and non-CSCs cells can also be resistant to chemotherapy and radiation therapy. They also reported that they found about a third of the total number of CSCs in glioma and breast cancer cell lines were in an inactive state and only became active after radiation. Because the activation of CSCs is "a direct response of the cancer cell population to treatment," they concluded that, when chemotherapy or radiation therapy causes CSCs to become activated at a greater rate than that of cancer cells being killed, "cure becomes impossible."

This explains why conventional cancer therapies, because they focus on tumor reduction and the elimination of cancer cells that are not cancer stem cells, yet fail to target and eliminate CSCs, are so often unable to prevent recurrences of cancer, many of which return in a more aggressive state than that of the original cancer. These recurrences are also cases of metastatic cancers, which account for approximately 90 percent of all deaths caused by cancer.

Current research into the nature of CSCs indicates that they possess the means to protect themselves from drugs that normally kill other cancer cells by targeting their genes. CSCs, in comparison to other cancer cells, also appear to be better able to repair damage to their DNA, thereby improving their ability to survive and resist traditional cancer treatments. They also are able to protect themselves because of their ability to maintain a low reactive oxygen species (ROS) environment, compared to differentiated cancer cells. Research suggests that this ability is critical for CSCs ability to survive and continue functioning during cancer treatments. In addition, because of the similarities between CSCs and normal stem cells, both chemotherapy and radiation aimed at killing CSCs are hindered in their ability to do so because of the severe side effects and toxicity they can cause to normal stem cells and other healthy cells, as well as healthy tissues and organs.

All of these traits of cancer stem cells explain why more effective approaches beyond the scope of conventional cancer treatments are required to meet and resolve the challenges cancer patients face.

Circulating Tumor Cells

During the process of metastasis, as tumors spread beyond their localized place of origin to invade other areas of the body, they can shed cancer cells into the bloodstream and lymphatic system. These cells are called circulating tumor cells (CTCs), sometimes also referred to a disseminated tumor cells (DTCs).

CTCs can also be spread as a result of surgery to remove tumors. (CTCs can be spread during needle biopsies, as well.) This highlights why there is no guarantee such treatments will work. Moreover, it can take months to years before patients who have been told they were cancer-free find out that they in fact never were. In such cases, CTCs within their bodies resisted treatment via a process called *micrometastasis* that evades detection by conventional cancer screening tests until visible tumors form.

It's for this reason that, after surgeries to remove or debulk tumors, cancer doctors usually recommend follow up treatments of chemotherapy, radiation, or both, even when they tell patients "We got it all". That's because, even though they may have completely removed the tumor, they recognize that CTCs are likely still present in the bloodstream. The purpose of chemotherapy and/or radiation is to try and kill off these CTCs before they can spread and cause further tumors to grow. But there is no guarantee that such treatments will work. And when they fail and cancer returns, it is often too late to save patients' lives, especially if the original treatment approaches continue to be relied upon.

Further compounding this problem is the fact that when CTCs are exposed to chemotherapy and radiation when cancer patients are treated initially, they often transform into new cancer cells that are distinctly different from the primary tumor cells, making them, like cancer stem cells, more able to resist the same type of treatments if they are administered later on. CTCs also exhibit distinct metabolic and gene functions, enabling them to become fully grown metastatic tumors, unless their metabolic function is shut down in time.

The presence and degree of CTCs in cancer patients has also been shown to affect survival rates. This was demonstrated in a study involving patients with colorectal cancer. The patients were divided into two groups: non-metastatic (stages 1-3) and metastatic (stage 4). Screening tests to detect CTCs were given to all of the patients, who were then followed during the course of their treatment period and for up to 53 months after their treatments concluded. The study found that detection of CTC in the blood of patients in both the non-metastatic and metastatic groups "was significantly associated with worse overall survival".

Similar findings occurred is a study of women with non-metastatic (stages 1-3) breast cancer. They too were screened for CTCs, which were detected in 73 of the 302 women who participated in the study (24 percent). As the researchers of the study noted, it is well-established that the presence of CTCs in women with metastatic breast cancer "correlate with poor prognosis" for survival. Their study demonstrated that the presence of one or more CTCs also "predicted early recurrence and decreased overall survival" for non-metastatic breast cancer patients. Please note that even a single CTC was found to increase the likelihood of a recurrence of cancer and decrease the likelihood of long-term survival.

Similar findings occurred in studies of men with prostate cancer. In one study, men with metastatic prostate cancer who had five or more CTCs per blood sample were found to have had a median survival rate of only 8.4 months, compared to men with less than five CTCs, whose median survival rate was four years.

In another study, blood samples were taken from men whose PSA levels rose after they had undergone surgery for prostate cancer. (PSA levels that continue to rise are considered to be an indication that cancer will recur.) Fifteen of the men received radiation treatments. Sixty percent of them in whom CTCs were found in their blood samples experienced a progression of cancer during radiation therapy, whereas none of the men whose blood samples did not contain CTCs showed any signs of cancer progression. Additional research confirmed that the presence of CTCs in blood samples of cancer patients post-prostate surgery results in less favorable outcomes of follow-up radiation therapy.

Other research shows that CTCs have characteristics similar to those of cancer stem cells, further explaining why they, too, can cause cancer recurrence and metastasis. For example, one study of CTCs detected in blood samples of patients with glioblastoma, a deadly form of brain cancer, found that the CTCs had the same negative effects as cancer stem cells. Another study of CTCs found in blood samples of patients with colorectal cancer revealed that the CTCs also had characteristics similar to cancer stems cells and functioned in the same way. These findings have led some researchers to theorize that it is only CTCs with CSC-like characteristics that are responsible for the cancer recurrences and metastases CTCs are known to cause. Lending weight to this speculation is the fact that, overall, the number of all CTCs found in blood samples of cancer patients is far greater than the incidence of cancer recurrences and metastasis among those patients unless the CTCs possess CSC-like properties.

Why Addressing CSCs and CTCs Is Crucial For Long-Term Remission

Now that you know how both cancer stem cells and circulating tumor cells can, and often do, cause recurrences of cancer, even after initial cancer treatments appear successful, you can understand why treatments that only focus on the primary tumor site are not enough to achieve lasting, long-term remission. This is borne out by statistics, which confirm that many times it is the spread of cancer to different regions in the body that is the cause of cancer deaths, not the original cancer. When cancer recurs, it is usually much more difficult to treat because many times it has metastasized before it is discovered. And CSCs and CTCs are often what cause the metastasis.

Unfortunately, the current conventional cancer treatment paradigm by and large still focuses on the primary tumor site and the genetic characteristics of its cancer cells, ignoring the fact that many times the cancer cells involved in metastasis have a different genetic makeup than the original cancer cells, and that these changes occur because the spreading cancer cells continue to differentiate.

This fact has also been confirmed by research. One study of metastatic breast cancer patients, for example, compared the genetic characteristics of the cancer cells taken from metastasis sites with the characteristics of cancer cells from the original breast tumors. Initially, the researchers found that more than 30 percent of the time, the genetic makeup of the metastasis cells was nearly entirely different than that of cells from the original breast tumors.

Further analysis revealed that none of the original breast tumors' genetic makeup was identical to that of the tumors formed by metastasis. These genetic changes, the researchers noted, help explain why metastatic cancer cells often behave differently and can be more aggressive, compared to cancer cells from the original tumor site. This and similar studies also help explain why treatments that appear to work for initial non-metastatic cancers produce poor outcomes when used to treat cancer that has metastasized. The risk of such problems happening can be greatly reduced by a more comprehensive and integrative treatment approach that simultaneously attacks both primary tumors and which also takes cancer stems cells and circulating tumors cells into account to stop them from spreading. The elements of such an integrative approach is the focus of Chapter 12.

A Silver Lining

For all of the risks posed by both CSCs and CTCs, the testing methods that have been developed to detect them can help improve treatment outcomes. This is particularly true of circulating tumor cells. A number of CTC testing methods not only enable cancer specialists to detect CTCs, but also aid in creating a treatment plan that has the highest likelihood of a successful, lasting outcome. Moreover, these tests can help practitioners gauge how well the treatments are working during the course of treatment, instead of taking a "wait and see" approach after treatments are completed. Research and clinical experience demonstrate that CTC testing can be a valuable tool for predicting how well cancer patients will respond to their treatments, and whether or not the treatments need to be altered early on to achieve better outcomes.

Just as importantly, CTC testing can also help predict the likelihood of cancer recurring in patients following the completion of their course of treatment because of the tests' ability to continue to screen for CTCs. Tests that screen for cancer stem cells are also helpful in this regard.

You will learn which of these testing methods I most recommend in the next chapter.

Keys To Remember

1. Targeting the initial cancerous tumor alone is most often not enough to prevent cancer from returning later. Conventional cancer treatments typically target fast growing cancer cells, leav-

ing circulating stem cells (CSCs) untouched. Chemotherapy and radiation can also make CSCs more aggressive.

2. When cancer recurs, it usually has metastasized to other areas of the body and is more difficult to treat.

3. Two prime factors that can lead to cancer recurrences and metastasis are cancer stem cells (CSCs) and circulating tumor cells (CTCs).

4. Both CSCs and CTCs have the capability to evade and resist cancer treatments that focus only on the original tumors. This allows them to spread elsewhere in the body, where they can lie dormant, sometimes for years, before triggering cancer recurrences.

5. Both CSCs and CTCs can develop resistance to chemotherapy and other cancer treatments. This is especially true of cancer stem cells.

6. Stem cells are the basic building blocks that form our bodies and all of its organs. They can transform into any type of cell that the body needs to regenerate itself. Stem cells can renew themselves indefinitely.

7. CSCs are a class of stem cells in cancerous tumors. They enable tumors to grow, regenerate, and spread. CSCs are the only type of cancer cells that are able to create cancer tumors.

8. Cancer treatments must be able to eliminate or silence all CSCs in order to have any hope of curing cancer. Conventional cancer treatment approaches fail to do this, whereas a comprehensive integrative approach makes sure to target CSCs in addition to the primary tumor.

9. Circulating tumor cells can be shed by tumors, and also be spread as a result of surgery and needle biopsies. CTCs travel through the bloodstream and lymphatic system.

10. Certain CTCs have characteristics that are similar to cancer stem cells. It is this class of CTCs, along with CSCs, that are most likely to cause cancer to recur and metastasize.

11. Often cells of recurring cancer and metastasis have different genetic characteristics than cancer cells of the original cancer tumors. This is a primary reason why the cancer treatments patients received when they were first diagnosed with cancer are often ineffective as treatments when cancer returns.

12. Screening for CSCs, and especially CTCs, can help health practitioners better determine the most appropriate types of treatments for their cancer patients, and monitor how well treatments progress, indicating whether or not the treatments need to be adjusted to ensure a better result.

Chapter 5

Know Your Risk

As Benjamin Franklin famously noted, "An ounce of prevention is worth a pound of cure." This is certainly true when it comes to cancer. The earliest possible detection of cancer greatly increases the chances of long-term recovery and a complete and lasting remission. Just as importantly, early detection makes treating cancer far less costly, compared to when it is detected later and has progressed.

The best solution for cancer is doing all that you can to prevent it from occurring. In order to best do so, you need to know the degree to which you are at risk for developing cancer, as well as knowing the tests that are available to you for both detecting cancer, and monitoring it during the course of treatment. That is the focus of this chapter.

To begin, please take a moment to answer Yes or No to each of the questions in this self-assessment questionnaire that I developed for my patients.

Cancer Risk Assessment

(**Important Note:** This questionnaire is designed to be used for educational purposes only. It is not intended to substitute medical evaluations or discourage regular medical check-ups or seeking medical advice to discuss concerning symptoms.)

Toxic Exposures

Regular exposure to toxins is a major risk factor for cancer. Common sources of such exposures include the following.

- **Home:** Do you regularly use commercial cleaning supplies, dish washer detergent, laundry soap, air fresheners and fragrances?

- **Yard/ Garden:** Do you maintain your yard and/or garden using chemical pesticides, especially glyphosate?

- **Personal Care/Beauty Products:** Do you regularly use commercial brands of cosmetics, soap, shampoo, deodorant, tooth paste, etc?

- **Food Consumption:** Are non-organic foods, sweets, canned foods, soda, commercial fruit juices (high because of their high sugar content) foods containing artificial ingredients, and hydrogenated oils regular parts of your meals?

(The chemicals contained in the above three categories can increase the toxic burden on your body, and in some cases are known carcinogens.)

- **Cookware/Food Storage Containers:** Do you cook primarily using aluminum, teflon-coated, and/or cast iron pans, and do you regularly store food in containers made of plastic?

- **Occupational Exposures:** Do you work in a profession known to have high toxin exposure rates, such as auto mechanic, commercial farmer, hair dresser, dentist, painter, construction, driver, or the airline industry (pilot, stewardess, maintenance)?

- **Environmental Toxins:** Do you live or work in a big city or on or in close proximity to factories or commercial farm land?

- **Addictions/Prescriptions:** Are you a smoker (including a user of marijuana) and/or a regular consumer of alcohol, and/or do you regularly use (at least once a week) over-the-counter or prescription medications, including antacids?

- **Electrosmog Exposures:** Certain electromagnetic frequencies (EMFs), and electromagnetic radiation (EMR) have been known for decades to increase the risk for cancer, although by and large this evidence continues to be ignored. Are you commonly exposed to sources of EMFs/EMR via regular cell phone use, computer/laptop/tablet use, Wi-Fi, smart meters, smart home devices such as Alexa, and/or is your home or workplace situated close to power lines and/or cell phone towers?
- **Dental:** Do you have dental amalgam (silver) fillings or root canals?
- **Home Water Supply:** Do you commonly drink, shower or bathe in municipal, unfiltered tap water, and do you regularly drink water (as well as other beverages) from plastic water bottles?
- **Signs Of Toxicity:** The following symptoms are physical indications of toxicity in your body. As above, please answer Yes if you suffer from or are prone to any of them in each category below.
- **Lungs:** Chest congestion, asthma or bronchitis, shortness of breath, difficulty breathing, chronic cough.
- **Weight:** BMI 25 or above or hip to waste ratio above 0.9 for men and above 0.85 for women.
- **Energy:** Fatigue or sluggishness, hyperactivity, restlessness, insomnia, startled awake at night.
- **Nose/Sinuses:** Stuffy nose, sinus problems, hay fever, sneezing attacks, excessive mucus.
- **Joints/Muscles:** Pain or aches in joints, stiffness or limited movement, pain or aches in muscles, recurrent backaches, feeling of joint/muscle fatigue or weakness.
- **Skin:** Eczema, psoriasis, frequent rashes, acne.
- **Colon/GI Tract:** Constipation, diarrhea, abnormal stool consistency, bloating, frequent flatulence, frequent heartburn.

- **Hormonal Imbalances:** Hypo- or hyperthyroidism, low testosterone, elevated estrogen. (**Note:** Hormonal imbalances are best determined by working with a health care practitioner skilled in the use of bioidentical hormone therapies.)
- **Emotional Issues:** Frequent feelings of anxiety, depression, worry, ADD, anger, or irritability
- **Immune Dysfunctions:** Allergies, recurring colds/flu infections.

Lifestyle and Other Risk Factors

Your lifestyle and related life choices can increase your risk for cancer, especially with regard to the following.

- **Exercise/Physical Activity:** Do you live a sedentary lifestyle and take less than a 20-minute walk twice weekly?
- **Hydration:** Do you drink less than half your weight in ounces of pure, filtered water per day, or fail to eat enough water-containing fruits and vegetables on a daily basis?
- **Sleep:** Do you fail to get enough sleep, regularly go to bed after 10-11 PM, suffer from insomnia, sleep apnea, restless sleep, sleep in a bedroom with Wi-Fi, electrical devices plugged in within eight feet of your bed, and/or sleep with a cell phone near your bed?
- **Hereditary:** Is there a history of cancer in your family that occurred within the last two generations?

Emotional Risk Factors

Various emotional factors can also increase the risk of cancer. In fact, researchers and physicians who work with cancer patients have determined that in many cases, an actual "cancer personality" can predispose a person to develop cancer. I can confirm that such a personality exists based on my own decades-long work as an integrative oncologist.

The following traits are common among people with a cancer personality. Once again, please answer Yes for each of the traits that describe you.

1. Being highly conscientious, dutiful, responsible, caring, hard-working, and usually of above average intelligence.

2. Exhibiting a strong tendency toward carrying other people's burdens and toward taking on extra obligations, often "worrying for others."

3. Having a deep-seated need to make others happy, tending to be "people pleasers."

4. Having a great need for approval from others.

5. Having a history of lack of closeness with one or both parents, sometimes, later in life, resulting in lack of closeness with spouse or others who would normally be close.

6. Harboring long-suppressed toxic emotions, such as anger, resentment and/or hostility. (Typically the cancer-susceptible individual internalizes such emotions and has great difficulty expressing them.)

7. Reacting adversely to stress, often becoming unable to cope adequately with such stress. (Usually experiencing an especially damaging event, or "life shock", about two years before the onset of detectable cancer. The patient is unable to cope with this traumatic event or series of events, which comes as a "last straw" on top of years of suppressed reactions to stress.)

8. Exhibiting an inability to resolve deep-seated emotional problems and conflicts, usually arising in childhood, often even being unaware of their presence.

9. Lacking a sense of purpose, lacking deep social connections (family, spouse, friends), and/or lacking a sense of fulfillment in your day-to-day life.

Grading Your Assessment Score

Once you've finished taking the above assessment, add up each Yes answer that you made. Then compare your risk to the grades below.

a. (low risk): 3 or less Yes answers.

b. (mild to moderate risk): 4-6 Yes answers.

c. (moderate to serious risk - strongly consider making lifestyle changes): 7-9 Yes answers.

d. (very high risk - strongly consider including detoxification and nutritional strategies along with lifestyle changes): 10 or more Yes answers.

In my experience, most people's scores fall into either category C or D, with the majority falling in D. If you find yourself in either category, don't be alarmed. As I made clear in this book's Introduction, cancer is not something to be feared. Rather, it is something we all need to be aware of and do our best to prevent. The best course of action starts with being honest about our individual risk factors, and then doing all that we can to reduce them. Showing you how to do so is the primary reason why I wrote this book.

Returning to the theme of prevention that began this chapter, regular cancer screening tests (annually, in most cases) are something I highly recommend. These types of tests fall into two main categories—blood markers, such as the various screening and diagnostic tests that I shared with you in Chapter 1, and diagnostic tests you are doubtless already aware of, such as CT scans, PET scans, and X-rays.

The remainder of this chapter discusses other cancer tests you need to know about, starting with three that you are most likely familiar with—colonoscopy, mammography (mammograms), and the PSA test used to screen for prostate cancer.

Colonoscopy

Colon cancer is the second leading cause of death by cancer in both men and women. For this reason, colonoscopy has for years been recommended by doctors as an important cancer screening method, especially for people 50 years and older.

During a colonoscopy, a long, flexible tube known as a colonoscope is inserted into and passed through the rectum and up through the large intestine (colon) and the bottom of the small intestine. At the tip of the colonoscope is a tiny video camera which enables a doctor to view the inside of the entire colon, looking for inflamed or swollen tissues and lesions, polyps, and other potential signs of cancer. Polyps and unhealthy tissues are usually removed during the procedure and sent to a lab to be biopsied.

Doctors typically recommend that all men and women undergo a colonoscopy when they turn 50 (even earlier for people at a higher risk for cancer, including a family history of the disease), and then, depending on the findings, to repeat the process every five to 10 years until age 75, after which the procedure is less advantageous.

Research shows that colonoscopy reduces the risk of being diagnosed with cancer of colorectal cancers (cancer of either the colon or rectum). Moreover, it is covered by insurance with, in most cases, no out of pocket expenses incurred by patients, making it widely available as a screening regardless of one's financial situation. (However, should the procedure result in a biopsy or removal of a polyp or abnormal tissue, it may no longer be regarded as a screening test, depending on one's insurance company, in which case a co-pay may be charged, although patients won't have to pay the deductible of their insurance policy.) In many hospitals, patients can even request a colonoscopy without a physician's order. Prior to the Covid outbreak of 2020, more than six million colonoscopies were performed annually in the US.

Until recently, colonoscopy was also assumed to reduce the risk of dying from colorectal cancers. However, a 2022 study published in the *New England Journal of Medicine* calls that assumption into question. The study involved nearly 85,000 men and women between the ages of 55 and 64, all of whom were presumed to be healthy. According to the study's authors, "The participants were randomly assigned in a 1:2 ratio either to receive an invitation to undergo a single screening colonoscopy (the invited group) or to receive no invitation or screening (the usual-care group). The primary end points were the risks of colorectal cancer and related death, and the secondary end point was death from any cause."

During a median follow-up of ten years, the researchers found that participants in the invited group who chose to have a colonoscopy at the start of the study reduced their relative risk of developing colorectal cancer over the following ten years by 18 percent, compared to those in the usual-care group who chose to forgo the procedure (0.98 percent vs 1.2 percent). However, the absolute risk reduction in the invited group was only 0.22 percent, which equates to only 22 more people in a population of 10,000.

More troubling to the researchers was the fact that the difference in deaths due to colorectal cancer in both groups was statistically insignificant (0.28 percent in the invited group and 0.31 percent in the other group, a difference of only three people in every 10,000). Moreover, the rate of all cause mortality in both groups was virtually identical, with 11.3 percent of the participants having died in the invited group by the study's completion, compared to 11.4 percent of people in the other group. "This relatively small reduction in the risk of colorectal cancer and the nonsignificant reduction in the risk of death are both surprising and disappointing…," the authors wrote. Compounding this fact is research that found that as many as 25 percent of all colonoscopies performed in the U.S. each year are unnecessary.

Like other medical procedures, colonoscopy is also not without risks, all of which need to be considered before undergoing this procedure.

One of the most common risks is that of infection, which is caused by improper sterilization and disinfection of the colonoscope between procedures. Colonoscopes are not disposable and must be properly sterilized before each use. Yet it is estimated that in the majority of cases, the instrument is cleaned using Cidex (glutaraldehyde). The effectiveness of Cidex as a means of sterilization has been called into question. A superior approach is to clean with paracetic acid, which is known to more thoroughly dissolve and eliminate potentially harmful proteins and other residues that can cause infection. If you choose to undergo a colonoscopy, be sure to confirm beforehand that the clinic or hospital uses paracetic acid, not Cidex.

While rare, in some cases colonoscopy can also cause perforation of the colon and gastrointestinal bleeding/hemorrhaging (4 in 10,000 cases and 8 in 10,000 cases, respectively, according to published studies). People most at risk are those with diverticulitis and other GI conditions, and those with adhesions in the GI tract due to previous surgery.

Another potential risk is dysregulation of the internal environment (microbiome) of the GI tract due to the prescribed bowel-cleansing liquid formula that needs to be consumed one day prior to the procedure (typically in the afternoon or evening, depending on the scheduled time of the colonoscopy). This liquid acts as a harsh laxative, causing the equivalent of diarrhea in order to flush out the contents of the colon, including healthy gut flora (bacteria) needed to ensure proper functioning of the GI tract.

Finally, prior to the procedure beginning, patients may be offered anesthesia. Although you may prefer to be completely sedated so that you are not conscious during your colonoscopy exam, I advise forgoing anesthesia altogether, or choosing only to be lightly sedated, due to complications that can arise as a result of full sedation.

Despite these risks, for most people, they are far outweighed by advantages colonoscopy offers, especially given that it is the most dependable way to screen for colon cancer, and enables physicians to remove polyps and abnormal tissues that may be found during the procedure so that they can be biopsied.

Alternatives To Colonoscopy: A number of other screening tests for colorectal cancer are also available as viable alternatives to colonoscopy. They include flexible sigmoidoscopy, virtual colonoscopy, and three at-home stool tests (fecal occult blood test, fecal immunochemical test, and a multi-targeted stool DNA test).

Flexible Sigmoidoscopy is similar to a colonoscopy in that it, too, involves the insertion into the GI tract of a tube (a sigmoidoscope) with a camera attached. The difference is that the scope only travels up through the rectum into lower part of the large intestine (colon), a distance typically of two feet that encompasses the rectum, sigmoid colon and most of the descending colon. Like a colonoscopy, a sigmoidoscopy can screen for polyps, swollen and inflamed tissues, and lesions, and also enables physicians to remove them for biopsy, but only within the area that is examined. It can also be used to screen for and remove internal hemorrhoids, and to look for signs of diverticulitis.

Compared to colonoscopy, sigmoidoscopy carries less risk of perforation and internal bleeding. It also usually can be administered without the need for anesthesia or pain medication, and is a quick procedure only requiring about 15 minutes to be performed.

Like colonoscopy, flexible sigmoidoscopy is recommended for men and women between the ages of 50 to 64, but more frequently (once every five years, compared to ten years for most colonoscopies).

Virtual Colonoscopy, also known as CT colonoscopy, involves the use of a CT scan or, in some cases, magnetic resonance imaging (MRI), to provide physicians with two- and three-dimensional images of the entire large intestine, from the rectum to the lower end of the small intestine. It, too, is capable of screening for polyps, signs of inflammation in the colon, and diverticulitis. It also does not require anesthesia, although the use of a bowel-flushing laxative is still required to be taken before the day before procedure. Its most obvious disadvantage is that it cannot remove any polyps or tissue abnormalities, should they be discovered. If that is the case, follow-up with an actual colonoscopy to remove them will likely be advised.

It, too, is recommended once every five years.

The **Fecal Occult Blood Test (FOBT)**, also known as the Hemoccult Test, is a simple stool test that screens for hidden (occult) blood in the stool, which can be an indication of polyps in the colon or rectum, as well as colon cancer. Because occult blood typically only passes in small amounts, the chemicals used in the FOBT are necessary to screen for it. It is conducted on a sample of collected feces and screens for hemoglobin, a primary component of human blood. A positive finding of hemoglobin will usually result in further diagnostic tests being ordered, such as a colonoscopy or sigmoidoscopy, in order to screen for potentially cancerous polyps or tumors in the colon or rectum. It can also used to screen for anemia.

FOBT is not always accurate, however, and false-positive readings can occur if patients consume iron-rich vegetables or red meats prior to testing. Aspirin, iron tablets, nonsteroidal anti-inflammatory drugs (NSAIDS), and large doses of vitamin C can also result in false-positive readings.

The **Fecal Immunochemical Test (FIT)** is similar to the FOBT test in that it can also be used to screen for hidden blood in stools, but it typically has a higher degree of sensitivity, making it more accurate. Moreover, unlike FBOT, foods do not interfere with FIT readings, reducing the likelihood of false positive readings.

Unlike FOBT and Fit, the **Multi-targeted stool DNA test (mt-sDNA)**, more commonly known as the Cologuard test, not only screens for hemoglobin present in hidden blood, but also for DNA mutations that can indicate the presence of colorectal cancer, as well as precancerous advanced adenomas (benign tumors that may turn cancerous, and which can also negatively affect various organs in the body).

Despite the convenience of the above at-home stool tests, because of how their sensitivity and accuracy vary, colonoscopy or sigmoidoscopy are still advised for people with a known higher risk for colorectal cancer, and definitely advised should the stool test results be positive. It is recommended that screening with these tests be conducted annually.

Mammograms

Breast cancer is the second leading cause of cancer deaths in women, behind only lung cancer. It strikes one out of every eight women during the course of their lives, and is now occurring in women much earlier than before. Research shows that 15 percent of all cases of breast cancer in the United States occur in women who are 45 or younger. When breast cancer strikes earlier in life it is usually more aggressive and more fatal than when it strikes older women. For these reasons, mammograms, along with breast self-examinations, are recommended by the National Cancer Institute (NCI), the American Cancer Society, and most conventional doctors as the best way for women to detect breast cancer.

Mammograms involve the use of X-rays that allow doctors to look for dense structures within the breast that can be an indication of a tumor. This form of detection is known as structural imaging. Research shows that mammograms are useful for detecting breast cancer in 80 percent of all women over the age of 50. However, that means that 20 percent of women age 50 or older can have breast cancer that is undetected by mammograms. And among younger women that percentage is even higher (as much as 40 percent).

Mammograms are also largely ineffective for detecting cancer located in the upper area of the breast and within the peripheral areas next to the chest wall. They can also miss signs of breast cancer among women who have large or dense breasts, and women who have had breast augmentation. Fibrocystic breast disease can often also prevent breast cancer from being detected by mammograms.

Despite these limitations, the American Medical Association, the American College of Radiology, the American Cancer Society, the National Cancer Institute, and other medical organizations, along with most conventional physicians, still continue to recommend that all women 40 and over receive annual mammograms.

I question these recommendations, based on a growing body of research that has examined the value of mammograms. For example, in 2010, the ineffectiveness of mammograms was highlighted by a study conducted by researchers in Norway. The study found only a 10 percent decrease in breast cancer deaths among women who regularly screened for breast cancer using mammography.

Commenting about this finding, two of the study's authors stated, "As we embarked on the project, we were aware of the controversies that have surrounded mammography screening...When we received the available evidence and contemplated its implications in detail, however, we became increasingly concerned...The relative risk reduction of approximately 20 percent in breast-cancer mortality associated with mammography that is currently described by most expert panels came at the price of a considerable diagnostic cascade, with repeat mammography, subsequent biopsies, and over-diagnosis of breast cancers—cancers that would never have become clinically apparent."

A 25-year Canadian study also documented mammography's failure to prevent breast cancer deaths. In addition, the study revealed a high incidence of over-diagnosis of breast cancer that resulted in unnecessary treatments. In the study, 89 835 women between the ages of 40 to 59 were randomly assigned to a group that received five annual mammography screenings, or to a control group that received no mammograms. The women in the mammography group aged 40 to 49, plus all of the women aged 50 to 59 also received annual physical breast exams, while the younger women in the control group received only a single exam. The authors of the study reported, "During the entire study period, 3250 women in the mammography arm and 3133 in the control arm had a diagnosis of breast cancer, and 500 and 505, respectively, died of breast cancer. Thus the cumulative mortality from breast cancer was similar between women in the mammography arm and in the control arm…After 15 years of follow-up a residual excess of 106 cancers was observed in the mammography arm, attributable to over-diagnosis."

The researchers concluded, "Annual mammography in women aged 40-59 does not reduce mortality from breast cancer beyond that of physical examination or usual care when adjuvant therapy for breast cancer is freely available," and reported that 22 percent of the "detected invasive breast cancers were over-diagnosed, representing one over-diagnosed breast cancer for every 424 women who received mammography screening in the trial."

Other published studies have documented similar findings. In addition, research also shows that women between the ages of 40 to 74 who undergo mammography on an annual or semi-annual basis can actually increase their risk of breast cancer due to the radiation they are exposed to during the procedure. (Similar risks also exist for both men and women who receive frequent X-rays, CT scans, and PET scans.) The risk is particularly pronounced in women with large breasts.

In light of this research, with the exception of younger women with a known higher risk for cancer, it may be more advisable for women to wait until they turn 50 to consider mammograms, and to schedule them every two years instead of annually. All women should also regularly (once a month) conduct self-exams of their breasts to screen for lumps and other potential signs of breast cancer. Instructions for how to conduct a breast self-exam are available at www.nationalbreastcancer.org/breast-self-exam.

As an alternative to mammography, you can also consider a radiation-free screening tool called thermography, discussed later in this chapter.

PSA Test

The PSA test is commonly recommended for men by many physicians. It measures the amount of a protein called prostate-specific antigen in the blood, and is used as a screening method for detecting both an enlarged prostate (benign prostate hypertrophy, or BPH) and prostate cancer. This protein is produced in the prostate gland, with PSA levels typically becoming elevated in cases of prostate cancer.

When the test reveals higher-than-normal PSA levels (4 to 10 ng/mL or higher), physicians often recommend a biopsy of prostate tissue to determine if cancer is present, particularly for levels 10 ng/mL or greater. However, such biopsies are not without risk. Not only can they be painful—with the pain lingering for days and even weeks—if cancer is present, biopsies can cause cancer stem cells and circulating tumor cells (see Chapter 4) to break off from the tumor to enter the bloodstream and circulate undetected to other areas of the body. Biopsy can also result in infection of the prostate gland, as well as bleeding.

Other limitations of the PSA test include the fact that PSA levels can rise due to BPH, not cancer, and prostatitis (inflammation of the prostate gland, usually caused by infection). Levels can also change in men as a natural consequence of aging. The results of the test can also be misleading, resulting in both false-positive (a diagnosis of cancer when it is in fact not present) and false-negative (undetected cancer) readings. Over-diagnosis of prostate cancer is another potential problem because some cases of prostate cancers detected by PSA tests never cause symptoms or are fatal. In cases of over-diagnosis, men may be advised by their physician to undergo an unnecessary prostectomy (surgical removal of the prostate gland), which is fraught with many, often long-term, complications, or unnecessary chemotherapy or radiation treatments.

These risks and limitations caused Richard J. Albin, PhD, who discovered PSA in 1970, to call upon physicians to stop relying upon it as a prostate cancer screening tool. He even co-wrote a book to this end, *The Great Prostate Hoax*, and pointed out that there is no normal reading for PSA levels. (The PSA test continues to be an accurate indicator for BPH, however, and since BPH can often be a precursor to prostate cancer, the PSA test still has some value.)

Alternatives to the PSA test include:

- **Digital Rectal Exam:** This test involves a medical practitioner inserting a gloved finger into the rectum to feel for any irregularities in the prostate that might be signs of a tumor. DRE is also used to test for signs of BPH.

- **Transrectal Ultrasound (TRUS):** TRUS is a form of ultrasound used to produce an image of the prostate gland and to check for enlargement and any abnormalities indicating cancer. It involves the insertion of a small probe into the rectum. The probe emits sound waves that create a picture of the prostate on a computer screen. Though the procedure is uncomfortable, it is also over quickly, usually lasting ten minutes or so. TRUS can also be used to guide biopsy should it still be necessary.

- **Mi-prostate score (MiPS):** MiPS is a urine test that is given after a PSA test or DRE indicates the possibility of prostate cancer. It scores the levels of three markers—blood PSA and the genes PCA3 (prostate cancer gene 3) and T2:ERG. Elevated levels of these three markers in urine are rare in men who do not have prostate cancer, but higher in men in with the disease. The higher the levels are, the more likely it is that prostate cancer is present. A urine test that measures levels of PCA3 alone can also be useful. It is more accurate than the standard PSA test because it is more effective for screening out the various noncancerous factors that can cause elevated PSA.

A number of other blood tests have also proven to be more accurate screening tools for cancer than the standard PSA test. They include the free PSA test, IsoPSA, the 4K score, and the prostate health index (PHI).

Whereas the standard PSA test measures the total amount of PSA in blood, which consists of two types—PSA bound to protein and unbound, or free, PSA, **the free PSA test** measures the levels of both types and provides physicians with a ratio between the two. The lower the level of free

PSA is, the more likely it is that cancer exists, since men with prostate cancer typically have low free PSA levels, compared to healthy men.

The IsoPSA test also measures both bound and free PSA levels, as well as the various proteins that PSA can bind to. It also determines the ratio of mature and immature PSA.

The 4K score assesses the results of four blood tests: total PSA, free PSA, intact PSA (inactive PSA molecules) and a gene called human Kallikrein 2 (or hK2), which is related to PSA, plus the results of a DRE, and the patient's age and whether or not he had a biopsy. The test creates an overall score that helps doctors predict if a biopsy is needed and, if cancer is found, whether the cancer is aggressive and requires treatment, or is a case in which watchful waiting with follow-up screenings is more appropriate. Studies have shown that the 4K score is far more accurate than biopsy alone for predicting whether prostate is aggressive and likely to metastasize or is of low risk.

PHI measures total PSA levels as well as two specific types of PSA proteins. Like the 4K score, it too can help physicians better determine the need for biopsy, and also gauge how aggressive cases of prostate cancer are should they be found.

Like the standard PSA test, none of the above alternative tests can completely confirm the existence of prostate cancer. Such confirmation requires a biopsy. However, they are all superior to standard PSA for determining if a biopsy is needed and therefore are tests all men should know about.

Other Cancer Screening Tests You Need To Know About

I've also found the following tests to be very helpful aids in guiding me in how best to treat my cancer patients. All of them are noninvasive and pose no risk of side effects. However, they also are commonly not used by most oncologists and other conventional physicians, so you may need to be proactive and seek them out on your own.

Thermography

Thermography is a safe and effective screening test for cancer and other purposes that has been in use for more than 50 years in both the United States and Europe. It is nontoxic and highly accurate, and, in contrast to mammograms, which are less effective at diagnosing breast cancer in dense breast tissue, thermography is not affected by tissue densities.

Thermography measures the emissions of infrared heat from various areas of the body. This is significant, since cancer cells and tumors emit more heat than normal cells and tissues do, and do so in a noticeably fluctuating, unregulated manner, compared to how heat is normally emitted by healthy cells and tissues. Thermography accurately detects these fluctuating heat emissions.

Thermography is particularly useful for detecting breast cancer, often up to five years earlier than mammography is capable of doing. Another major advantage of thermography is that it is free of the discomfort associated with mammograms. There is no compression, no direct contact with the body, and no exposure to radiation. Instead, once the body reaches a steady temperature state that is compatible with the special temperature conditions of the thermography room, a person is positioned in front of the thermography camera so that all surfaces of upper torso, including the underarms, can be imaged. The images are captured in real time and then transmitted to a computer for analysis. The computer allows doctors to isolate differences in surface body temperature and vascularity.

After the images are analyzed, they are graded using a standardized system based on five categories. Depending on the results of the exam, further tests may be ordered should there be any indication of breast or other abnormalities. (It's important to note that neither thermography nor mammograms can definitively determine whether or not breast cancer is present in patients. Subsequent testing is always necessary for confirmation.) A normal reading provides doctors with a baseline reading that they can compare to follow-up thermography readings as part of an annual health check-up.

As noted earlier, mammograms fail to detect breast cancer 20 percent of the time. By contrast, breast thermography successfully detects indications of breast cancer 90 percent of the time, and has the added benefit of being able to do so up to eight to ten years earlier than mammography.

Because thermography can detect variations in surface body temperature throughout the entire body, it is also useful for detecting prostate and other cancers, as well as other diseases, including inflammatory breast disease, fibromyalgia, gastrointestinal disorders, thyroid issues, hiatal hernias, and even early warning signs of heart disease and stroke.

Given the errors, false negatives, and radiation exposure dangers that are so common to mammography, thermography is one of my preferred methods for breast cancer screening, at least initially. If cancer is detected, mammograms can then be used to pinpoint the location of breast tumors.

Although thermography has been approved by the Food and Drug Administration (FDA) since 1982, you may need to seek out providers of thermography on your own, since many physicians still fail to consider its use. See the Resources section of this book for a list of organizations that can help you do so.

Dry and Darkfield Blood Analysis

No doubt, you are familiar with examination of blood using standard microscopy (also known as Bright field microscopy because of the type of microscope that is typically used). While this form of blood analysis can be useful, it is also limited in terms of what it can reveal about a person's health. Two lesser known types of microscopy that provide more comprehensive findings are dry blood analysis and darkfield microscopy, both of which I use to guide my treatments of my patients with cancer and other disease conditions.

Dry Blood Analysis: This form of microscopy originated in Germany in the early 20th century. Today, it is used in hundreds of clinics worldwide.

Another name for dry blood analysis is the mycotoxic oxidative stress test (MOST). During this procedure, a drop of blood is placed a glass slide and then exposed to ambient air (air free of air-borne pollutants). As the layers of the blood dry, they go through a natural process of spinning, leaving unique characteristics of the blood sample. Review of these samples using a bright field microscope allows for evaluation of this information.

A dry blood drop can be likened to a hologram of the human body, with its different layers, or rings, representing different parts of the body. Wherever abnormalities appear in the blood drop, they indicate where dysfunctions may be occurring. In addition, practitioners skilled in the use of dry blood analysis can use it to determine a timeline of when the dysfunctions first began and the underlying factors that are causing them.

Darkfield Microscopy: Unlike conventional electron microscopy, darkfield microscropy enables physicians to observe microscopic living organisms, including blood cells, as well as the presence of disease-causing microorganisms.

To perform this task, physicians place a drop of a patient's blood on a slide under a specially adapted microscope, which then projects the magnified image of the blood (usually a magnification of 1500 times) onto a video screen to reveal the blood's internal environment and the shape and motion of the blood's components, including its cells.

By contrast, conventional microscopy reveals very little about the true condition of the blood.

For example, doctors using conventional microscopy will often seek to obtain a total white blood count (WBC) of immune cells known as neutrophils. A WBC that falls within the normal range can lead them to assume that their patient is healthy. Using darkfield microscopy, physicians are able to easily see if the neutrophils have abnormalities consistent with cancer and other disease states. In addition to revealing distortions in the shapes of the cells themselves, darkfield microscopy also shows whether or not cells are circulating properly. It can also detect free radical damage and reveal if there is cell leakage from within the cellular walls due to cell-wall deficiencies.

All of these factors, while not providing definitive proof of cancer, nonetheless are indications that cancer or other disease may be present. Once they are observed, physicians can then order follow-up tests. In this way, cancer can often be detected much earlier than conventional screening tests usually allow for. Equally important, once cancer treatments begin, continued darkfield blood analysis can provide physicians with solid indications of whether or not their treatment approach is working based upon whether or not there are positive changes occurring as follow-up blood samples are observed. Unfortunately, darkfield microscopy is rarely used by conventional physicians and oncologists despite the fact that it can be an important tool for detecting signs of cancer in the bloodstream.

The Cancer Profile© Test

This test is available from American Metabolic Laboratories in Florida and was developed by the late Emil Schandl, PhD. It incorporates multiple tests which, combined, provide a far more accurate indication of whether or not a person's biochemistry is shifting towards an unhealthy state than if the tests were done separately. The test measures levels of thyroid-stimulating hormone (TSH), an indicator of thyroid function (low thyroid function, or hypothyroidism, can predispose one to developing cancer); DHEA-S, a hormone produced by the adrenal gland that serves as an indicator of adrenal and immune function and is a marker for cancer; *gamma-glutamyltranspeptidase* (GGTP), an enzyme marker for overall liver function (healthy liver function is essential for protecting against cancer); and the cancer markers CEA (*carcinoembryonic antigen*), PHI (*phosphohexose isomerase enzyme*), and HCG (*human chorionic gonadotropin*), the last of which is measured using two different methods to ensure the best possible accuracy.

Based on his many years of research, Dr. Shandl observed that the substances his Cancer Profile test measures tend to become elevated at least 10 or more years before cancer can be detected using conventional screening tests. Because of this long timeline, looking for shifts in biochemistry such as those the Cancer Profile measures can help patients avoid cancer before it gains a foothold inside their bodies, using highly effective approaches such as the dietary, nutritional, and other therapies that you will learn about later in this book.

The Cancer Profile Test involve two statistical measures—sensitivity and specificity. Sensitivity refers to the probability that a test will show a positive result when cancer exists, while specificity refers to the probability that a negative test result will occur when no cancer exists. A test that has high sensitivity and high specificity is far more useful than tests for which one or both of these measures are lower. Many conventional cancer marker tests, including many that you learned about in Chapter 1, fall into this latter category. Dr. Shandl developed the Cancer Profile test for precisely this reason. He wanted to ensure a high level of accuracy, which cannot be achieved when doctors rely on only one marker alone. For example, despite the fact that numerous scientific studies show that HCG levels in the body become elevated when cancer cells are present in the body, other studies have found that tests that screen for HCG alone often fail to detect such increases in elevations, usually because, even though the levels have risen, they may not have done so at levels high enough to be detected. As a result, HCG screening tests by themselves account for approximately 30 percent false negative results. Similarly, other studies have shown that screening for either CEA or PHI alone can also lead to false negative results, whereas when both of these markers are measured, the overall accuracy of such testing increases significantly.

The combination of markers included in the Cancer Profile will usually detect cancer with far more accuracy and usually much earlier than conventional cancer tests. Testing has shown that the Cancer Profile has an overall accuracy rate of between 87 and 97 percent, depending on the type of cancer that a person may be developing, which exceeds the rates of many other cancer screening tests.

Another benefit of the Cancer Profile test is that can also be used to monitor how well cancer treatments are working. This is important because no cancer treatment works 100 percent of the time. By using the Cancer Profile test to monitor how well their treatments are working, physicians can quickly know whether they are on the right track or whether they need to change what they are doing before it is too late.

In addition, if surgery is necessary to remove cancerous tumors, the Cancer Profile can be used prior to surgical procedures to provide patients and their physicians with a benchmark to determine whether or not the surgery was successful. Following surgery, a follow-up Profile test can be given. If surgery was successful, the Profile will confirm that by showing lowered levels of the cancer markers it measures. If the markers stay at the same level as before, or continue to rise, then doctors will know that their patients need additional care.

Just as importantly, physicians can use the Cancer Profile to monitor how well their patients who are in remission are maintaining their health. By using the Cancer Profile, physicians they can see how well their cancer patients are doing and, if necessary, take appropriate action should indications of cancer recurrence appear.

You can learn more about this yourself by visiting: americanmetaboliclaboratories.net. Your doctor can order the test for you, or you can do it yourself by contacting American Metabolic Laboratories directly. After you receive your results, you can also schedule a free phone consultation with one of the lab's trained representatives.

As with other blood screening tests for cancer, however, the Cancer Profile by itself cannot definitively prove that cancer is present. Such confirmation can only be obtained with further testing methods.

Galleri® Test

The Galleri test is another effective tool for detecting early signs of cancer signals. It works by screening for abnormalities in the methylation patterns of cell-free DNA (cfDNA) in the bloodstream. If found, the abnormalities are then analyzed using the test's proprietary next-generation sequencing (NGS) and algorithm technology.

All cells shed DNA into the bloodstream and make use of DNA methylation to regulate gene expression, including the oncogenes you learned about in Chapter 1. When methylation patterns of cfDNA become abnormal they can trigger changes in gene expression that initiate cancer and contribute to tumor growth. These changes in cfDNA methylation patterns act as cancer signals and provide information about where in the body the signals originated.

When a cancer signal is detected, the Galleri test can identify the origin of the signal with a high degree of accuracy, as well as helping to guide the next steps to a confirmed diagnosis. Though the test alone cannot confirm cases of cancer, research shows that it can detect indications of numerous types of cancer and is highly accurate in predicting the origin of cancer signals.

The accuracy of the Galleri test was clinically validated in a 2021 study of over 4,000 participants, all of whom had previously been determined to either have cancer (2823 participants) or who were cancer-free (1254 participants). Specificity, sensitivity, and cancer signal prediction accuracy of the test were all measured, with the participants followed up on one year later. The study showed that the Galleri test was able to detect cancer signals for over 50 different types of cancer, and that its specificity for cancer signal detection had an accuracy rate of 99.5 percent. In addition, the test's overall ability to accurately predict the origin of the cancer signals had a true positive rate of between 87 to 90.2 percent.

The Galleri test should be ordered by a physician. Results of the test are usually available within 10 business days following test manufacturer's receipt of the specimen sample. The test is not recommended for anyone 21 years or younger, however, or for pregnant women. It should also not be used for patients currently undergoing cancer treatments.

For more information, visit www.galleri.com.

Chronic Inflammation Test

As you learned in Chapter 2, chronic, systemic inflammation is a significant cause and driver of cancer. Therefore, being able to most effectively measure levels of inflammation in the body is an important step for both preventing cancer, and to assess the degree of inflammation that is affecting cancer patients, as well as monitoring how well inflammation is being reversed during the course of treatment.

In addition to the inflammation measurement tests and markers that I shared with you in Chapter 2, when treating cancer patients I also rely on what is known as the Chronic Inflammation Test. Unlike these other tests, the Chronic Inflammation Test is a urine test that measures levels of a substance called 11-Dehydro Thromboxane B2, as well as urinary creatinine levels, to calculate a ratio between the two. Elevated levels of 11-Dehydro Thromboxane B2 have been shown to be strongly associated with cancer, as well as Alzheimer's disease, diabetes, heart disease, and stroke. The 11-Dehydro Thromboxane B2 level, in turn, provides a measurement of thromboxane A2 production associated with inflammation in the body. The activation of the thromboxane A2 pathway is a major component of inflammation biochemistry in the body.

A major advantage of the Chronic Inflammation Test is that urine collection can be conducted at home. A collection kit can be ordered for this purpose, with the urine specimen then sent for analysis to Creative Clinical Concepts (CCC), the company that provides the test. In many states, consumers can order the test by themselves; in other states, a physician's order is necessary. As of this writing, the test is not available to residents of New York and Rhode Island.

For more information about the test, visit https://chronicinflammationtest.com.

Conclusion

Having finished this chapter, my hope is that you have a better understanding of the risk factors for cancer you may need to address based on your answers to the Cancer Risk Assessment. I recommend that you revisit the Assessment periodically to gauge the progress you make as you work to reduce any risks that you identified.

I also hope you better understand the benefits, limitations, and risks of the commonly recommended cancer screening tests I discussed, and recognize that, just as there are many options for treating cancer besides surgery, chemotherapy, and radiation, there other diagnostic options that are also available to you. Should you or any of your loved ones ever develop cancer, these tests can guide you to make the most informed decisions regarding the best course of treatment. When used appropriately, they have the potential to be lifesavers.

Chapter 6

The Importance of Addressing Your Spiritual Health

It's an unfortunate fact that fear, anxiety, and, very often, a sense of hopelessness, are among the first emotions that typically arise in people who are told that that have cancer. A cancer diagnosis can be overwhelming, both for cancer patients and for their families and other loved ones. Feelings of powerlessness and questions such as "Why me?" are common responses, as well. The support loved ones provide cancer patients, however well-intentioned it may be, can also often fall short simply because, unless they themselves have journeyed through cancer, they have no idea of the full extent of the challenges cancer patients face.

It is precisely in these moments of fear and despair that many cancer patients realize and admit to themselves that they cannot overcome cancer on their own, or even with the help of their oncologists and other health care providers. For many cancer patients, this admission can be a turning point, one that leads them to call on God to help them.

This is what happened to Lori G, the long-term cancer survivor you were introduced to in this book's Introduction. As Lori shared, asking for

God's help and being willing to accept it can marshal patients' inner resources in ways that were previously unknown to them. This, in turn, can provide them with the strength and will power to meet their challenges with resilience and a deep commitment to do "whatever it takes" to get well again, combined with faith in God as the true source of all healing. This is the formula that makes it possible for miracles to occur.

Having witnessed this formula in action many times over, I can attest to how pivotal it is for improving the likelihood of full recovery from cancer and other life-threatening diseases.

This is why I encourage all of my patients, regardless of what health challenges they may be facing, to place their spiritual health first, knowing that, if they do so, their physical, mental, and emotional issues will improve, as well.

The reason for this was explained in an article entitled *Cancer: Religion and Spirituality*, written by Andrew W. Kneier, PhD and Rabbi Jeffery Silberman. In it, they stated, "A life-threatening disease such as cancer makes us confront realities and questions that cause us to step back from our lives and reflect on the meaning and implications of the illness.

"Our perspective on these realities and questions emerges in large measure from our religious, spiritual, or philosophical orientation, and it influences how we experience the illness— its meaning, how we feel about it, and how well we come to terms with it. A religious perspective can help us as we grapple with these issues and seek to keep our bearing through the mental and emotional turmoil that comes with having cancer."

Somewhere between your body and mind lies your inner knower— that part of you that senses the truth and importance of the experiences that you have in your life. It seeks to join your mental, emotional, and physical aspects into a sum that is greater than its parts. You can call this your soul, your Higher Self, or whatever other name you choose. This core self at the deepest level of your Being is what you need to tap into in order to better manage your mind, emotions, and body to banish the effects of stress, enhance your health, and truly heal disease.

As the National Cancer Institute (NCI) points out, "Spiritual and religious well-being may help improve health and quality of life in the following ways:

- Decrease anxiety, depression, anger, and discomfort.
- Decrease the sense of isolation (feeling alone) and the risk of suicide.
- Decrease alcohol and drug abuse.
- Lower blood pressure and the risk of heart disease.
- Help the patient adjust to the effects of cancer and its treatment.
- Increase the ability to enjoy life during cancer treatment.
- Give a feeling of personal growth as a result of living with cancer.
- Increase positive feelings, including:
  - Hope and optimism.
  - Freedom from regret.
  - Satisfaction with life.
  - A sense of inner peace.

Spiritual and religious well-being may also help a patient live longer."

The rest of this chapter explains how crucial spiritual health is when dealing with cancer, and provides you with what I've found are the best approaches for deepening our connection with God to receive Divine guidance.

What Is Spiritual Health?

To me, spiritual health, while often the most overlooked aspect of healing, is actually the ultimate goal of medicine because of how it leads to a heightened awareness of the Divine Spirit or Life Force referred to by all religions and spiritual traditions. It isn't important what name you give it. What matters is that you come to know and attune yourself to its guidance in all areas of your life, especially if you have cancer. Doing so will reduce your feelings of stress, anxiety, depression, and fear, and provide you with a greater capacity for loving yourself and others unconditionally. It will also help you reconnect to your special talents and gifts and use them to fulfill your life's purpose, which can be a further powerful factor for healing.

In many respects, another name for Spirit is *unconditional love*. This includes unconditional love for yourself. Learning to love yourself unconditionally is one of the most effective ways I know of for developing a deeper awareness of and relationship with God. Yet, for many people, it is also one of their most difficult challenges because of how they tend to judge themselves, focusing on perceived shortcomings, regrets, and so forth.

Such self-judgments are often much harsher than how they judge others, and can include recriminations towards themselves for getting sick. It's not uncommon for some patients with cancer to believe that somehow they are to blame for having cancer, or that they did something wrong that caused it. Such beliefs foster or exacerbate fears, anxiety, and anger, creating additional stress which, in turn, can weaken immune function.

By contrast, learning how to accept and forgive yourself can alleviate stress, making it easier for healing to occur. In addition, the more that you become able to love, forgive, and accept yourself, regardless of your present circumstances, the more likely you are to develop a deeper awareness of God supporting you throughout your journey through cancer.

Becoming spiritually healthy helps restore ease throughout your whole person (body, mind, and spirit) as your conscious awareness of your connection with the Divine deepens and you discover that there is a higher power for you to draw upon, and that you are not alone. Spiritual health also entails social health, leading to a deeper connection with family, friends, and community. Our relationships provide us with some of the greatest opportunities to grow spiritually, and for teaching us how to receive and give unconditional love. The teachings of Jesus, Buddha, Moses, Mohammed and other great spiritual teachers through history illustrate this point. At their core, their messages are the same: *Place God first in all that you do, and love your neighbor as you love yourself.* The more that we are able to do so, the more that we experience unconditional love, joy, gratitude, and a personal relationship with God or Spirit, along with a stronger, more positive connection to our loved ones and our community.

Spirituality and Religion: While religious beliefs and practices can improve spiritual health, it is not necessary to be religious or a member of a religion to experience your connection with God. There are many ways to be spiritual, none of which are dependent on a specific belief system. How people define spirituality varies. While spiritual practices often involve a belief in God and participation in religious services and practices, there are also other ways to experience a connection to Spirit, as well as to the rest of humanity.

Although non-religious people who devote time for spiritual practices such as prayer, meditation, and charitable acts share many common traits with people who are religious, there are certain differences between both groups. For example, non-religious people who engage in spiritual practices tend to do so by themselves, without adhering to specific sets of rules or beliefs. Very often, their focus is on discovering and creating more meaning in their lives. Religious people, by contrast, typically adopt specific beliefs and religious customs, spend time reading from and studying religious texts, and practice their beliefs in a community of like-minded people in churches, temples, mosques, and other places of worship. Both approaches offer many benefits. What's most important is discovering what approach works best for you and then committing yourself to it.

Assessing the State of Your Spiritual Health

(**Disclaimer:** The following questionnaire is for educational purposes only and is not intended to be a substitute for medical advice given by health care professionals. Consult your physician or other health care professional before commencing any medical treatment.)

To help determine the state of your spiritual health, answer the following questions and total your score. Score each response with a number between 0 to 5.

0 = Never or almost never
1 = Seldom (once or month or less)
2 = Occasionally (2 to 4x/month)
3 = Often (2 to 4x/week)
4 = Regularly (more than 4x/week)
5 = Daily (every day).

1. How often do you actively engage in spiritual or religious practices? _____
2. How often do you pray or meditate? _____
3. How often do you rely upon your intuition or "turn within" to receive inner guidance? _____
4. How often do you engage in creative activities that fulfill you and make use of your talents? _____
5. How often do you move beyond your "comfort zone" to grow and learn? _____
6. Do you have faith in God or a Higher Power? [Rate on a scale of 0-5] _____
7. Are you free of anger towards God? [Rate on a scale of 0-5] _____
8. How often do you "count your blessings" and express gratitude for them? _____
9. How often do you spend time in nature? _____
10. How often do you spend time nurturing yourself and your family? _____

11. Are you able to put your self-interest aside when deciding the best course of action for yourself and others? [Rate on a scale of 0-5] _____

12. How often do you experience joy and laughter? [Rate on a scale of 0-5] _____

13. How able are you to forgive yourself and others? [Rate on a scale of 0-5] _____

14. Do you have one or more close friends? [Rate on a scale of 0-5] _____

15. Do you or did you have a close relationship with your parents? [Rate on a scale of 0-5] _____

16. If you have experienced the loss of a loved one, have you fully grieved that loss? [Rate on a scale of 0-5] _____

17. Has your experience of pain enabled you to grow spiritually? [Rate on a scale of 0-5] _____

18. How often do you volunteer your time to help others or donate to charitable causes? _____

19. Do you feel a sense of belonging to a group or community? [Rate on a scale of 0-5] _____

20. How often do you experience feelings of unconditional love? _____

Scoring:

90-100 Optimal
80 - 89 Excellent
70 - 79 Good
50 - 69 Fair
0 - 49 Poor.

Common Health Benefits of Spiritual Practices

Research continues to document the many ways that spiritual and religious practices benefit those who engage in them on a consistent basis. Common health benefits of spiritual practices include:

- Better overall health
- Improved mental and emotional health and greater overall psychological well-being
- Fewer and less intense instances of anxiety and depression
- Lower incidence of hypertension (high blood pressure)
- Fewer instances of stress and greater ability to handle it should it occur.
- Fewer instances of pain
- Decreased incidence of disease and improved (reduced) recovery times should disease occur
- Improved immune function
- Reduced risk of hospitalization
- Greater motivation to stay physically fit and improved ability to maintain healthy weight.

Other common benefits include:

- A greater resilience to stress and an improved ability to cope with life challenges
- An improved ability to deal with negative emotions
- More positive feelings and experiences on a regular basis, along with a deeper sense of gratitude
- A deeper connection to family members and friends

- A greater sense of meaning in and satisfaction with one's life and current circumstances
- A reduced fear of death.

Overall, this is true for both men and women, regardless of their age, race, and other social circumstances.

People who regularly engage in spiritual practices has also been shown to typically live longer, be happier, have more rewarding family lives and relationships, and experience less feelings of isolation and loneliness.

Further substantiating the importance of spirituality to both health and illness are the findings of researchers from Harvard T.H. Chan School of Public Health, and Brigham and Women's Hospital that confirmed that a high level of spirituality is associated with better health outcomes in both currently healthy people, and people suffering from illness.

The researchers conducted a systemic review of studies and articles with evidence addressing spirituality in serious illness or health that were published between January 2000 to April 2022, all of which "were graded as having low, moderate, serious, or critical risk of bias." Over 370 studies and 215 health outcomes articles published within that time period met the researchers' criteria for inclusion. These studies were then assessed by panel of experts in both medicine and spirituality. The panel consisted of members of various religious faiths, as well as atheists and people who identified as "spiritual but not religious" to determine the studies' relevance for health care.

Based on their review and assessment of the studies, the experts "proposed 3 top-ranked implications of this evidence for serious illness: (1) incorporate spiritual care into care for patients with serious illness; (2) incorporate spiritual care education into training of interdisciplinary teams caring for persons with serious illness; and (3) include specialty practitioners of spiritual care in care of patients with serious illness."

In addition, the experts recommended incorporating "patient-centered and evidence-based approaches regarding associations of spiritual community" to improve patient health outcomes, and increasing awareness among physicians and other health care professionals of the evidence supporting the "protective health associations of spiritual community, and an overall recognition of spirituality "as a social factor associated with health in research, community assessments, and program implementation."

"This study represents the most rigorous and comprehensive systematic analysis of the modern day literature regarding health and spirituality to date," lead study author Tracy Balboni, stated. "Our findings indicate that attention to spirituality in serious illness and in health should be a vital part of future whole person-centered care, and the results should stimulate more national discussion and progress on how spirituality can be incorporated into this type of value-sensitive care."

Co-author Tyler VanderWeele added, "Spirituality is important to many patients as they think about their health. Focusing on spirituality in health care means caring for the whole person, not just their disease."

"Overlooking spirituality leaves patients feeling disconnected from the health care system and the clinicians trying to care for them," concluded fellow co-author Howard Koh. "Integrating spirituality into care can help each person have a better chance of reaching complete well-being and their highest attainable standard of health."

Spirituality As A Component of Cancer Care

The above health benefits of spirituality and religion are of particular importance for cancer patients due to all of the uncertainties that can arise following a diagnosis of cancer. Research specific to cancer and spirituality confirm this, showing that spiritual and religious practices provide cancer patients with feelings of comfort and support, as well as, in many cases, guidance and direction about their best course of action. Many of these studies focused on the power of prayer, such as one study involving 32 men and women with cancer receiving treatment at various oncology and radiation clinics. As the study authors wrote, "Prayer is a valuable internal resource, which can lessen the effect of cancer."

Another study demonstrated how one's concept of God affected cancer patients' mental health both during and after treatment. Researchers compared the attitudes of faith among both current cancer patients and survivors of cancer and the influence on their mental health behaviors to mental health. Nearly 160 participants were involved in the study, most of whom were women with breast cancer. They were evaluated for their concepts of God, such as whether they perceived God as stern or loving, as well as how often they prayed, and their mental health status. This study found that mental health "was positively related to a concept of a loving God and negatively related to the concept of a stern God" regardless of "the goal of treatment (cure vs. chemotherapy/palliation), frequency of prayer, intrinsic faith motivation, or physical pain. Viewing God as loving was strongly related to better mental health, even in the presence of a poor prognosis or pain."

In another study, researchers explored whether religion, and specifically prayer, can play a role in increasing life expectancy in cancer patients. The 96 participants in this study were described as "malignant patients" who were receiving chemotherapy. All of them were Muslims living in Iran who prayed multiple times each day. Based on the study's results, the researchers wrote that "cancerous patients can overcome their illness through praying, and they can also triumph [over] cancer through self-confidence, and control it by getting more knowledge of their disease and become more hopeful about their future.

"The outcome of this research showed that the amount of praying was almost higher than the usual, and it also revealed that there was a significant relationship between praying and life expectancy. This result could be related to the culture of our people. The life expectancy went up as praying became more prevalent... The people who believe in spirituality and use the spiritual method to treat themselves are less entangled with stress, anxiety, and mind disorders and, because they accept the existence of their illness, they can become more tolerant and more compatible [with their treatment]"

A scientific review of peer-reviewed studies of cancer patients in diverse populations from around the world that examined the importance of spirituality in cancer care produced similar results. The researchers who conducted this review stated that its results "suggest that it may be helpful for clinical oncologists to be aware of the prevalence of the use of spirituality in their individual practice. Patients should routinely be asked about the use of spiritual medicine as part of every cancer patient's evaluation."

Yet another study on the effects of spiritual health on cancer patients concluded that "cancer patients with a higher degree of meaning/peace in their lives were able to tolerate severe physical symptoms and enjoy their lives."

In 1997, a study was conducted to "determine the relationships among spiritual well-being, religiosity, hope, depression, and other mood states in elderly people coping with cancer and if differences in hope, depression, and other mood states exist between those elderly with high and low intrinsic religiosity and spiritual well-being."

This study involved 100 men and women with cancer who were receiving treatment in two acute care facilities in the Midwest. Their median age was 73, and 62 percent of them were dealing with breast, colon, or lung cancer. Each participant was evaluated based on a religiosity index, a spiritual well-being scale, a depression scale, a hope scale, and an overall profile of the mood state scale. The researchers found that "significantly higher levels of hope and positive moods existed in elderly patients with high levels of intrinsic religiosity and spiritual well-being" and that "religiosity and spiritual well-being are associated with hope and positive mood states in elderly people coping with cancer."

Research has also demonstrated that spiritual and religious beliefs can improve the coping ability of patients with malignant melanoma. One such study investigated the role of spiritual and religious beliefs in 117 melanoma patients. The researchers found that greater reliance on spiritual and religious beliefs among the patients correlated with "an active rather than passive form of coping," leading the researchers to suggest that spiritual and religious beliefs "provide a helpful active-cognitive framework for many individuals from which to face the existential crises of life-threatening illness."

Similar results have also been found among women with breast cancer who hold strong spiritual or religious beliefs.

These are just a sampling of many scientific studies that attest to the power of spiritual and religious beliefs and practices to aid patients in their journey through cancer. Now let's turn our attention to some of the most practical and effective practices you can use to improve your spiritual health and cultivate and deepen your relationship with God.

Prayer

Mahatma Gandhi once stated, "Prayer is not an old woman's idle amusement. Properly understood and applied, it is the most potent instrument of action." A growing body of research—literally thousands of scientific studies so far— into the effects of prayer on health bears this out.

Prayer, in one form or another, is the most common form of spiritual practice performed by most people around the world, and the majority of people who pray report a greater sense of well-being compared to people who don't engage in prayer. Surveys consistently show that approximately 90 percent of all Americans pray, and that about 70 percent believe that prayer can result in better physical, mental, and emotional health. Many people who pray also report that prayer provides them with a sense of peace, and often guidance related to whatever life issues they may be dealing with. Through prayer, it is not uncommon to feel inspired and guided to take specific beneficial actions that might otherwise be ignored.

People who pray regularly also report that doing so leaves them feeling consoled, encouraged, and connected to a power greater than themselves. And when they are sick, prayer helps them admit and give voice to their pain and feelings of grief and loneliness, expressing them in ways that leaves them comforted, with a sense that God is listening to them.

One of the first modern-day researchers to examine the beneficial effects of prayer was Herbert Benson, MD, who is best known as the author of *The Relaxation Response*. During the course of his investigations, he discovered that regular prayer, and even the simple repetition of spiritual phrases such as "The Lord is my shepherd," "Shalom," or "Hail Mary," stimulates feelings of relaxation, thereby reducing stress, enhancing immune function, and providing many other physiological and psychological benefits. Dr. Benson noted, however, that the degree of benefit depends on by the degree of faith on the part of the person praying.

Among the many other health benefits that praying regularly has been shown to offer are a lower incidence of disease compared to people who don't engage in spiritual practices, as well as faster recovery rates and better coping ability during sickness. Research shows that praying regularly also correlates with lower levels of depression and anxiety.

In addition, prayer often leads to significant reduction in pain. This fact was demonstrated by a medical study of an 83-year-old, chronically ill woman who suffered from a rare form of neuropathy related to her diabetes. Various pain management treatments, including lumbar epidural steroid injections, had been tried to alleviate her pain, all of which had failed. Praying, however, often relieved her pain. As she explained to her doctor, "Some people are sick and have pain and it gets the best of them. Not me. Praying eases pain, takes it away. Sometimes I pray when I am in deep, serious pain. I pray, and all at once the pain gets easy . . . I believe in God. He's my guide and my protector."

It's also worth noting that this woman, despite her condition and the fact that she resided in a nursing home, regularly attended church services and had "a strong social support network through church."

People who pray have also been shown to score higher on life-purpose indexes. This is of particular importance for people dealing with cancer. Multiple studies involving large numbers of participants followed over a period of years have consistently demonstrated that people with a strong sense of purpose live longer and maintain their cognitive abilities to a greater extent than people who lack a life purpose. Having a strong sense of life purpose has also been shown to reduce stress levels and inflammation, and lower the risk for developing chronic, degenerative disease. This is true, regardless of age, gender, race, and nationality.

In one study, nearly 7,000 men and women between the ages of 50 and 61 were followed over a period of five years after they first completed a questionnaire and were given a life purpose score based on their responses. At the end of the study, the participants who had the lowest life-purpose scores were found to be twice as likely to have died than those with the highest scores.

Discovering and committing to your life purpose is discussed in more detail in Chapter 7.

Proposed Theories As To How and Why Prayer Works: Although prayer in relationship to healing has been studied for decades, scientists have yet to definitely determine the means by which praying can be such an effective healing aid. Currently, four possible mechanisms of action have been proposed based on an analysis of studies on prayer:

1. Prayer, as Herbert Benson discovered, elicits the body's relaxation response.

2. Prayer acts as a placebo response. Though the placebo response is often dismissed by critics, particularly those with a materialistic mindset, research dating back decades has shown that placebo can provide as much as 50 to 70 percent of the therapeutic benefit attributed to pharmaceutical drugs and various surgical procedures. So, even if prayer's benefits were only due to placebo—which I personally do not believe—that is no reason to discount prayer's value.

3. Prayer elicits positive emotions, such as calm, peace, joy, faith, trust, and love. All such emotions have long been associated with improved overall well-being.

4. Prayer acts as a channel of divine or "supernatural" intervention. This possible mechanism of action of prayer is the one that many scientists have the most trouble accepting because it goes far beyond the scope of established science. Yet, to me, based on my personal experience in my own life and in working with thousands of patients over the course of my career, it is the primary reason why prayer can be such a powerful aid for healing. As prayer researchers Marek Jantos and Hosen Kait pointed out in one of their published studies, "the most common reason why people turn to prayer is their belief in a divine being that transcends the natural universe and hear and responds to prayer." I've witnessed the proof of how that belief is rewarded many times over.

Whichever of the above mechanisms of actions best explains the power of prayer doesn't really matter. What matters is that prayer *is* an effective healing aid, which is why I encourage my patients to make it a part of their daily life, just as I do in my own life.

How To Pray Most Effectively: There are many ways to pray, both for yourself and for others. For some, prayers from their religious upbringing may be most appropriate. Other people may choose to make prayer a time of personal conversation with God. Even spending time in nature and in contemplation can be a form of prayer. Simply taking the time to acknowledge all you have to be grateful for and giving thanks can be effective as well.

Interestingly, research shows that the most effective types of prayer are those that take the form of an active conversation with God without necessarily petitioning for healing. As one study found, "Devotional prayers involving an intimate dialogue with a supportive God appear to be associated with improved optimism, wellbeing and function. In contrast, prayers that involve pleas for help may, in the absence of a pre-existing faith, be associated with increased distress and possibly poorer function."

Meditation

Decades of research has established that meditation, like prayer, offers many mental, emotional, and physiological benefits. These include stress-relief, improved immune and cardiovascular function, relaxation, and decreased pain. The regular practice of meditation can also lead to new insights about life issues, heightened creativity, inspiration, greater compassion for others, and a greater connection to one's own inner guidance. This last benefit is one of the principal reasons why meditation in non-Western countries has been practiced for thousands of years. In those cultures, meditation is primarily considered to be a spiritual practice to deepen one's awareness of and connection to God.

Meditation is sometimes referred to as the practice of mindfulness, meaning being "present in the moment". Numerous studies have confirmed the many health benefits that mindfulness meditation can provide, including:

- Reducing anxiety, depression, and stress
- Improving blood pressure levels
- Reducing both acute and chronic pain
- Improving overall sleep quality
- Reducing symptoms of post-traumatic stress disorder (PTSD)
- Improving weight management and eating behaviors .

Other research demonstrates that mediation helps improve overall mental and emotional health, increases attention span, enhances self-awareness, and may even reduce memory loss related to aging, including in Alzheimer and dementia patients.

In addition to the above benefits, studies also show that certain types of meditation can result in increased positive feelings and actions toward oneself and others, and cause people who regularly meditate to become kinder and more compassionate over time. This is particularly true of a kindness-based form of mediation known as *metta*. One study involving 50 college students, for example, found that practicing metta meditation three times per week improved positive emotions, interpersonal interactions, and understanding of others after only four weeks.

To practice metta mediation, sit comfortably with your spine straight, yet relaxed. Close your eyes and take a few deep breaths. Then silently repeat the following a few times:

- May I be safe.
- May I be happy.
- May I be healthy.
- May I be filled with love and kindness.
- May I find peace.

After a few moments, bring your attention to those you care about and silently repeat:

- May you be safe.
- May you be happy.
- May you be healthy.
- May you be filled with love and kindness.
- May you find peace.

You can then shift your attention other people that you normally have neutral feelings about, or even dislike or have issue with, repeating the same phrase as you think of them.

Finally, focus your attention on the entire world and everyone in it, repeating the same phrase.

Throughout this meditation, allow whatever emotions may come up for you as you continue to gently breathe.

Meditation and Cancer: Research specifically focused on cancer patients who practice meditation also confirms meditation's benefits. For instance, an analysis of 29 studies involving 3,274 total participants, most of whom were women with breast cancer, found that cancer patients who practiced meditation exhibited "significantly reduced psychological distress, fatigue, sleep disturbance, pain, and symptoms of anxiety and depression".

Another scientific analysis of 124 studies published between 2008 and 2014 further documented the health benefits of meditation for cancer patients. The selected studies addressed one or more aspects of cancer management: cancer prevention, and stress, pain, fatigue, cachexia, sleep disorders related to cancer, as well as mediation's effects on caregivers of cancer patients, radiation therapy, and cost-effectiveness".

One of the analyzed studies compared women who regularly mediated to women who did not. Urine samples were collected from all of the women in both groups to measure a urinary marker for melatonin. This study showed that women in the meditation group had higher levels of melatonin than the women who did not meditate. "This is significant," the authors wrote, "since melatonin has been shown in multiple studies to have anti-cancer properties as well as other biologic functions important in maintaining health and preventing disease such as immunomodulation and hematopoiesis [formation of blood or blood cells in the body]."

Other findings from the analyzed studies showed that the regular practice of meditation resulted in "significant improvements" in:

- cancer pain tolerance
- reduced cancer-related fatigue
- restful sleep
- cancer-related digestive problems
- depression scores
- fear and stress reduction related to a cancer diagnosis
- natural killer (NK) cell activity (NK cells are an important component of the immune system and play a vital role in detecting and killing cancer cells and tumors)

- T cell activity (T cells are another vital class immune cell cancer-fighters)
- levels of tumor necrosis factor α interleukin-6, both of which are markers for immune function restoration
- reduced anxiety levels among prostate cancer patients, as well as improved "uncertainty intolerance, and significant increases in mindfulness, global mental health and post-traumatic growth"
- tolerance to radiation therapy
- reduced levels of cachexia symptoms (cachexia is characterized by unhealthy weight loss and loss of muscle mass, both of which are common cancer symptoms)
- "self-kindness, self-judgment, common humanity, over-identification, mindful observation, acting with awareness skill sets and self-compassion"
- self-care and coping ability
- "patient and caregiver capacity to respond to the emotional challenges that often accompany advanced cancer"
- reductions in "proinflammatory gene expression and inflammatory signaling" in premenopausal women with breast cancer.

Another of the analyzed studies involved 57 adults with colorectal cancer. Prior to beginning their initial chemotherapy treatments, all participants had their salivary cortisol levels measured. They were then divided into three groups. The first group received chemotherapy alone, the second group received chemo and education about cancer, and the third group received chemo, cancer education, and guided instruction in mindfulness meditation. "Saliva samples were collected at the start of chemotherapy and at subsequent 20-minute intervals during the first 60 minutes of chemotherapy. More than twice as many patients in the mindfulness group versus the controls showed a cortisol rise suggesting that mindfulness practice during chemotherapy can reduce the hypothalamic pituitary axis (HPA) blunting profiles typically observed in cancer patients."

In addition, several of the analyzed studies found that meditation and mindfulness practices are more cost-effective compared to traditional approaches to manage stress and improve quality of life issues among cancer patients.

Another important benefit of meditation is its ability to improve cognitive function in cancer patients. Impaired cognitive function is another fairly common symptom caused by cancer, as well as various by related factors, such as stress, chemotherapy ("chemo brain"), impaired hormone activity, the body's proinflammatory response, and cancer-related fatigue. Research has shown that meditation can be "particularly effective in alleviating cancer-related cognitive impairment."

There are a variety of meditation techniques. Meditation can be performed while sitting, lying down, or while walking. Some people also prefer chanting a word or phrase that has spiritual significance to them. What all meditative techniques have in common is conscious breathing and a focus on what is happening in each present moment. This enables the mind to let go of thoughts, judgments, and past and future concerns. As with prayer, choosing the meditation technique that you are most comfortable with will provide the greatest benefit.

A simple way to get started is to sit comfortably erect with your eyes closed, while paying attention to your breathing. Observe yourself inhaling and exhaling, allowing whatever thoughts you have to pass you by. In the beginning of your practice, you will find your mind wandering. Each time this occurs, gently refocus on your breath.

As you breathe, you can also silently repeat a word, or *mantra*, such as love, peace, or Jesus. Eventually, you will experience your thoughts "slowing down". Be patient and don't force matters. Try to sit for 10 to 20 minutes once or twice a day, but if you find yourself too distracted or pressed for time, end your session, instead of sitting restlessly. With commitment and consistent practice, the benefits of meditation will become more apparent to you.

Regularly Attending Worship Services

As demonstrated by the 83-year-old woman cited earlier in this chapter, who found prayer and church attendance to be the most effective means of relieving pain, participating in worship services on a regular basis can also provide important health benefits, while also being a means to deepening one's faith and connection to God.

Studies show that people who attend worship services once a week or more tend to commit more time to self-care practices such as exercise and healthy eating compared to people who do not do so. They are also less prone to smoke or to quit if they do smoke. They typically also abstain from alcohol or drink only in moderation, and are better able to maintain stable, loving marriages, as well as healthier relationships with friends and family members.

Studies also have found that many people do not adopt healthy lifestyle choices until they begin to regularly attend religious or other worship services. One reason for this is because of the positive support they receive and friendships they form as a result of their attendance. These social benefits make it easier for people to commit to improving their health.

Perhaps most significantly, regular worship service attendance has been shown to significantly improve people's ability to live longer. This fact was confirmed by data from 1992 to 2012 that was supplied by 74,534 women who participated in Nurses' Health Study, one of the largest long-term investigations into the risk factors for major chronic diseases in women.

The study analyzed data from answers to questionnaires the women completed every four years. Over 14,000 of the women attended religious services more than once per week, while over 30,000 attended once per week. Nearly 18,000 women never attended religious services, while just over 12,000 attended less than once per week. During the study period, 13,537 of the women died, including nearly 4,500 from cancer and over 2,000 from heart disease. Overall, the researchers found that the women who attended religious services an average of twice a week were 33 percent less likely to die, compared to those who never attended services. The study also found that even occasional churchgoers had a mortality risk that was 13 percent lower than non-churchgoers.

Commenting on the study, Tyler VanderWeele, one of its lead authors, stated that it demonstrated that religious service attendance in and of itself is what actually causes the better health outcomes, rather than other factors.

"Because the nurses answered questionnaires periodically over a long time frame, the researchers were able to look at whether a change in service attendance led to a change in health," he said. "They found numerous benefits associated with attending services. Women who started going to services then became more likely to quit smoking and less likely to show signs of depression, for instance—even when the researchers controlled for a long list of other variables, from age and exercise habits to income and other non-religious social engagement. The effect of religious attendance, they found, was stronger than that of any other form of participation in a social group like a book club or a volunteer organization."

Since this study was published, subsequent studies have revealed similar, and even more impressive findings, such as a study by researchers at Vanderbilt University that found that men and women between the ages of 40 and 65—the specific target group of the study—who regularly attend church or other worship services can reduce their risk of death by as much as 55 percent. The study was based on analysis of data collected on over 5,000 people that tracked their church attendance along with such variables as socioeconomic status and health insurance coverage.

Based on these and similar studies, I hope you can understand why regularly attending religious services can be one of the most significant and important steps you can take to not only express and deepen your faith, but also to improve and maintain your health, and to find the nurturing support you may need while dealing with cancer or any other serious life challenge.

Practicing Forgiveness

"To err is human; to forgive, divine." These words, written centuries ago by the English poet Alexander Pope, go to the heart of spiritual development and health. Practicing forgiveness opens up our hearts, making it easier to deepen our connection with God. It is also mentally, emotionally, and physically liberating because of how forgiveness releases stress, tension, and related feelings of upset and anger. This, in turn, ushers in more positive emotions which are proven to boost immunity. If you think back to a time when you forgave someone or were forgiven by others you will remember how relieved and good you felt afterward. Harnessing those same feelings during times of illness can go a long way to speeding recovery.

Since, as Pope pointed out, all of us err at various times in our lives, without forgiveness we could not sustain are most precious relationships with others, or be truly capable of giving and receiving love. Moreover, being unwilling to forgive locks us into limited and unhealthy patterns from our past, preventing us from moving forward without the baggage of recrimination and its associated stress.

For many people, forgiving others is often easier than forgiving themselves. This tendency can be exacerbated when dealing with cancer. It's not uncommon for cancer patients to blame themselves, thinking they did something wrong that caused their cancer. Such thoughts and beliefs—as will be explained in more detail in Chapter 7—not only do not serve us, they can be harmful because of the stress and immune suppression they can cause, as well as a loss of hope for recovery.

The first step in learning how to forgive yourself is to recognize and accept that, whatever may have been true of you in the past, you are always doing the best you can at all times, based on your level of awareness at the time. As are everyone else, including those people in your life whom you may need to also forgive. Again, "to err is human". Forgiveness enables us to better connect with God and our own spiritual nature, while not forgiving ourselves or others keeps us "stuck" and saps our energy.

The more that you can accept whatever past actions you may still feel angry, upset, or guilty about, the more you will be able to forgive yourself. And the more you are able to forgive yourself, the more you will also find your are able to forgive others. And vice versa. Always keep in mind, too, that when you forgive others, you are forgiving *them*, not excusing or condoning their actions.

To begin a practice of forgiving yourself, I recommend that you make a written inventory of your past actions and the issues you still have about them, doing so honestly and without judgment. (Judgment, especially self-judgment, is often a major impediment to forgiveness.) Then, choosing one action at a time, review what you did, said, or thought, while simultaneously allowing yourself to fully feel whatever emotions may come up as you do so. Then ask yourself if you can let go of that moment from your past. If the answer is Yes, ask yourself if you can forgive yourself for it. If that answer is also Yes, tell yourself that you forgive yourself and continue to do so until you feel your emotions shift to something more positive. Eventually, you will know that the issue has been healed.

If your answer is No to either of the above questions, ask yourself why. What keeps you from doing so? Is there a lesson for you still to learn from your past action? Is there a reason you are still unable to forgive yourself? Be gentle with yourself as you ask such questions. Eventually, the answers will come, guiding you to deeper levels of self-acceptance and further healing of your past. Once you feel the positive shift taking hold of you, move on to the next item on your inventory list.

You can also work with this same process as you practice forgiving others.

A Forgiveness Prayer: Another forgiveness practice that you can use on behalf of yourself and others comes from the Huna tradition, a teaching said to have originated in ancient Hawaii that was introduced to the modern world at large by Max Freedom Long (1890–1971). Within the Huna tradition is a forgiveness practice known as Ho'oponopono (a Hawaiian term meaning *correction*), which was modernized by the Huna healer Morrnah Simeona (May 1913 –February1992), and later popularized by her student, Ihaleakala Hew Len (April 1939 – January 2022).

Morrnah Simeona stated, "If we can accept that we are the sum total of all past thoughts, emotions, words, deeds and actions, and that our present lives and choices are colored or shaded by this memory bank of the past, then we can begin to see how a process of correcting or setting aright can change our lives, our families, and our society." The forgiveness prayer she taught is based on the idea that we are responsible for everything in our world, both internal and external, and that therefore, we can correct, or heal, all of it.

The Ho'oponopono prayer is practiced by first directing one's attention to whatever you feel is in need of correcting, while always taking full responsibility for it. Then, keeping your focus on what you want to forgive, you verbally or mentally repeat the following phrase:

- I love you.
- I'm sorry.
- Please forgive me.
- Thank you.

You can direct this prayer to yourself, to others, to events and issues in your life, and even, in the case of cancer, to your body and the cancer cells and tumors that are affecting it. When practiced daily for at least a few minutes, many people report that this practice offers many benefits.

There are, of course, many other ways that you can practice forgiveness. What is important is that you find the method that you are most comfortable with and make it a part of your overall self-care routine.

Practicing Gratitude

We've all heard the saying, "Count your blessings." It's an excellent piece of advice, because when we pause to reflect upon all we have to be grateful for we experience more positive emotions. Acknowledging the blessings in your life also goes hand in hand with practicing forgiveness, and can further strengthen your connection with Spirit. In addition, when you choose to practice gratitude, you will likely start to attract further positive experiences to be grateful for. As the saying goes, "Like attracts like."

Although the idea of feeling grateful when you have cancer or face other serious life challenges may seem unreasonable, practicing gratitude during such times, even if only for a few moments, can often generate feelings of inner peace.

Becoming more aware of all that you have to be grateful for requires attention and practice.

One effective way to cultivate feelings of gratitude is to spend a few moments in quiet reflection when you wake up each morning. Before rising out of bed, close your eyes and give thanks for another day of life, as well as for family members and friends with whom you share your life. Also give thanks for your personal achievements and anything else in your life that makes you happy. Calling your blessings to mind each morning, and silently expressing gratitude for them, will instill in you a sense of enthusiasm and appreciation that you can carry with you throughout the rest of your day.

Another way to get in the habit of practicing gratitude is by writing down the events of the day for which you feel grateful in a journal before you go to bed at night. Once you finish your list, take time to read it over and say a prayer of thanks to God for all that you wrote down.

I find that patients who commit to these simple exercises of morning reflection and/or keeping a nighttime gratitude journal develop a deeper level of equanimity and cheerful optimism that increases over time, making them more resilient and more committed to overcome their life challenges. They also come to more deeply recognize that they are not alone, and that God's guidance and support is with them every step of the way along their journey. This can make all the difference in their recovery.

In concluding this chapter, I want to emphasize that your spiritual health is ultimately the most important factor that determines how well you are able to care for yourself and meet and triumph over whatever life challenges you may face. The more that you commit to being spiritually healthy, the more you will find yourself letting go of fear, worries, and stress. You will also strengthen your ability to give and receive love regardless of your circumstances because you will be deepening your awareness of God's presence in your life and all of the love, guidance, and support that entails.

Chapter 7

Optimizing Your Mindset, Beliefs, and Emotions

When dealing with cancer, creating and maintaining a positive, resilient mindset and addressing fears, limited beliefs, and persistent negative emotions is essential because your thoughts, emotions, and beliefs have a profound influence on your health, both positively and negatively.

This fact has repeatedly been confirmed by research in the field of psychoneuroimmunology (PNI), more popularly known as mind/body medicine. But long before such research first began to be conducted, its findings were already well-known by various luminaries throughout history, including the famed humanitarian and Nobel Laureate Albert Schweitzer (January 1875 –September1965), who wrote, "The greatest discovery of any generation is that human beings can alter their lives by altering the attitudes of their minds."

In this chapter, you will learn why optimizing your mindset, healing your emotions, and examining and, if necessary, correcting your beliefs can go a long way towards supporting and hastening your recovery from cancer, or any other serious life challenge you may be facing. More importantly, you will learn how to most effectively do so using the same techniques that I share with my patients.

How Your Thoughts, Emotions, and Beliefs Affect Your Health

Although research into the link between the mind and body in relationship to overall health did not begin to gain acceptance among conventional medicine practitioners until the 1960s and 70s, which was when the field of PNI was first established, the concept of mind/body medicine dates back thousands of year. Not only is it a central tenet of tradition Chinese medicine (TCM) and Ayurveda in India, both of which originated approximately 3,000 years ago, it was also recognized by Hippocrates (460 – 370 BC), the father of Western medicine, as well as other Western healers throughout the centuries, including Galen (130 – 200 AD), Paracelsus (1493 – 1541), Samuel Hahnemann, the founder of homeopathy (1755 – 1815), and many others. But it was not until the 1960s that the field of PNI began to take root in the West.

Two of the pioneers in this field at that time were Elmer Green, Ph.D., a psychologist and physicist then working at the Menninger Foundation in Topeka, Kansas, and his wife, Alyce Green, both of whom helped establish biofeedback therapy as a proven clinical tool after they became the first researchers to use biofeedback to help treat various medical conditions.

Another pioneer was Candace Pert, PhD. In 1972, Pert discovered and was able to quantify the existence of the opiate receptor, a molecule occurring on the surface of cells in the brain and throughout the body. Pert dubbed this and other receptor molecules, which are known as neuropeptides, "messenger molecules" and "molecules of emotion". Her discovery led to further research that proved neuropeptides are capable of altering mood, pleasure, and pain. More importantly, research by Pert and others found that endorphin and other neuropeptides, which were previously thought to be present only in the brain, actually are located throughout the body, including within the immune and endocrine (hormone) systems.

This discovery also demonstrated that emotions directly influence neuropeptide activity. Emotions such as calm, compassion, happiness, and joy have been shown to cause neuropeptides to more positively impact various physiological functions, including improving immunity. So-called negative emotions, by contrast, are now known to decrease immune function and increase the risk of disease. They are also capable of reducing the amount of neuropeptides present in cellular receptor sites, thereby opening the way for viruses that share the same sites to more easily invade cells.

Another pioneer in the mind/body field was O. Carl Simonton, MD. His work is particularly noteworthy for cancer patients. In 1971, Simonton began teaching cancer patients guided visualization exercises and documented the fact that making use of visualization helped his patients to stabilize, and in some cases completely recover, from cancer by harnessing the power of their imaginations. You will learn more about Simonton's work later in this chapter.

As a result of the work of the Greens, Pert, Simonton, and many other researchers, various mind/body medicine techniques are now used in many major hospitals and taught in a number of medical schools across the United States and other countries. And ongoing research continues to show how mind/body techniques can help prevent and reverse disease and improve health.

Among the disease conditions now known to be influenced by thoughts and emotions are addiction, asthma, back pain, bronchitis cancer, cardiovascular disease, colitis and other gastrointestinal conditions, diabetes, eczema, endocrine disorders, fatigue, headache, heart disease, hypertension, immunological conditions, migraine, peptic ulcer, psoriasis, rheumatoid arthritis, and even obesity due to the tendency to overeat that unhealthy emotions can cause.

Additional research demonstrates that:

- Emotions such as anger, anxiety, depression, grief, hopelessness, loneliness, and sorrow can significantly impair immune function and be co-factors in a number of chronic disease conditions, including heart attack and other cardiovascular conditions and hypertension. (Cardiovascular conditions are especially susceptible to anger, both when it is inappropriately expressed and when it is repressed.)

- Chronic stress has a broad suppressive effect on immune function, and can diminish natural killer (NK) cell function, thereby exacerbating chronic conditions, including cancer.

- Stress and anxiety can trigger increased cortisol production by the adrenal glands, causing chronic fatigue, compromised immune function, and reduced ability of cells to repair themselves.

- Repressed anger can be a contributing factor in sinusitis.

Conversely, research has found that saliva levels of immunoglobulin A (IgA), a protective immune system antibody, increase in response to laughter, humor, compassion, and caring, and decrease in response to anger.

Still other studies demonstrate that feelings of joy and exhilaration produce a measurable increase of a neuropeptide that produces effects similar to the anticancer drug interleukin-2, and that these same emotions improve tissue repair and enhance circulation.

Perhaps most significantly, multiple studies have shown that people who are habitually pessimistic tend to die earlier, compared to people who are optimistic by nature. This is true of both men and women in both categories regardless of other factors in their lives.

Other research demonstrates that optimistic feelings help protect older adults from stroke and heart failure and also help protect against cancer, respiratory failure, and premature aging and associated co-morbidities.

Research also shows that optimistic people "view desired goals as obtainable, so they often confront adversities in active manners resulting in perseverance and increased goal attainment".

Studies indicate that positive thoughts and emotions and an optimistic outlook on life directly and positively affect the body's neuroendocrine and immune systems. Indirectly, such thoughts and emotions are associated with healthier and more protective life choices and behaviors, as well as more adaptive and resilient coping strategies in response to life challenges.

Emotional Characteristics Common to Cancer Patients: In addition to depression and chronic stress, the most common emotional characteristics of cancer patients are anxiety, fear, grief, hopelessness, indecisiveness, loneliness, and low self-esteem and lack of self-worth. Many cancer patients also live isolated lives and lack meaningful personal relationships. Other emotional issues that can act as co-factors in the cancer process include bigotry, hostility, resentment, and selfishness. Limited and faulty beliefs can also play a significant role in how patients respond to their cancer treatments. For example, many people, upon being diagnosed with cancer, automatically assume the worst, even when there is no reason to do so. As a result, they can unconsciously sabotage their ability to recover even when they receive the most appropriate and effective types of cancer treatment.

Chronic, unresolved emotions have also been shown to significantly affect the immune system by lowering the immune response. This is of utmost importance when it comes to preventing and treating cancer since a healthy immune system is essential in both cases. Therefore, it is vitally important that all of us, whether or not we have cancer, take care to properly manage and express our emotions and to do all that is necessary to heal and recover from any unexpected shocks or traumas we may have endured.

The following checklist of questions can help you to determine if unresolved and improperly expressed emotions are affecting you. Answer each question truthfully. The more Yes answers you give, the more likely it is that you need to start addressing your emotions and beliefs in order to stop them from compromising your health.

- Have you endured an unexpected shock or trauma within the last three years (death of a loved one, divorce, break up of a relationship, loss of your job, etc)?
- Do you regularly experience bouts of sadness or grief?
- Do you regularly experience bouts of anxiety or depression?
- Are you experiencing lingering feelings of anger or resentment towards anyone or anything?
- Do you suffer from low self-esteem?
- Do you lack meaningful relationships in your life?
- Do you feel lonely?
- Are you pessimistic by nature?
- Do you harbor regrets over experiences from your past?
- Do you feel as if you are cut off from support from others and have to do everything on your own?
- Are you prone to compromise so as not to hurt others' feelings even when doing so means giving up on your own desires and dreams?
- Do you believe that life is a struggle filled with hardships?
- Are you pessimistic about the future and the way things are going in the world?
- Are you an "all work and no play" type of person?

Improving Your Mental and Emotional Well-Being by Managing Stress

People who live long and healthy lives typically have learned how to effectively cope with and manage stress. Even when faced with significant life challenges, including cancer, they are able to meet such circumstances with resilience and maintain their mental and emotional equanimity.

To understand why managing stress is so vital to your health, you need to know about the autonomic nervous system (ANS), that part of your body's central nervous system that regulates all of the functions in your body that occur without you being consciously aware of them. This includes the activities of your heart, brain function, hormone production, digestion, circulation, immune system processes, and so forth.

The ANS is comprised of the sympathetic and the parasympathetic nervous systems. The sympathetic nervous system oversees your body's performance, as well as its production of energy, and is in charge of the "fight, flight, or freeze" mechanisms in the body that are triggered by stress.

By contrast, the parasympathetic nervous system is responsible for conserving your body's energy and oversees the physiological mechanisms of rest, recovery, and repair. It is also the part of the ANS that triggers and oversees your body's "relaxation response", producing feelings of calm, peace, and contentment.

Both the sympathetic and parasympathetic nervous systems play many vital roles in keeping you alive and healthy. However, in today's stress-filled world, most people are in what is known as a sympathetic-dominant state, meaning that even though they are usually unaware of it, their bodies are in a hyper-vigilant state of chronic stress that results in an excessive expenditure of energy, chronic tension, and eventual poor health. Sympathetic dominance also triggers stress-related thoughts and emotions, such as worry, anger, fear, or depression.

Ideally, sympathetic dominance should only occur when you need a rapid influx of energy, such as during physical activity or in the face of acute emergencies. Otherwise, you want to be in a healthy state of calm relaxation, which is what occurs when the parasympathetic nervous system is dominant.

Research has shown that people in a state of parasympathetic dominance are generally healthier and live longer than people who are in a sympathetic dominant state. They are better able to deal with stress and unforeseen life challenges. By learning how to master stress, you can assist your parasympathetic nervous system in carrying out its many important tasks.

In addition to affecting the ANS itself, stress also directly impacts the body's vagus nerve network and the hypothalamus-pituitary-adrenal axis.

The Vagus Nerve: The vagus nerve is primary nerve of the parasympathetic system responsible for nerve impulses to the heart. It consists of a network of approximately 100,000 nerve fibers in the body. It connects the brain to the body, running from the brainstem, through the neck and down into the heart, lungs, GI tract and other major organs. Its primary function is to activate the parasympathetic nervous system, slowing and relaxing the heart, regulating the immune system (including its inflammatory response), improving digestion, and initiating the body's other rest and repair mechanisms. When the vagus has a healthy tone, the effects of stress in the body diminish and are replaced by feelings of calm.

A number of effective self-care techniques that you can use to stimulate the vagus nerve are discussed later in this chapter.

The Hypothalamus-Pituitary-Adrenal (HPA) Axis: This axis directs the functioning of the hypothalamus and the pituitary and adrenal glands in response to stress and any other threats, both real and perceived, you may face. The hypothalamus, located in the brain, causes the HPA axis to initiate the "flight, fight, or freeze" response when stress occurs. Once this happens, the adrenal glands release elevated levels of cortisol and other stress hormones into the blood stream. This, in turn, constricts the blood vessels that supply oxygen and nutrients to the body's cells and organs in order for more blood is made available to nourish the tissues of the arms and legs, since it is primarily these extremities that the body uses to fend off external attacks and to get out of harm's way.

Prior to this response, blood is concentrated in the visceral organs (kidneys, liver, and stomach and other organs of the GI tract) responsible for digesting and metabolizing foods and nutrients, excretion, and various other functions that provide for proper cell growth and production of cellular energy. As blood is directed to the tissues of the arms and legs, the visceral organs temporarily cease functioning at 100 percent, which impairs all growth-related activities in the body.

In addition, if this response is sustained, the HPA axis causes the adrenal glands to suppress immune function in order to conserve the body's energy reserves via the adrenal glands' increased production of stress hormones. A chronically suppressed immune function increases susceptibility to disease, including heart attack and cancer. (Unmanaged stress can not only cause cancer, it has also been shown to accelerate the growth and spread of cancer cells.)

Assessing How Stressed You Are

In order to most effectively manage stress, you first must become better aware of the types of stress to which you are most commonly exposed.

Stress and its associated triggers typically fall into one or more of the following categories:

- **Physical stress:** Common causes of physical stress include allergens, temperature (too hot or too cold), physical inactivity, illness, physical pain or trauma, and lack of restorative sleep.

- **Emotional stress:** Causes of emotional stress include suppressed or inappropriately expressed emotions, such as anger, anxiety, depression, fear, and guilt; divorce or other breakups; death; suffering on the part of those you care for; chronic illness (yours or someone you love); lack of nurturing relationships/friends; and unresolved life issues from the past.

- **Environmental stress:** Stressors in this category include nutritional deficiencies; exposure to allergens, chemicals and other environmental toxins; fluorescent lights; and electomagnetic radiation (EMR) from computer and computer printers, cell phones, and various household appliances, such as so-called smart meters and smart TVs.

- **Social stress:** Common causes include relationship issues with a spouse or significant other, family members and friends; issues with co-workers; unpleasant neighbors; job promotions or demotions; financial issues; and politics.
- **Spiritual stress:** Common causes include not knowing your life's purpose, fear of death and/or the afterlife, lack of faith, and a variety of other existential issues, all of which can cause or worsen a spiritual crisis.

Take a moment to evaluate any stressors you may currently be experiencing within each of the categories above, writing them down so that you can review them later to gauge how well you are improving your ability to deal with them.

The following list of symptoms can also help show you how well you are coping with stress. Review this list and check off all symptoms that you may currently be experiencing.

- Anger that persists
- Anxiety/worry that persists
- Back, neck or shoulder pain/stiffness/tension
- Biting your nails
- Change in your sense of taste
- Difficulty concentrating
- Difficulty swallowing
- Digestive problems
- Fatigue that is persistent
- Headaches
- Heartburn that persists
- Heart palpitations/racing heartbeat
- High blood pressure

- Indecisiveness
- Insomnia
- Itchy or "burning" skin
- Loss of appetite
- Nausea
- Nervous exhaustion
- Persistent feelings of loneliness, sadness, and/or unworthiness
- Oversleeping
- Sexual problems
- Shortness of breath
- Stiff or painful muscles and/or joints

Add up the number of items you checked on the list above. This will give you a better idea about how well, or poorly, you are coping with stress.

(**Disclaimer:** As with the questionnaires in this book, the above checklist is for educational purposes only and is not intended to be a substitute for medical advice given by health care professionals.)

Distorted Thinking Patterns

Often, it isn't the events in our lives that cause stress, but how we think about and react to them. Many times, the events themselves are neutral. As Shakespeare wrote in *Hamlet*, "There is nothing either good or bad, but thinking makes it so."

Thoughts that cause stress are often forms of distorted thinking. This means seeing things not as they are, but as we choose to think or interpret them. The most common distorted thinking patterns are:

- **Polarized thinking:** Thinking characterized by seeing things in absolutes. People whose thinking is polarized tend to see things as "black or white" and "good or bad," without any "grey areas" or a middle ground. Polarized thinkers are usually unable to view anything and anyone without automatically judging that events and people are good or bad, regardless of objective reality. Not only does polarized thinking prevent us from developing a broader, and therefore less stressful, perspective of the people and events we encounter in our lives, it can also make it very difficult to accept ourselves without similar judgments.

- **Emotional reasoning:** Thinking pattern characterized by a belief that whatever we feel must be true. While feelings certainly can be valuable clues to what is true in our lives, automatically accepting your feelings as true is often inadvisable.

- **Negative thinking:** Thinking focused on the negative details related to the events and people we encounter, to the point where all positive details are filtered out. This leads to a distorted magnification of the negative details, making them worse than they actually are. People who are negative thinkers tend to willfully refuse to see "the bright side" of people or events.

- **Personalization:** Thinking characterized by the belief that everything people do or say is some kind of reaction to you. People who think in this manner take everything personally, perceiving slights, insults, and other negative intentions from people even when that is not the case.

- **Victim thinking:** Victim thinking is common in people who view themselves as helpless when it comes to certain people or events. People who think in this way believe they have no control over what happens to them, when in fact they do. Victim thinking prevents them from recognizing their ability to take control of their lives.

- **Blameful thinking:** People who think from a blameful perspective hold themselves or others responsible for every problem that comes their way, even when neither they nor others are to blame.

Usually, blaming also prevents them from moving on from past situations and from taking responsibility for their present experiences.

- **"Should have" thinking:** People who think from a "should have" perspective tend to have a list of ironclad rules about how they and other people should act. People who break these rules anger them. Additionally, they feel guilty if they violate the rules themselves.

All of the above types of distorted thinking create "lose-lose" situations that can turn neutral, and even positive, situations and social interactions into stressful ones.

All of us fall into these types of thinking patterns from time to time. What matters most is becoming conscious of when you do so, so that you can choose to move out of them.

Once you identify any distorted thinking patterns that you are prone to, review the list of stressors that I asked you to create above. As you do, ask yourself what patterns of distorted thinking might be involved in the stressors that are most common in your life. Then ask yourself if the stressors would have the same effects on you if the way you think about them wasn't distorted.

Take your time with this exercise and be honest with yourself as you go through it. You may be surprised to discover that at least some of your stressors on your list needn't be stressful at all.

Reframing Distorted Thinking Patterns and the Stressors in Your Life: The first step in effectively dealing with distorted thinking patterns is to realize that they are occurring. If you completed the exercises above, you've already begun that process. (If you haven't, stop reading now and go back and do them before continuing further.)

You can take this one step further using a method known as reframing. Reframing is a process that will help you to see things in a different way than you have seen them in the past. More specifically, reframing helps to remove the judgments that are the principal causes of distorted thinking patterns.

You can use reframing with any situation that throws you out of balance and causes stress, whether it's a cancer diagnosis, a relationship issue, something work-related, or an unexpected event.

There are three steps in the reframing process. The first step is to simply recognize and admit to distorted thinking when you find yourself doing it. Then, instead of automatically reacting to the situation that triggered it, take a moment to notice how your thoughts are contributing to what you are feeling. Then recognize that you have a choice in how you are responding to the situation at hand. You can also take a few deep breaths to help calm yourself and relax. This will prepare you for step two.

As you contemplate the situation that is triggering your stress, take time to consider all the possible ways you can deal with it. Look at each potential response that you come up with and ask yourself which one is most appropriate for you. Which one best serves you and brings you peace of mind? Then choose accordingly.

The third step is practice. Distorted thinking habits do not occur overnight. Usually they are ingrained, unconscious patterns that have been with us for most of our lives. Therefore, it is unrealistic to assume you can get rid of them without some effort. The more you practice consciously examining your thought patterns, the more you will develop the ability to choose how you want to think about—and therefore respond to—people and situations that in the past triggered stressful reactions within you. Awareness is the key.

Once again, take a look at the list of stressors you wrote down when performing the exercises above. Select a person or situation on your list that in the past has caused you a high degree of stress. Once you have made your selection, spend time writing down all of the possible ways in which you could have responded differently to that person or situation. Your aim should be to discover for yourself the response that best serves you and which leaves you with the least amount of stress.

Be honest with yourself as you perform this exercise. Since you don't have to share what you write with anyone but yourself, there is no reason for you to ignore all possible responses that occur to you. There is not a right or wrong way to do this exercise. Simply allow yourself to think of as many possible responses to the stressor you've selected as you can. This will help you discover the best solution to the stressor. After that, it's just a matter of practicing applying it so that the person or situation no longer affects you in the same way.

The rest of this chapter provides you with other effective self-care methods you can use to further optimize your mindset and beliefs, followed by therapies that are also very valuable in this regard.

Stimulating the Vagus Nerve

Research shows that a number of easy-to-perform self-care exercises help to stimulate the vagus nerve. By regularly performing them, you can help maintain healthy vagus nerve function and reduce the effects of stress, while also deriving a variety of vagus nerve-related health benefits, such as improved mood, better digestion, pain relief, enhanced immune function, greater calm, and reduced feelings of anxiety and depression.

Diaphragmatic Breathing: Diaphragmatic breathing can be performed at any time and is especially beneficial whenever you find yourself feeling stressed or tense. The key is to breathe slowly and deeply from your belly in a gentle, relaxed manner. Inhale and exhale through your nose, not your mouth. Exhaling twice as long as you inhale improves this exercise because exhalation increases parasympathetic nervous system function.

A diaphramatic breathing technique known as box breathing is another effective way to stimulate the vagus nerve and counteract stress and tension. It is performed by inhaling for a count of 4, then holding your breath for another count of 4, then exhaling for a count of 4, and then holding your breath for a count of 4, and then repeating the process for a few minutes. Repeat as many times as you need throughout the day.

Humming and Singing: These activities stimulate the vagus nerve because they all involve your vocal cords, which the vagus nerve runs through. Performing them for a few moments multiple times a day is an easy and enjoyable way to increase vagal nerve tone. You can also obtain similar benefit by chanting a word or phrase out loud.

Gargling: Gargling for a minute or two in the morning and before bed after you brush your teeth activates the back muscles of the throat, which the vagus nerve also runs through. Using a solution of warm water and salt, slightly tilt your head back and gargle. While gargling, your eyes may tear up. This is a sign that your throat muscles are being fully activated.

Cold Exposure: Cold exposure causes the body to activate the vagus nerve in order to reduce the body's sympathetic stress response. In addition to strengthening the vagus nerve, research shows that cold exposure provides a variety of other health benefits, including improved blood and lymph flow, improved heart function, increased energy, and improved metabolic and immune function.

You can easily achieve cold exposure by drinking cold water with ice, splashing your face and neck with cold water, sucking on an ice cube, and taking cold showers.

Laughter: Laughing is the most enjoyable way to stimulate the vagus nerve, as well as causing a flood of positive emotions. The importance of laughter to health is discussed in more detail below.

Prayer and meditation (see Chapter 6) also improve vagus nerve function, as do activities such as yoga, receiving a massage, spending time in nature, and spending time with loved ones or pets.

Working With Affirmations

Affirmations are positive messages that you repeat to yourself either verbally or in writing. Over time, they affect the unconscious mind by "reprogramming" it with the thought you consciously select to positively influence your behavior. In the process, they can unleash and stimulate healing energies in all areas of your life.

One of the early pioneers in the use of affirmations was Emil Coue (1857-1926). His work with the imagination and "conscious auto-suggestion" was a primary aspect of the free health clinic he operated between 1910 and the mid-1920s. Coue encouraged his patients to notice their thoughts and emotions, and to deal with negative thoughts by placing their attention on something happier or more positive. He also instructed patients to verbally repeat his famous affirmation, "Every day in every way I am getting better and better," twenty times a day upon awaking and just before going to bed.

Coue believed that illness, as well as other life events, was the direct result of how we think, and that listening to repeated suggestions of illness is enough to cause the actual illness to manifest. He taught that feeding the unconscious with positive suggestions can lead to healing and created a series of positive suggestions for specific disease conditions, instructing his patients to daily repeat them. Coue successfully treated a variety of chronic disease conditions in this manner, including constipation, asthma, tuberculosis, varicose ulcers, and fibrous tumors.

Because of their simple nature, the greatest challenge in working with affirmations is to suspend judgment long enough to allow them to produce the results you desire. In addition, it helps to feel your affirmations as you recite or write them, since this brings more energy to the experience. Make the process as vivid and real as possible.

The following guidelines will help you gain the most benefit when you work with affirmations:

- Always state your affirmation in the present tense and keep it positive. Don't use negative sentences, such as "I no longer suffer from migraines". Instead, use positive affirmations, like "I am pain-free".

- Keep your affirmations short and simple, no longer than two or three sentences.

- Write or say each affirmation ten to twenty times once or twice a day, ideally upon awakening each morning and before going to bed.

- Whenever you experience yourself thinking or hearing a habitual negative message, counteract it by focusing on your affirmation.

- Repeat your affirmations in the first, second, and third person, using your name in each variation. First person affirmations address any mental conditioning you have given yourself, while affirmations in the second and third person helps to release the conditioning you may have accepted from others. In each case, write out or repeat the affirmation ten times.

As you practice affirmation exercises, bring your emotions into the process, and involve as many of your senses as you can in order to experience how the goal that you are working on would look and feel *as if* it were your current reality. For example, your affirmation might be "I am completely healthy and full of vibrant energy." Imagine what that would look like and feel for you.

Make a commitment to practice your affirmations for at least 60 days or well beyond the time you begin experiencing the results you desire.

Guided Imagery and Visualization

Research confirms that it is possible to improve health by using guided imagery and visualization techniques. Numerous studies also confirm that regular practice of imagery and visualization techniques can produce greater feelings of peace and relaxation, enhanced creativity, greater fulfillment in relationships, improved professional success, and improved ability to reshape negative habit patterns. All such techniques harness the power of your thoughts and imagination. Combining them with affirmations can enhance their effectiveness.

In 1971, the aforementioned radiation oncologist O. Carl Simonton, MD, first discovered the benefits guided imagery and visualization can offer cancer patients while treating a 61 year-old man with a "hopeless" case of throat cancer that had caused drastic weight loss (he only weighed 98 pounds at the time), and left him struggling to breathe and swallow. Because of the severity of his condition, his doctors were worried that the radiation treatments he was scheduled to receive would cause his condition to deteriorate further. This concern led Simonton to create a guided imagery exercise for the man to follow throughout the course of his treatments, performing it three times a day for five to 15 minutes each time.

In the exercise, the man visualized the radiation treatments as "bullets of energy" striking and killing the cancer cells in his body. He imagined the cells shrinking and withering away, and visualized himself becoming healthy again. As a result of diligently performing this exercise, the man experienced only minor discomfort while receiving radiation, and within two months, he was completely cancer-free.

This outcome led Dr. Simonton to develop guided imagery and visualization exercises as self-care tools for his cancer patients. Those who used them experienced better response rates to their cancer treatments, better recoveries, and in many cases, complete remissions.

One of the most famous cases of recovery from cancer attributed to the use of imagery is that of Garret Porter. When Garret was nine years old, he was diagnosed with an inoperable brain tumor. Working with Patricia Norris, PhD, another pioneer in mind/body techniques and the daughter of Elmer and Alyce Green, Garrett created an imaginary scenario based on *Star Trek*, his favorite TV show. In conjunction with radiation treatments and biofeedback therapy, Dr. Norris taught Garrett to visualize a Star Trek spaceship shooting beams of energy at his tumor and imaging the tumor dissolving. Garrett faithfully practiced this visualization every day for a year. At the end of that year, to the astonishment of his doctors, his tumor had completely disappeared, and he was still cancer-free nearly 50 years later.

Dr. Norris taught that a positive attitude that is realistic and optimistic rather than based on falsely positive wishful thinking is the best approach when practicing guided imagery and visualization exercises. She also made the following recommendations:

1. Ask your body to show you the unconscious imagery it is holding.
2. Allow yourself to receive the imagery from your body.
3. Create a conscious visualization of what you want. Give this back to your body.
4. Create an audio of this visualization and play it to yourself every night before you go to sleep.
5. Gain feedback through your achievements.
6. Be confident that you are helping yourself to heal through the use of your thoughts and imagination.
7. Keep "talking" and "listening" to your body to receive more insights.

Journaling

Journaling involves writing down your thoughts and feelings and recording noteworthy events of your daily life. Keeping a journal can help you analyze problems and challenges you may face, discover your limiting beliefs, and identify habitual yet unconscious behaviors that no longer serve you. It can also help you become more aware and appreciative for all that you have to be grateful for. It is also a way to tap into your intuition and for becoming more aware of the spiritual guidance you may receive from God (see Chapter 6).

People who keep a journal often report that doing so helps them become better able to achieve their goals, including goals related to their health. Journaling is also valuable for people who have difficulty expressing their emotions. In their journals they have the opportunity to write out and resolve what they are feeling without having to worry about others judging them.

Research has also found that journaling helps people process trauma, including post-traumatic stress disorder (PTSD), and that it can reduce feelings of anxiety and depression.

The most common form of journaling is keeping a diary. Three other forms of journaling are:

- **The Gratitude Journal:** This type of journaling was discussed in Chapter 6, including my recommendations for how to gain the most benefit from it.

- **The Stream-Of-Consciousness Morning Journal:** This method was popularized by Julia Cameron, author of *The Artist's Way*. After you wake up each morning, write down whatever thoughts come into your head and continue to do so until you fill up three pages of paper. Don't edit yourself, just write all the thoughts that occur to you. Cameron claims that this exercise helps people rid themselves of "mental debris," allowing them to become better able to then focus on and accomplish their goals during the rest of the day.

    A variation of this technique is to write for 15 minutes and then read over what you wrote, underlining any thoughts that you find negative. Then rewrite each of them as a positive affirmation (see above). For example, if you wrote, "I'm feeling tired and I wish I didn't have to get up and go to work," your rewrite might read, "I am naturally energetic and enjoy my job." Do this for each sentence you underlined.

- **The Illness Dialogue:** The mental or emotional components of cancer and other illnesses aren't always readily apparent. This form of journaling helps to uncover the "hidden" meaning or message of any illness you might be dealing with so that you can better understand possible underlying causes and "messages" behind your symptoms.

    You can perform an illness dialogue by asking yourself, "If this illness (or pain) could speak, what would it say?" Then write down the first impression that comes to you. Once again, don't edit yourself. Write whatever occurs to you, even if it seems ludicrous or upsetting. Then read your response and ask yourself the first question that presents itself. Then write down your next response. Repeat the process until no further questions occur to you or you feel that you have the answer that can help you. Most likely you will need to repeat this exercise for a few days or more before your questions are resolved, but the rewards of doing so can be well worth it.

Cultivating Laughter

It is often said that "Laughter is the best medicine." One of the most famous examples proving this point is that of Norman Cousins, who recovered from a life-threatening arthritic condition by watching hours of Marx Brothers movies, reruns of *Candid Camera*, and other comedies while taking high doses of vitamin C. As he documented in his book *Anatomy of an Illness*, laughing regularly caused his pain to lessen, until eventually his illness disappeared altogether. Cousins developed this method of dealing with his illness after his doctors had determined there was nothing that could be done for it.

The work of Patch Adams, MD, founder of the Gesundheit Institute in Arlington, Virginia, also documented laughter's therapeutic effects had his patients.

Joyful laughter offers many of the same benefits as gentle exercise. Laughing exercises the facial muscles, shoulders, diaphragm, and abdomen. It also decreases anxiety and stress and can improve our outlook on life, which is very useful when we get sick. Research shows that laughter also boosts endorphin levels, increasse circulation, and enhances immune activity.

Like any skill, cultivating laugher takes practice, but the more you look for opportunities to laugh throughout the day, the more you will be giving your health a boost.

Discovering and Committing To Your Life Purpose

As you learned in Chapter 6, having a strong sense of life purpose is another proven factor for reducing the risk of disease and for promoting a longer, healthier lifespan. Not everyone is aware of their life purpose, however, and in some cases, even if they are, they do not honor and commit to it.

If you are unsure of what your life purpose might be, here are some suggestions that can help you discover it.

1. Take time to identify what you most care about, both in your personal life, in your community, and even the world at large. Once you have identified your cares in each of these areas, ask yourself what changes you think would lead to improvements in each of them and why you think those changes would make a difference.

   Now take time to consider what practical steps you could take to help bring those changes about. As you do so, notice which of your answers most excite you or that you have the most passion about.

2. Take time to write down an inventory of your talents and gifts. Don't edit yourself as do this exercise.

   Also ask yourself these questions: What are you good at? What do you most enjoy doing? What do you most appreciate about yourself? What activities in your life are most meaningful for you? Connect your talents that you first wrote down to the answers to these questions. Again, notice what most excites you as you do so.

3. Reflect back upon the dreams and ambitions you had for yourself when you were younger, especially as a child and early teenager, before you took on your current adult responsibilities.

   Many people defer pursuing their dreams as they move into adulthood due to the obligations they incur as they earn their living, get married, start a family, and so forth. But if their childhood dreams are genuine, they don't die; they are still there, waiting to be fulfilled.

This fact often becomes apparent to cancer and other patients when given a poor prognosis for recovery. It's not uncommon for them to commit to fulfilling their dreams as best as they are able in the time remaining to them. And once they make that commitment, many of them go on to disprove their doctors' prognoses, regaining their health as they go about making their dreams come true. You needn't wait to get sick to do the same.

4. Get out of your "comfort zone" and try new things. While old habits may indeed "die hard", they can also often stand in the way of further growth and self-discovery. It's human nature to develop and stick to routines that make us comfortable, but moving beyond such routines from time to time can lead to new experiences that are both fulfilling and potentially even life-changing in many positive ways. Seeking out new experiences and trying new things can often bring more clarity about one's life purpose.

    Are there activities that you've often thought about engaging in? Places you'd you like to travel to? People you would like to meet? If so, be willing to "go after them". As you do, you will likely discover how your talents and skills also come into play, helping you discover things about yourself that provide more meaning in your life and that potentially make a positive difference in others.

    Obviously, when faced with a serious, debilitating illness like cancer, one's attention is primarily focused on simply getting better, and rightly so. However, even under such circumstances, taking time to explore the answers as to *why* they want to get better can be a powerful incentive that mobilizes patients' will and commitment to do "whatever it takes" to get healthy so that they can achieve the goals they set for themselves once their health is regained. This is why I encourage my patients to set clear goals for themselves. Doing so provides them with "something to live for", and that can make all the difference in their recovery.

In addition to the above self-care approaches, I have found that the following therapies are also valuable aids for optimizing one's mental and emotional state and detecting and correcting limiting beliefs.

Bach Flower Remedies

Flower essence therapy is a system of healing that has been proven to help relieve stress and resolve unhealthy emotional states in order to help bring about healing, both emotionally and physically. It was developed by the English physician Edward Bach (September 1888 – November 1936) in the early 20th century.

Bach® Flower Remedies are the most well-known flower essences. Bach discovered and formulated them after observing that his patients suffering from physical illnesses habitually exhibited unhealthy emotional states such as anger, anxiety, depression, fear, guilt, jealousy, resentment, and shyness. Based on these observations, Bach realized that it was his patients' negative emotional and mental states that were the primary obstacle to them becoming well again.

A deeply spiritual man, Bach was intuitively guided to investigate the healing properties of the wildflowers native to his English countryside. After testing thousands of plants, he identified 38 flowers and distilled out their essences according to a specific process he developed. He found that these flower essences improved people's underlying emotional states, resulting in recoveries from their physical illnesses. Based on his findings, Bach wrote, "True healing involves treating the very base of the cause of the suffering. No effort directed to the body alone can do more than superficially repair damage. Treat people for their emotional unhappiness, allow them to be happy, and they will become well."

Bach Flower Remedies are available at most health food stores as well as online. They are nontoxic and have no side effects, do not interfere with other medications or supplements, and can be used without professional guidance.

Selecting and Using Bach Flower Remedies: Bach intended for his remedies to be used for self-care. To determine which essences to use, be honest about whatever emotions, thoughts, and behaviors are negatively affecting you, then choose the essence or essences that best match your mood and behavior.

Dr. Bach's 38 remedies and their indications for use are as follows:

- **Agrimony:** Suffering covered by a cheerful or brave facade. Distressed by argument or confrontation, may seek escape from pain or worry with addictive behavior through the use of food, drugs, cigarettes, or alcohol.
- **Aspen:** Vague fears or anxiety of unknown origin. Apprehension, foreboding.
- **Beech:** Critical, intolerant, or easily finding fault. May overreact with annoyance or irritability to the shortcomings of others.
- **Centaury:** Overly anxious to please, weak willed, or easily exploited/dominated by others. May neglect own needs to serve others. Avoids confrontation, difficulty saying No. **Cerato:** Lacks confidence in own judgment. Little trust in inner guidance. Constantly seeks advice of others, therefore vulnerable to being misguided.
- **Cherry Plum:** Fear of losing mental or physical control, of doing something desperate or violent. Tantrums, suicidal thoughts, impulse to do something thoughtless or known to be wrong. Fear of letting go. May be near nervous breakdown.
- **Chestnut Bud:** Failure to learn from experience, repeats inappropriate patterns. Difficulty correcting mistakes.
- **Chicory:** Loving, but possessive, emotionally needy, easily hurt or rejected.
- **Clematis:** Lacks concentration, daydreams. Halfhearted interest in present circumstances. Inactive, ungrounded. Trouble achieving goals.

- **Crab Apple:** Cleansing remedy when feeling toxic, contaminated, or unclean. Ashamed of self-image. Fear of being contaminated. Need for cleanliness. Can be used to assist detoxification, if needed.

- **Elm:** Overwhelmed by responsibilities. Normally capable, now doubts ability to perform tasks. Temporary feelings of inadequacy due to overload. Difficulty prioritizing.

- **Gentian:** Mild despondency or discouragement due to setback, difficulty, or failed expectation. Negativity reverses easily with positive events or successes.

- **Gorse:** Helplessness, hopelessness, sense of futility. Convinced situation will not improve; may not be willing to try remedies.

- **Heather:** Self-centered, self-obsessed, or self-absorbed. Seeks the companionship of anyone who will listen to them. Constant chatterer, poor listener, unhappy if left alone.

- **Holly:** Strongly felt negative feelings such as hatred, envy, jealousy, suspicion, revenge, or wrath.

- **Honeysuckle:** Dwelling in the past: old traumas, nostalgia, homesickness, regrets for happier times. Little expectation of future happiness.

- **Hornbeam:** Mental fatigue and tiredness; procrastination. Weary before day or task begins. Difficulty starting.

- **Impatiens:** Impatience, irritability, restlessness, or frustration with slow moving people and events. Quick in thought and action, requires all things to be done without delay. May prefer to work alone.

- **Larch:** Lacks self-confidence despite being capable. Feels inferior. Anticipates failure; may refuse to make effort to succeed.

- **Mimulus:** Everyday fear of known things such as heights, public speaking, pain, water, illness, flying, poverty, other people, being alone, etc. For the shy, nervous, or timid personality type.
- **Mustard:** Sudden deep gloom, depression, melancholia, or heavy sadness with no known cause.
- **Oak:** Struggling on despite difficulties. Does not give up even if ill or overworked. Strong sense of responsibility and determination. Difficulty resting when exhausted.
- **Olive:** Complete mental and physical exhaustion, sapped energy with no reserve, for example, after a long personal ordeal or illness.
- **Pine:** Guilt or self-reproach, feeling unworthy or undeserving. May blame self for another person's mistakes. Not satisfied with own achievements.
- **Red Chestnut:** Fear for the well-being of others, fearing the worst will happen to loved ones.
- **Rock Rose:** Nightmares. Terror or any great fear or panic.
- **Rock Water:** Self-denial. Strict, perhaps rigid, adherence to a living style or to religious, personal, or social disciplines.
- **Scleranthus:** Difficulty in deciding between two choices, seeing value in both. Uncertainty.
- **Star of Bethlehem:** Great unhappiness, grief, loss, trauma, after-effects of shock. Helpful after bereavement.
- **Sweet Chestnut:** Unbearable anguish, has reached the limits of endurance. Dark night of the soul, facing the abyss.
- **Vervain:** Fixed ideas, over-enthusiasm. Attempts to teach, convert, convince, save the world. Champion of justice. Energetic, intense, or driven.
- **Vine:** Overly strong-willed, capable, may become dictatorial or tyrannical. May disregard rights or needs of others. May be power-hungry or merciless.

- **Walnut:** Protection from negative influences or pressures and from the effects of change. Stabilizes emotionally during periods of transition: puberty, adolescence, menopause, aging, job change, new home, relationships, etc. Breaks links to past; facilitates freedom to move forward.

- **Water Violet:** Loners, quiet, aloof, self-reliant. They go their own way and leave others to go theirs. Prefers to bear health or other challenges alone.

- **White Chestnut:** Persistent unwanted thoughts. Mental arguments, worries, or repetitious thoughts that prevent peace of mind and disrupt concentration.

- **Wild Oat:** Career uncertainty, unfulfilled ambition, or boredom with present status and course in life. Although capable and talented, is unclear on which of many paths to take. Frustration or dissatisfaction may result.

- **Wild Rose:** Resigned or apathetic. Indifferent to life's circumstances. Will surrender to health or other problems. Rarely complains. Little effort to improve things or find joy. Emotionally flat or dull.

- **Willow:** Resentful or bitter toward life, blames others. Self-pity. Sees self as victim.

- **Bach Rescue Remedy:** In addition to the above remedies, you can also use Bach Rescue Remedy®, an all purpose stress relief formula. It contains Cherry Plum, Clematis, Impatiens, Rock Rose, and Star of Bethlehem essences, and can be an effective aid in times of emergencies, as well as everyday stress. It is particularly useful for promoting calm during accidents and other acute emergency situations, physical trauma, family upsets, and episodes of hysteria.

Heart Rate Variability

The overall status of a person's autonomic nervous system can be determined using a diagnostic test known as heart rate variability (HRV). During this test, sensors are attached to a person's chest to record the heartbeat, first while the person is lying down for a few minutes, and then for a few additional minutes when the person is standing. The results are then plotted, or graphed, to reveal levels of both sympathetic and parasympathetic nervous system activity. High heart rate variability reading readings indicate better overall health and a high, positive parasympathetic score. High HRV scores have also been shown by researchers to be an accurate indicator of positive emotions.

An increasing number of physicians now offer HRV testing to their patients during office visits. There are a number of HRV systems that are also available for home use. You can even download HRV apps onto your smart phone or tablet.

Applied Psycho-Neurobiology (APN)

Applied psycho-neurobiology (APN) is a practical process of healing the impact of an emotionally difficult event. It was developed by Dietrich Klinghardt, MD, PhD, and requires working with a health care professional trained in its use, such as myself. Dr. Klinghardt developed APN based on his deep understanding of psycho-neuroimmunology and neurobiology.

During an APN session, the practitioner first engages in a dialogue with the patient's subconscious mind. Through the use of relevant questions and biofeedback testing, the practitioner is able to quickly uncover unresolved psycho-emotional conflicts and trauma that a patient is dealing with, most often unconsciously. The patient is then guided to a deeper understanding of the limiting beliefs that she or he formed in an attempt to resolve these conflicts and trauma. Finally, this process uncouples, or disconnects, the autonomic nervous system from the unresolved psycho-emotional conflict, replacing them with freeing beliefs.

APN also measures slight changes in specific muscles as indicators for the state of the autonomic nervous system. The autonomic nervous system and the specific test-muscle are the delicate testing instrument. The changes after a successful treatment can be confirmed by Heart Rate Variability testing.

APN treatments are performed with the patient laying on a massage table. Session times range from 30 to 60 minutes. At the end of each session, patients usually find that they are more relaxed and aware of their conflict's resolution. It is also common for them to continue to notice improvements in their health and general well-being in the days and weeks after an APN treatment.

Anyone can benefit from APN. It is a safe and efficient way to uncover and resolve long-standing emotional traumas, false negative beliefs, and unresolved emotional conflicts. I strongly recommend it, especially for people dealing with cancer or any other chronic health issue. By combining other methods of healing with applied APN, the return to health will be quicker and the results will be more permanent.

To learn more about APN, contact my office.

Tension & Trauma Releasing Exercises (TRE(R))

Scientists over the past few decades have discovered that past traumatic events and their effects are stored within the body's cells as cellular memories. Just as your brain records what happens to you every moment, your cells absorb the impact of everything you experience, as well as the responses and interpretations you make about your experiences. Unless the cellular memories are healed, a trauma response can reoccur any time that the cellular memories are triggered. Usually, this triggering process happens automatically and we aren't even conscious of it. The implications of this fact are crucial and should not be overlooked because the trauma from your past will continue to negatively affect you until it is released.

Recognizing this fact led David Berceli, PhD, to develop what he calls Tension & Trauma Releasing Exercises (TRE) after spending 15 years living and working in war-torn countries in Africa and the Middle East as a certified clinical social worker and field traumatologist. During that time, while sheltering behind a wall in a building being shelled by mortar fire, he observed how he and everyone else in the room contracted their shoulders and hips as if to curl into a ball each time that a mortar exploded. This posture, he realized, was an instinctual (unconscious) and universal response to danger, as well as to other types of trauma, and that each time it happened it caused tension to build up and be stored in muscles.

Berceli also realized that releasing that tension could provide various health benefits, and set about analyzing the most effective ways of doing so, using his additional skills as a certified massage therapist and bioenergetics therapist. The result of his analysis led to the development of TRE.

TRE is a simple yet innovative series of exercises that help the body to release deep muscular patterns of stress, tension, and trauma by safely activating a natural reflex mechanism of muscular shaking. As the shaking occurs, muscle tension is released, inducing calm in the nervous system that shiftss the body into a more balanced and relaxed state of well-being.

One of the significant advantages of TRE is that it enables stored tension and trauma from past events to be released without any need to "revisit" and relive the events themselves. As the tension and stored trauma is released, the cellular memories associated with the events that caused them are released, as well.

TRE trainers and their clients consistently report that the TRE exercises offer a wide range of health benefits, including reduced feelings of anxiety, depression, and worry; reduced stress; improved energy and endurance levels; reduced back and muscle pain; increased flexibility; improved sleep; improvements in personal and work relationships; greater emotional resiliency; and relief and healing from old injuries and chronic medical conditions.

TRE exercises are easy to learn and can be performed any time that you feel a need to release stress and trauma and restore your physical, mental, and emotional equilibrium. Detailed instructions are available through Dr. Berceli's books, DVD, and an app that is available for both iPhone and Android systems. You can also work directly with a certified TRE provider, either one-on-one or in a group workshop. For more information, visit traumaprevention.com.

Another important factor that influences our mental and emotional states is what is known as the microbiome, the inner environment of the gastrointestinal tract. In the next chapter, I explain why and also discuss the diets and nutritional supplements that are known to be most effective for preventing and helping to reverse cancer.

Chapter 8

Optimizing Your Gut Health With Diet and Nutrition

One of the most important steps you can take to most effectively prevent and reverse cancer is to consume only those foods and beverages that support optimal health. But that step alone is not enough if what you consume is not fully digested. Unfortunately today, impaired digestion is a chronic health problem for many American, even among people committed to an organic lifestyle. In this chapter, you will learn the reasons why, as well why the health of your GI tract (your gut) is so vital to your overall health.

You will also learn the dietary "do's and don'ts" that must be followed in order to improve and maintain your health, especially if you are already dealing with cancer. Just as importantly, you will also learn about the most effective anti-cancer diets and how to determine which one is most appropriate for you.

Your Gut: The Overlooked Key to Good Health

Your body's gastrointestinal (GI) tract consists of hollow tube known as the alimentary canal that is between 26 and 32 feet long. It begins at your mouth and ends at your anus, and also includes the pharynx, esophagus, stomach, small intestine and large intestines, and the rectum.

One of the main functions of the GI tract is to provide your body with the nutrients it requires to maintain its health. It is assisted in this digestive process by the liver, gallbladder, and pancreas. Additionally, and of equal importance, the GI tract is also responsible for preventing unhealthy substances from being absorbed into your body. These interrelated functions are accomplished in three ways: the movement of food along the alimentary canal that occurs as muscles in the GI tract push food particles forward; the secretion of gastric juices by the stomach, pancreas, and liver, which enables food particles to be broken down; and the absorption of the fluids and nutrients contained in food by the small and large intestines.

In addition to its primary roles in digestion and elimination of wastes and toxins, the GI tract is also home to the enteric nervous system located in the linings of the esophagus, stomach, and small and large intestines. Brimming with neurotransmitter proteins, the enteric nervous system acts very much like your body's "second brain" because these proteins transmit nerve impulses from nerve cells to other cells, enabling your body to properly perform its many functions. These proteins produced by GI tract cells are identical to neurotransmitter proteins in the brain. In fact, there are more neurotransmitters in the gut than there are in the brain. The gut also contains one of the largest concentrations of mood-altering neurotransmitters, including serotonin, 90 percent of which is produced in the gut, not in the brain, as is commonly believed. Research has shown that enteric nervous system's neurotransmitter network mimics actual brain function, enabling it to operate independently, learning, remembering, and producing so-called "gut feelings."

All of these processes are part of the overall operation of the body's autonomic nervous system that you learned about in Chapter 7. The nerve endings attached to linings of the GI tract provide nerve impulses that stimulate the operation of the various organs and glands within the body. The type of stimulation that the ANS is able to provide to organs and glands is a direct reflection of the health of the GI tract. The gut wall also houses 70 percent of the cells of the immune system.

Healing the digestive system and the gut is one of the first and most important steps to improving overall health, and absolutely crucial for anyone dealing with cancer. Sadly, this fact is often overlooked by many oncologists and other physicians.

How Disease Occurs in the Gut: Healthy gastrointestinal function largely depends on the health of the lining of intestinal walls which, in turn, depends on a coating of "friendly" bacteria in the gut. (As many as 500 distinct species of bacteria exist within the GI tract, creating a population of approximately 100 trillion combined bacteria in the gut, a number that is ten times greater than the total number of cells in the body.) These friendly bacteria, also known as *flora*, form a protective shield that prevents harmful toxins, bacteria, viruses, and other microorganisms from penetrating the lining of the intestinal walls to enter the bloodstream, while at the same time allowing the passage of vital nutrients and fluids through the GI lining into the blood, which transports them to the body's tissues and organs. These bacteria are also critical for overall immunity, including optimal function of natural killer (NK) immune cells.

Exposure to food-borne toxins and other harmful substances impairs flora. When such exposures occur, white blood cells within the gut lining get activated to attack and eliminate the toxins. In cases of short-term exposures, this usually resolves matters before GI problems can arise. But when such exposures become chronic, as is the case with many people today, the prolonged activity of these white blood cells irritates the gut lining, causing it to become inflamed.

Ongoing exposures to toxins, combined with the irritation and inflammation, damages the defensive capacities of the friendly flora, impairs digestion, and results in the intestinal walls becoming increasingly permeable. The greater this degree of intestinal permeability, the more toxins, undigested and abnormal proteins, and other harmful substances are able to pass through the gut lining into the bloodstream. This is known as "leaky gut syndrome," a condition that is increasingly common today, yet still often undiagnosed or ignored.

Left unchecked, leaky gut causes a proliferation of harmful substances in the gut, setting the stage for disease to occur, first within the GI tract itself, and then potentially in other areas of the body. During this process, healthy bacteria are forced to contend with unhealthy bacteria, leading to a condition known as *dysbiosis*, which is characterized by the growth of harmful flora in the lower colon, where they are normally kept in check by friendly bacteria, into other areas of the GI tract and into the bloodstream. Further damage is also caused by the spread of free radicals that are produced as a side effect of the chronic inflammation in the GI tract. The end result is an overall disruption and impairment of gut function, leading to weakened digestion and poor absorption of essential nutrients. This creates a vicious circle in which the body is not only under attack from toxins and other harmful substances within the gut, but also suffering from impaired immune, hormonal, and neurological functioning because of a lack of sufficient nutrients. These same nutritional deficiencies also result in greater susceptibility to infectious disease, autoimmune conditions, and other health risks, including cancer, heart disease, and stroke. All of these risks are further exacerbated by the toxins and pathogens passing into the bloodstream due to leaky gut.

The toxins, undigested food particles, and other harmful substances that escape from the GI tract to enter the bloodstream can also shut down different parts of the body's blood-brain barrier to both directly and indirectly affect the brain. When this happens, it can lead to anxiety and depression, autism, attention deficit disorder (ADD), bipolar disorder, and even schizophrenia, as well as other brain-related conditions.

Other conditions caused or made worse by impaired gut health include acne and other skin conditions, allergies, bad breath (halitosis), bloating after meals, candidiasis and thrush, colds (especially recurring colds), cold sores, constipation, cystitis, diarrhea, ear and eye infections, eczema, fatigue, flatulence, poor sleep, sore throat, and stomach and other gastrointestinal tract conditions, among others. Sugar and other unhealthy food cravings are also typical, as is longer than normal healing times.

The Gut Microbiome: Bacteria, both "good" and "bad", are not the only microorganisms that the GI tract is home to. Also present are other microbes, including viruses, yeasts and other fungi, and other protozoa, as well as their genes. In a state of good health, all of these microbial species coexist in a state of symbiosis that is beneficial to both the human body and the microbes themselves. Collectively, they exist within an environment known as the *microbiome*.

Medical science's view of the GI tract and the microorganisms it contains has changed in recent decades due to ongoing discoveries about the microbiome. One shocking discovery scientists have made is that more than half of the human body is actually not human at all. According to the latest scientific evidence, only 43 percent of our bodies' total cell count is comprised of human cells. The larger amount (57 percent) consists of cells of the microorganisms that live on our skin, inside our mouth and nasal passages, and, primarily, within our gut.

Scientists have also discovered that the genome of the microorganisms that exist within the microbiome far exceeds the human genome in size and number. The human genome consists of 22,000 different types of genes, whereas the microbiome contains between two to 20 million genes comprising a second genome within our bodies that augments and directly influences the human genome.

In light of these discoveries, scientists are finding that health is greatly dependent on having a balanced microbiome, and that an unhealthy microbiome is a primary cause of chronic inflammation and a wide variety of diseases.

In addition, scientists now know that the microbiome is also responsible for calorie extraction from foods that supplies the body with energy, as well as for synthesizing certain vitamins and amino acids. Because of the various health-supporting roles it plays in the body, some scientists even refer to the microbiome as one of the body's organs, with its health depending on how well the microorganisms it houses co-exist and interact. But when that balance is disturbed, dysbiois occurs, increasing the risk of illness.

Because the microbiome is an alive and dynamic environment, the number of various species it contains can fluctuate on a daily, weekly, or monthly basis depending on a variety of factors, especially diet. Other factors that can affect the microbiome for good or bad include the use of antibiotics and other medications, stress, environmental toxins, and exercise or the lack thereof.

To conclude this overview of the gut, I'd like you to imagine your gut as a city.

A thriving, efficient city has many systems working together in harmony, such as the transportation (digestive) system that gets people (nutrients) where they need to go (into the bloodstream to be transported to your body's cells, tissues, and organs), and the waste removal system (elimination) that keeps the streets clean (elimination of waste by-products, toxins, etc).

Now imagine that one of those systems starts to break down.

Suddenly, the whole city is thrown into chaos.

The same is true for your body. When your gut is not functioning correctly, it causes a ripple effect of dysfunction throughout your entire body, leading to many problems. This is why it's essential to heal the gut. When we do, we restore harmony to the whole body, enabling it to function optimally. Once the gut is healed, the body's detoxification pathways can operate more effectively, toxins are eliminated more efficiently, and food is properly digested and metabolized, resulting in better assimilation of the nutrients they contain, leading to enhanced immune, hormonal, and other overall body function. This is why healing the gut is vital for overall health and well-being, and most especially for helping to prevent and heal cancer.

The Link Between Poor Gut Health and Cancer

While the exact mechanisms by which poor gut health impacts cancer risk are still being investigated, there is no doubt a link between the two. And this link is only becoming more apparent as research progresses.

Two of the most obvious reasons have to do with weakened immunity and inflammation. As discussed above, poor gut health has been linked to a weakened immune system, the body's primary line of defense against cancer, both in terms of detecting and eliminating cancer cells before they can take hold in the body, and for fighting cancer if it does occur. Given that the GI tract is the home of at least 70 percent of the immune system, it should be obvious that optimizing gut function will improve immunity, making doing so an essential element of overall cancer treatments. Yet, as I mentioned earlier, addressing and healing the gut is far too often not a component of conventional cancer care. Moreover, both radiation and chemotherapy are known to further disrupt gut health and weaken immune function, making their use a double-edged sword.

The dietary eating habits of most Americans is a major cause of inflammation in the gut, triggering leaky gut syndrome and eventually causing inflammation outside of the gut, as well. As you learned in Chapter 2, chronic inflammation is a primary cause of cancer, as well as most other serious, degenerative disease conditions, and increases the risk of infection, which in turn causes even more inflammation. This vicious circle often first occurs in the gut before spreading to other areas of the body.

Numerous studies have confirmed that chronic inflammation and infectious microbes in the gut can directly and indirectly cause various types of cancer. For example, inflammation in the gut has been linked to an increased risk of pancreatic cancer, and research show that various harmful gut bacteria are associated with an increased risk of colorectal cancer. Other research has found links between the following types of cancer and infectious agents:

- Bile duct and bladder cancers and abnormal *E. coli* and other bacteria known to cause urinary tract infections (UTIs).

- Brain cancer and *Borrelia bergdorferi*, the principal cause of Lyme disease.

- Breast cancer and elevated levels of *E. coli* and *Staphylococcus epidermidis*, and diminished levels of "friendly" bacteria, such as *Lactobacillus* and *Streptococcus*. Human papilloma virus (HPV) has also been linked to breast cancer.

- Cervical cancer and human papilloma virus (HPV).

- Colorectal cancer and elevated levels of *E. coli, fusobacterium*, and other types of bacteria, along with a reduced supply of a specific strain of *Clostridium*, a bacterium known to help control glucose levels in the gut.

- Esophageal cancer and *Porphyromomas gingivalis* and *Tanerella forsythia*, both of which are common causes of gum disease that are carried into the gut via swallowing.

- Liver cancer and hepatitis B virus (HBV), hepatitis C virus (HCV), and *Porphyromomas gingivalis*. *Opisthorchis viverrini*, a parasitic flatworm (fluke) has also been shown to be a cause of cancer in the liver's bile ducts. It typically enters the body as a result of eating raw or undercooked fish.

- Nose and throat cancer and Epstein-Barr virus (EBV).

- Penile cancer (cancer of penis) and human papilloma virus (HPV).

- Prostate cancer and *Bacteriodes massiliensis* and *Helicobacter hepaticus*, as well as reduced levels of the healthy bacteria *Eubacterium rectalie* and *Faecalibacterium praunitzii*.

- Stomach cancer and *Helicobacter pylori* (*H. Pylori*).

- Vaginal cancer and cancer of the vulva and human papilloma virus (HPV).

Various infections have also been linked to certain types of lymphoma. For example, human t-cell leukemia/lymphoma virus type 1 (HTLV-1) is known to be a cause of an aggressive type of non-Hodgkin lymphoma called **adult T-cell leukemia/lymphoma** (ATLL), while Kaposi sarcoma-associated herpes virus (KSHV), also known as human herpes virus-8 (HHV-8), has been linked to primary effusion lymphoma. And gastric MALT lymphoma, which occurs in the stomach lining, has been linked to *H. pylori.*

Infections have also been shown to play a role in the development of lung cancers, ovarian cancer, and cancer of the fallopian tubes. Accumulations of various bacteria that form in the gut and known as biofilms have also been linked to various types of cancer.

The human immunodeficiency virus (HIV), which is said to be the cause of AIDS, can also cause cancer, although not directly. Still, it is a risk factor to screen for because of how it weakens immunity. According to the National Cancer Institue (NCI), "People infected with HIV have increased risks of a number of cancers, especially Kaposi sarcoma, lymphomas (including both non-Hodgkin lymphoma and Hodgkin disease), and cancers of the cervix, anus, lung, liver, and throat."

Because of the ongoing discoveries related to the microbiome, researchers in recent years have begun to shift their focus away from individual infectious agents to the roles that the microbiome itself plays in the development of cancer, as well as in cancer prevention. As the authors of the published study *Gut Microbes, Diet, and Cancer* wrote, "An expanding body of evidence supports a role for gut microbes in the etiology [causes] of cancer. Previously, the focus was on identifying individual bacterial species that directly initiate or promote gastrointestinal malignancies; however, the capacity of gut microbes to influence systemic inflammation and other downstream pathways suggests that the gut microbial community may also affect risk of cancer in tissues outside of the gastrointestinal tract. Functional contributions of the gut microbiota that may influence cancer susceptibility in the broad sense include (1) harvesting otherwise inaccessible nutrients and/or sources of energy from the diet (i.e., fermentation of dietary fibers and resistant starch); (2) metabolism of xenobiotics [chemical substances not naturally produced in the body], both potentially beneficial or detrimental (i.e., dietary constituents, drugs, carcinogens, etc.); (3) renewal of gut epithelial cells and maintenance of mucosal integrity; and (4) affecting immune system development and activity. Understanding the complex and dynamic interplay between the gut microbiome, host immune system, and dietary exposures may help elucidate [make clear] mechanisms for carcinogenesis and guide future cancer prevention and treatment strategies."

Echoing that message, the authors of a 2022 research review entitled *The Potential of the Gut Microbiome to Reshape the Cancer Therapy Paradigm*, wrote, "Ultimately, the importance of gut bacteria in cancer therapy cannot be overstated in its potential for ushering in a new era of cancer treatments. With the understanding that the microbiome may play critical roles in the tumor microenvironment, holistic approaches that integrate microbiome-modulating treatments with biological, immune, cell-based, and surgical cancer therapies should be explored."

This is why addressing the microbiome as a whole is so important for preventing and helping to reverse cancer. The rest of this chapter provides you with the information you need to begin doing so on your own.

Unhealthy Foods To Avoid

The most important factor that determines the health of your gut and microbiome is your diet. What and how you eat is something you have complete control over. By choosing to adopt healthier eating habits you will not only improve your overall health, but also significantly reduce your risk of cancer and most other illnesses.

Just as there is no single "magic bullet" cure for cancer, there is also no such thing as a one-size-fits-all diet that is most appropriate for everyone, especially for people dealing with cancer. Genetically and biochemically, we each have unique dietary and nutritional needs. However, there are certain dietary guidelines that apply to all of us, especially when it comes to unhealthy foods we would all do well to avoid.

Broadly speaking, the foods and beverages that need to eliminate from your diet fall into the following categories.

Genetically Modified Foods (GMOs): Now rebranded and labeled as bioengineered (BE) foods, GMOs are increasingly prevalent within America's food supply and the number of different foods that are becoming genetically modified continues to grow. Once limited to plant foods, GMOs are now found in animal food products, as well, such as GMO salmon.

Although the FDA and the US Department of Agriculture (USDA) continue to insist that GMO foods are safe for human consumption, this fact has never been established with long-term human safety studies. Moreover, animal studies indicate GMOs may cause or increase the risk of cancer and other serious diseases.

The DNA GMO foods contain are foreign to the body and cannot be effectively digested when consumed. Avoiding GMO foods requires diligence, however. It also means avoiding certain nonorganic foods altogether, such as corn and soybeans, 90 percent of which are genetically modified if grown in the US. Corn and corn-derivatives such as corn starch and corn syrup are also common additives in most canned, boxed, and other types of packaged and processed foods. In addition, GMO corn and soybeans are both used to feed livestock, poultry, and farm-raised fish by most commercial meat, poultry, and fish producers due to how inexpensive they are.

Nearly all cottonseed grown in the US is also genetically-modified and is also used to feed livestock for the same reason. This is one reason why you should always choose meats and poultry derived from grass-fed, pasture-raised animals, and also opt for wild-caught fish that are low in mercury.

Meats, Poultry, and Fish Laced With Antibiotics and Growth Hormones: All conventionally raised livestock and poultry in the US today are injected with growth hormones and antibiotics before they are slaughtered, as are many farm-raised fish. Even cow's milk and other dairy products from conventionally raised cows likely contain growth hormones, including IGF-1, which is known to increase the risk of cancer. Conventionally raised livestock also have higher levels of stress hormones which flood their system before they are slaughtered. All of these harmful substances enter your body whenever you eat foods derived from animals and fish raised this way. Avoid consuming such foods whenever possible.

Foods Laced With Pesticides and Herbicides: Billions of pounds of pesticides and herbicides are sprayed on conventionally grown food crops in the US, and are also used on the feed given to conventionally raised livestock and poultry. These substances, when ingested, are a primary cause of leaky gut syndrome because of how they perforate the GI tract's inner lining.

Like GMOs, chemical pesticides and herbicides have never been tested for long-term human safety. One of the most harmful and prevalent pesticides is glyphosate, the main ingredient in RoundUp and other commercial weed killer products. Unlike other pesticides and herbicides, many of which, at least to some extent, can be washed off from conventionally grown fruits and vegetables, glyphosate penetrates inside food crops and cannot be washed off. Eating glyphosate-laced foods wreaks havoc in your body and increases your risk for certain cancers.

The use of glyphosate is now so prevalent that human population studies have found that virtually all Americans have glyphosate residues in their bodies. Glyphosate has also been found in 70 percent of our nation's drinking water and even in the air we breathe.

You can find lists of foods with the lowest amount of pesticide/herbicide content at the website of the Environmental Working Group (EWG.org), starting with their free annual report *Shopper's Guide To Pesticides in Produce*™. EWG also provides other resources that can help you make healthier food buying choices. When possible, choose to buy and eat organic foods and food products.

Processed Foods: Processed foods are any foods that contain artificial food additives and preservatives. They include all packaged foods, fast foods, and nonorganic snacks. While preservatives can and do preserve the shelf life of such foods, their chemical nature can trigger inflammation, damaging cellular DNA, and disrupting hormone balance. The same is true of artificial food additives.

One of the most common preservatives is monosodium glutamate (MSG), which is also labeled as "textured protein", "soy protein isolate", or "natural flavoring", and other seemingly innocent terms. Other common preservatives and additives are aspartame (Equal and NutraSweet), saccharin (Sweet'N'Low), sodium nitrate, sucralose (Splenda), BHT, BHA, potassium bromate, carrageenan, food dyes, and other so-called natural food colorings.

Nonorganic Dairy Products: Nonorganic milk, butter, and other dairy products contain high levels of antibiotics, growth hormones, and pesticides. They also create excess mucus in the intestines, lungs, and sinuses, and cause chronic acidity and inflammation.

Farm-Raised Fish/Fish High in Heavy Metals and Other Toxins: While fish can be a healthy addition to your overall diet, it's important to avoid consuming fish high in mercury and other heavy metals and toxins, and to avoid farm-raised fish because of the antibiotics, food dyes, and other harmful substances they contain. You can obtain a list of fish with the lowest levels of mercury and other heavy metals in *The Smart Seafood Buying Guide*, a free report by the Natural Resources Defense Council. It is available at www.nrdc.org/stories/smart-seafood-buying-guide.

Iron-enriched Foods: While iron plays many important roles in the body, including being essential for the production of hemoglobin in red blood cells, too much iron can cause oxidative stress and be toxic. Both excess stored and unbound levels of iron tend to rise as we age. This is especially true for middle-aged men and postmenopausal women.

Research has shown that even mild cases of iron overload can increase the risk for cancer, diabetes and metabolic syndrome, heart attack and heart failure, hypothyroidism, liver disease osteoarthritis, osteoporosis, and in some cases premature death. Iron overload has also been linked to neurodegenerative diseases such as Alzheimer's, Parkinson's, Huntington's, epilepsy and multiple sclerosis. For these reasons, it is not advisable to consume iron as a supplement, whether alone or as an ingredient in multivitamin/mineral formulas.

Foods high in iron include cereals, dark and red meat, poultry, eggs, dark green leafy vegetables, black-eyed peas, chickpeas, other dried beans, beets, raisins, dates and apricots. If you are at risk for iron overload, consume these foods sparingly. In addition, you can reduce excess iron levels by donating blood a few times each year, and exercising regularly.

Sugar and Simple/Refined Carbohydrates: Sugar and simple/refined carbohydrates are staples of the standard American diet. Sugar intake weakens the immune system and increases the risk of infection. Among its other harmful effects, it causes excessive insulin production, increases the production of harmful triglycerides, increases the buildup of fat in the body, and promotes systemic yeast overgrowth (candidiasis) and other types of fungal infections. Sugar in all of its form is also a primary fuel source for cancer cells and tumors.

Sugar is a common ingredient in packaged foods and commercial beverages in the forms of fructose, sucrose, corn syrup, lactose, and maltose. Canned, processed, or cured foods are also typically high in sugar.

Simple/refined carbohydrates act in much the same way that sugar does in the body. Common types of these foods are white breads, pastas made from white flour, instant mashed potatoes, white rice, chips, and sugar laden commercial cereals.

Foods That Cause Fungal Infections: As you learned in Chapter 3, researchers have now linked fungal infections with cancer. Various foods can be a primary cause of such infections and exacerbate them when they are already present. In addition, fungi in the body produce poisonous substances called mycotoxins that further weaken immune function and overall health. Fungi and mycotoxins are major triggers of leaky gut syndrome.

In addition to the sugars and simple/refined carbohydrate foods mentioned above, other fungal-causing foods to consider eliminating from your diet include breads and pasta, corn and corn products, fruits with high sugar content, grains, legumes (beans), mushrooms, peanuts and peanut-containing products, pistachios, potatoes and yams, and all foods containing yeast. Alcohol, margarine and other butter-substitute products, and commercial salad dressings should also be avoided. Two of the best anti-fungal diets are the GAPS diet, created by Natasha Campbell-McBride, MD, and the Kaufmann diet, created by Doug Kaufmann. You can find out more about them by visiting www.gapsdiet.com and www.knowthecause.com, respectively.

Hydrogenated Oils and Omega-6-Rich Vegetable Oils: While certain fats are essential for good health, others, such as many vegetable and seed oils, trans-fatty acids and hydrogenated fats, are common risk factors for cancer and other diseases. Trans-fatty acids and hydrogenated fats are commonly found in margarine, cooking fats, commercial peanut butter, commercial cereals, and packaged foods.

Unlike trans- and hydrogenated oils and fats, omega 6 essential fatty acids (EFAs) are vital for good health when taken in the correct amounts, as are omega-3 EFAs. Without enough EFAs, your body cannot adequately produce enough energy, regulate hormone production and proper nerve function, maintain brain health, and maintain the proper functioning of the musculoskeletal system.

As I discussed in Chapter 3, for much of human history, the dietary balance between omega-3 and omega-6 fatty acids was approximately 1:1. Today, that ratio has been skewed to between 1:8 to as much as 1:25. Research has found that at least nine percent of the total amount of calories consumed by the average American today comes from polyunsaturated fats high in omega-6 fatty acids, and that omega-6s begin to create chronic inflammation and oxidation in our bodies when they exceed four percent of total daily caloric intake.

Most people consume excessive levels of omega-6 oils because of how widely used the vegetable oils that contain them has become. These include canola oil, corn oil, cottonseed oil, grapeseed oil, peanut oil, rapeseed oil, rice brain oil, safflower oil, soybean oil, sunflower oil, vegetable oil, and wheat germ oil. Such oils are staple ingredients in many canned and packaged foods and are also used by most restaurants and other dining establishments in the United States.

Use omega-6 oils sparingly, if at all, when you cook or bake at home, and check the labels of canned and packaged foods when you go shopping. For cooking, use coconut oil, olive oil, or ghee.

Sodas and Other Unhealthy Beverages: Soda should be eliminated from your diet, including so-called diet soda. Other beverages you should avoid are commercial, nonorganic fruit and vegetable juices (which are high in sugar and sodium, respectively), commercial sports drinks, nonherbal teas, and alcohol.

In addition to the above categories, you should also do your best to avoid foods and beverages packaged in plastic because the plastics they contain leaches into food and beverages to then enter the body when the foods and drinks are consumed. This includes foods sold in plastic wraps or in plastic food containers.

Unfortunately, because of the high amounts of plastic currently polluting our oceans, seafood now often contain plastic residues called microplastics, which are also harmful. If you enjoy eating fish, consider avoiding seafood and replacing it with freshwater fish, which aren't as apt to contain microplastics. Healthy choices include bass, perch, trout, walleye, and wild caught salmon.

Plastic contaminants are also commonly found in canned food and plastic bottles. These contaminants include bisphenol A (BPA) and bisphenol S (BPS), along with a class of chemicals called phthalates, which are also used in food packaging. All of these substances disrupt the body's endocrine (hormone) functions because of how they mimic estrogen. They also poison insulin receptors in the cells, and increase the risk for serious illnesses, including cancer.

To safeguard your health, avoid canned and other plastic-stored food and don't drink from plastic bottles. To store foods and liquids, use glass, porcelain or stainless-steel containers instead of plastic containers.

Eating The Rainbow: The Health Benefits Of Different Colored Foods

One of the healthiest steps you can take to improve your diet is to include a variety of different colored vegetables in each of your meals, as well as eating different fruits away from meals. (Why fruits should be eaten away from other foods is explained later in this chapter.) Eating this way will help to ensure that you are supporting your health with the wide array of nutrients that fruits and vegetables contain.

Among these important nutrients are a group called polyphenols that possess potent antioxidant properties that help prevent body's cells and tissues from becoming damaged because of oxidation.

Scientists have identified over 8,000 different types of polphenols in plants. Most of them are concentrated in the outer sections of fruits and vegetables (the peel, rind, and skin), but they occur in other parts of plants, as well. Polyphenols are responsible for many plant qualities, including their color, flavor, scent, and taste. They also help to keep plants strong and healthy by protecting them from harmful bacteria and fungi, as well as from insects and ultraviolet light. Research has found that polyphenols are also responsible for many of the health-promoting properties that fruits and vegetables provide when we eat them.

One of the main reasons why polyphenols are so important to good health is because they act as catalysts that enable other nutrients to properly do their job. Additionally, unlike most other nutrients, the health benefits polyphenols provide are broad in scope, including their ability to simultaneously regulate a wide variety of different cell functions. By contrast, nutrients such as vitamins, although they are also vital for good health, typically serve very specific and limited functions in cellular metabolism.

The best way to obtain a wide range of polyphenols from your diet is to eat a variety of different colored fruits and vegetables each day. Researchers and physicians such as Gabriel Cousens, MD, and David Heber, MD, have for many years pointed out the importance of eating in this way, yet the vast majority of Americans fail to do so. In fact, according to Dr. Heber, founder of the UCLA Center for Human Nutrition, the standard American diet is almost entirely "brown and beige" in color, consisting of foods that are not only lacking in vital nutrients, including polyphenols, but are also high in unhealthy refined starches, sugars, and fats. This fact alone goes a long way to explaining our nation's health crisis.

The extent to which most Americans fail to eat a full range of colorful foods—significantly increasing their risk for developing diet-related diseases such as cancer, diabetes, and heart disease—was revealed in *America's Phytonutrient Report* published by the Nutrilife Institute in 2010. The report highlighted the importance of the color of fruit and vegetables to bridge the nutrient gap common in Western diets and most specifically the standard American diet (SAD). According to the report, 88 percent of Americans do not eat enough blue and purple fruit and vegetables, while 86 percent fail to eat the minimum number of vegetables in the white range. In addition, approximately 75 percent of Americans do not consume an adequate number of green, yellow, or orange fruits and vegetables.

To get in the habit of eating a greater variety of different colored foods each day, remember to "eat the rainbow." By this I mean try to ensure that all of your meals contain an array of different colored foods. Doing so will enable you to more easily obtain a wider supply of the nutrients your body needs. In addition, you will also be supply your body with the fiber it needs to also stay healthy. (Most Americans only obtain about one-third or less of the fiber necessary for optimum gut health from their diet.)

What follows are categories of different colored fruits and vegetables, along with some of the polyphenols they contain:

- **Blue/Purple Group:** Fruits and vegetables in this group are rich in polyphenols called anthocyanins that have been shown to protect cells from damage due to their high antioxidant qualities. Anthocyanins can also help reduce the risk of developing blood clots, certain cancers, heart disease, and stroke. Research has also found that regularly eating blue/purple foods is linked to healthy aging and improved memory, in part due to the polyphenol known as resveratrol that they contain. Foods in this category include blackberries, blueberries, eggplant, figs, grapes (purple), plums, prunes, and raisins.

- **Green Group:** Fruits and vegetables in this group derive their color from chlorophyll, and are also rich in polyphenols such as indoles, isocyanates, leutin, sulforophane, and zeaxanthin. Among the benefits these polyphenols provide are protection against vision problems, including cataracts and age-related macular degeneration; protection against certain types of cancer; and protection against birth defects. Foods in this group include green apples, artichokes, asparagus, avocado, broccoli, bok choy, Brussels sprouts, green cabbage, cucumbers, grapes, green beans, green onions, green peppers, kale, kiwi, lettuce, peas, spinach, and zucchini.

- **Orange/Yellow Group:** These foods are rich in carotenoids and cryptothaxin. Carotenoids help support immune function and healthy mucous membranes, and reduce risk for cancer, heart disease, and macular degeneration. Cryptothaxin has also been shown to help protect against heart disease, and is also important for proper communication of the body's cells with one another. Foods in this group include apricots, apples (yellow), butternut squash, cantaloupe, carrots, corn, grapefruit, lemons, mangos, nectarines, oranges, papaya, peaches, persimmons, pumpkins, rutabagas, sweet potatoes, tangerines, and yellow squash.

- **Red/Purple Group:** Food in this group are also rich in anthocyanins, as well as lycopene, which has been shown to help protect against certain types of cancer, especially breast and prostate cancer, as well as heart disease. The polyphenol ellagic acid is also found in this food group. Ellagic acid acts like an antioxidant and can inhibit aromatase, an enzyme that converts pre-estrogen to active estrogen, the hormone that fuels 80 percent of all breast cancers. Foods in this group include apples (red), beets, cabbage (red), cherries, cranberries, grapefruit (pink), pomegranates, radishes, rhubarb, red peppers, red potatoes, strawberries, tomatoes, and watermelon.

- **White Group:** Fruits and vegetables in this group derive their color from polyphenols called anthoxanthins. White fruits and vegetables are a good food source for quercetin, a powerful antioxidant that also acts as a natural anti-histamine and anti-inflammatory agent. Research shows that quercetin may help to prevent cancer, especially prostate cancer. Certain foods in this group, such as garlic and white onions, also contain allicin, which can help reduce the risk of developing high blood pressure and cholesterol, heart disease, and stomach cancer. Foods in this group include cauliflower, garlic, ginger, jicama, mushrooms, onions, parsnips, potatoes, and turnips.

Ideally, you should try to eat foods from each of these food groups every day.

Other Healthy Eating Action Steps

To further improve your diet and overall eating habits, do the following:

1. Choose to eat organically grown fruits and vegetables whenever possible.
2. Eat wild caught fish and free-range meats and poultry food free of hormones and antibiotics.
3. Vary your meals to ensure you obtain a wide variety of nutrients, and to also minimize the risk of developing food allergies and sensitivities. Try to space out the same meals you enjoy to at least every four days.

4. Include healthy fats in your meals. Such fats help produce energy in the body, protect against inflammation, maintain healthy body temperature, build cell membranes, assist in transporting oxygen, aid in the absorption of fat-soluble vitamins, and help nourish nerves, mucous membranes, and the skin. Food sources of healthy fats include avocado, organic butter, coconut, whole eggs (preferably pastured), fatty fish (anchovies, herring, mackerel, sardines, wild-caught salmon), olives, nuts and seeds (almonds, macadamia nuts, walnuts, chia seeds, pumpkin seeds), and unsweetened, full fat, organic yogurt. Healthy fats are also found in coconut oil, flaxseed oil, ghee, extra virgin olive oil.

5. Eat fermented foods. Doing so will help your GI tract replenish healthy, immune-supporting bacteria because of the hundreds of different strains of friendly bacteria they contain. Fermented foods include kimchi, miso, organic pickles, sauerkraut, and tempeh.

6. Limit your caffeine intake (one to two cups of coffee per day).

7. Limit your salt intake, and choose Celtic or sea salt, both of which are rich in iodine and health-supporting co-factor minerals.

8. Avoid drinking with your meals. Drinking while eating dilutes stomach acid and digestive enzymes, impairing digestion. Drinking cold beverages while you eat also causes the blood vessels in your GI tract to constrict, negatively impacting their ability to absorb the nutrients food contains. If you must drink with your meals, choose warm water with lemon or organic, herbal tea.

9. Chew your food thoroughly to help ensure it is completely digested. Ideally, keep chewing until each bite of food is almost liquid before you swallow it.

10. Drink adequate amounts of healthy water to ensure that your body stays hydrated. Water is the medium through which all of

your body functions occur. Many people are chronically dehydrated and don't know it.

To help determine if you need to drink more water monitor your urine. It should be clear and almost colorless, like unsweetened lemonade. If you are slightly to moderately dehydrated, your urine will generally be yellow. If you are severely, or chronically, dehydrated, your urine will appear orange or dark-colored and rust-like. (**Note:** Urine can change color due to the use of vitamins and other nutritional supplements, often appearing bright yellow when such supplements are used.)

Do your best to only drink pure, filtered water, avoiding tap water because most tap water contains toxins, such as chlorine and fluoride (both of which have been linked to cancer despite being approved as tap water additives by government regulatory agencies), as well as various other contaminants.

11. Add more garlic and onions to your diet, both of which have been shown to provide anticancer and immune-boosting benefits. The anticancer benefits garlic and onions provide are due to a compound they contain called allium (*allium sativum* in garlic and *allium cepa* in onions). Research has shown that diets high in garlic and onions lower the risk of a number of cancer, including breast, colorectal, kidney (renal), ovarian, and prostate cancers, as well as cancers of the throat (esophagus, larynx, and pharynx).

12. Add more spice to your diet. Various spices are known to have anticancer properties, as well as supporting healthy digestion and overall gastrointestinal tract function. These include cinnamon, garlic powder, ginger, and turmeric.

13. Drink organic, green tea. The anticancer properties of green tea and its main active ingredient, *epigallocatechin gallate* (EGCG), have for decades been extensively studied by scientists all over the world. This research has shown that both green tea and

EGCG extract can prevent and delay the onset of cancer and to help prevent the onset of secondary cancers and the recurrence of cancers in cancer patients once they have achieved remission.

Green tea and EGCG have also been shown to inhibit the self-renewal and expression of transcription factors in human cancer stem cells (CSCs). CSCs, as you learned in Chapter 1, are a major cause of cancer recurrence and metastasis.

When drinking green tea, be sure to only use brands that are certified organic. This is important, because many brands contain green tea grown and harvested in China that are often laced with heavy metals and other harmful ingredients.

The Anticancer Benefits of Cruciferous Vegetables: Ongoing research suggests that making cruciferous vegetables a staple food group in your diet can also help prevent cancer. Vegetables in this category include arugula, bok choy, broccoli, broccoli rabe, Brussels sprouts, cabbage, cauliflower, collard greens, daikon root, horse radish, kale, kohlrabi, mustard greens, radish, rutabaga, turnips, and watercress. All of these vegetables are rich in fiber and various essential nutrients, such as calcium, carotenoids (beta-carotene, lutein, zexanthin), folate (a B vitamin that repairs DNA damage), and vitamins C, E, and K, as well as minerals and other plant compounds that support health on a cellular level.

Cruciferous vegetables also contain sulfur-containing chemicals known as glucosinolates. According to the National Cancer Institute (NCI), "During food preparation, chewing, and digestion, the glucosinolates in cruciferous vegetables are broken down to form biologically active compounds such as indoles, nitriles, thiocyanates, and isothiocyanates. Indole-3-carbinol (an indole) and sulforaphane (an isothiocyanate) have been most frequently examined for their anticancer effects.

"Indoles and isothiocyanates have been found to inhibit the development of cancer in several organs in rats and mice, including the bladder, breast, colon, liver, lung, and stomach. Studies in animals and experiments with cells grown in the laboratory have identified several potential ways in which these compounds may help prevent cancer:

- They help protect cells from DNA damage.
- They help inactivate carcinogens.
- They have antiviral and antibacterial effects.
- They have anti-inflammatory effects.
- They induce cell death (apoptosis).
- They inhibit tumor blood vessel formation (angiogenesis) and tumor cell migration (needed for metastasis)."

Human studies indicate that cruciferous vegetables may also reduce the risk of certain cancers, including breast cancer, colon (but not rectal) cancer in women (but not men), lung cancer, and prostate cancer.

"A few studies have shown that the bioactive components of cruciferous vegetables can have beneficial effects on biomarkers of cancer-related processes in people," according to the NCI. «For example, one study found that indole-3-carbinol was more effective than placebo in reducing the growth of abnormal cells on the surface of the cervix. In addition, several case-control studies have shown that specific forms of the gene that encodes glutathione S-transferase, which is the enzyme that metabolizes and helps eliminate isothiocyanates from the body, may influence the association between cruciferous vegetable intake and human lung and colorectal cancer risk."

Another reason why cruciferous vegetables can protect against cancer is because they are rich sources of a nutrient indole known as diindolylmethane, or DIM, which is produced in the body from indole-3-carbinol after cruciferous vegetables are digested and metabolized.

According to integrative physician Isaac Eliaz, MD, an expert in the use of nutrition and nutritional supplements to prevent and help reverse cancer, "Research shows that DIM controls a number of key proteins associated with inflammation, immunity, cancer formation and cellular behavior, as well as hormone metabolism. Importantly, DIM is shown to limit angiogenesis, the process that that creates blood vessels to feed the tumor. In addition, DIM also supports apoptosis.

"DIM also supports the immune system, helping to increase defenses against cancer, as well as infections and other assaults. One way DIM strengthens immunity is by helping the body produce more interferon-gamma, which directly stimulates the immune response."

DIM's anticancer benefits are also due to its effects on estrogen metabolism. "When estrogens get broken down, they can turn into either beneficial estrogen metabolites, acting as antioxidants, or they can become problematic estrogen metabolites associated with cancer and other chronic health conditions," Eliaz adds."This relationship with estrogen also makes DIM a potent detoxifier. Many harmful estrogen metabolites are toxins that are consumed or enter the body through skin, inhalation or other routes of exposure.

"These estrogen-mimicking chemicals, also known as endocrine disruptors, are commonly found in plastics, body care products, environmental pollutants, and numerous other everyday sources. The estrogen-like nature of these compounds tricks the body into allowing them to attach to estrogen and other hormone receptor sites, and wreak havoc. Ongoing exposure to estrogen mimics disrupts normal cell signaling and interferes with essential biological processes. But thankfully, DIM helps to remove these harmful estrogen-like compounds, and supports healthy hormone balance in both women and men."

Food Allergies and Sensitivities

Even when the above healthy eating guidelines are adopted, their benefits can be negated by food allergies and sensitivities (a milder form of food allergies), both of which are quite common today. Ironically, the foods that people are most often allergic or sensitive to are usually the foods they crave most. When they eat such foods they may initially feel satisfied and experience an improved mood. Later on, however, they may start to experience a wide range of symptoms that neither they nor their doctors suspect are caused by the foods they eat. In some cases, such symptoms can take as long as four days to manifest, which is one of the reasons they are likely to be misdiagnosed.

The following are often telltale warning signs of food allergies and sensitivities.

Physical Symptoms: dark circles, swelling or wrinkles under the eyes; vascular headaches; faintness or dizziness; sleepiness soon after a meal; insomnia; frequent waking during the night, or premature waking followed by an inability to return to sleep; runny or stuffy nose; postnasal drip; excessive mucus; watery eyes and/or blurred vision; ringing of the ears; earaches; recurrent ear infections (particularly common among children); sinusitis; sore throats, hoarseness or chronic coughing; gagging; heart palpitations; chest congestion; mucus or undigested food in the stool; nausea; vomiting; diarrhea; constipation; bloating after meals; flatulence; abdominal pains or cramping; extreme thirst; coated tongue; anal or vaginal itch; hives or rashes; dermatitis; brittle nails and hair; dry skin; dandruff; skin pallor; muscle ache; weakness and fatigue; arthritic symptoms or joint pain; symptoms of PMS; frequent or urgent urination; and obesity.

Psychological Symptoms: anxiety or panic attacks; depressions; crying jags; aggressive behavior; irritability; mental dullness or lethargy; confusion; excessive daydreaming; restlessness; poor work habits; inability to concentrate; slurred speech; and indifference or lack of enthusiasm for life.

The most common food allergy culprits are foods such as chocolate, corn, milk and dairy products, peanuts, shellfish, soy and soy products, and wheat. Nightshade vegetables such as eggplant, peppers, and potatoes are other common triggers of allergies and sensitivities, as are tomatoes, but any food can potentially be a cause. The more often foods are eaten on a regular basis the more likely it is that food allergies can follow. For this reason, many health practitioners recommend not eating any food more than every four days. Eating in this manner is known as a "rotation diet." Following a rotation diet can lessen the risk of food allergies and sensitivities, and help prevent you from developing them in the future.

Lectins: Foods containing lectins are another source of food allergies and sensitivities and a cause of other health problems. Lectins are a type of sticky proteins that bind to carbohydrates in plants order to protect the plants from threats by predators. Lectin-containing foods include all beans, grains, eggplant, lentils, peas, peppers, potatoes, taro, tomato extracts (but not tomatoes themselves), wheat, wheat germ, and fruits such as artichokes, jackfruit, limes, mango, and watermelon. Certain spices, such as allspice and cinnamon also contain lectins.

When lectin foods are consumed, they can trigger a wide range of symptoms, including bloating, chronic fatigue, celiac disease, irritable bowel syndrome, sinus problems, and weight gain, as well as overall impairment of immune function.

Lectins cause these health issues because of how they bind to carbohydrate molecules located on the surface of red blood cells (RBCs). Lectins often bind to multiple red blood cells at the same time, causing them to clump together and preventing them from entering the capillaries to provide oxygen to other cells, since RBCs can only travel through capillaries in single file. As a result, because oxygen delivery to other cells is diminished, the cells aren't able to produce energy efficiently. In addition, lactic acid begins to build up in the body's tissues, leading to impaired metabolic function that can cause disease.

To reduce the risk of lectin foods causing RBC clumping, consider taking digestive enzymes 30 minutes before or with meals. Cooking beans and legumes overnight, or even for one hour in a pressure-cooker, can reduce the harmful effects of these foods on red blood cells.

Food Preparation and Food Combining

How you cook foods can impact your gut health for better or worse. The best cooking methods are baking, boiling, sautéing and steaming foods. Grilling and frying should be used sparingly because they can create toxic substances called advanced glycation end products, or AGEs, which have been linked to accelerated aging and many chronic degenerative diseases.

If you do choose to grill or fry, use healthy oils that do not quickly oxidize, such as ghee or organic, cold-pressed, unrefined coconut oil.

In general, the less that foods are cooked, the more the nutrients they contain that will be available for your body to use, especially vital enzymes and certain vitamins, as these can be destroyed when foods are cooked at high temperatures.

The cookware you use is also important. Avoid using aluminum, stainless steel, and most nonstick pots and pans. Better cookware options include ceramic metal cookware, and porcelain and glass (Pyrex and Corning) products.

How food is combined in meals is also important. Improper food combining is one of the primary factors that cause gas, flatulence, heartburn, an upset stomach, and other gastrointestinal problems. What's worse, the resulting poor digestion can also contribute to malnutrition, even when you eat healthy foods.

The principle of food combining is based on how the foods you eat are digested. When you eat foods high in proteins, such as meat, fish, or poultry, your body will digest it in the stomach. To do so effectively, your stomach needs to create a temporary highly acidic environment (a pH between 1-3).

By contrast, digestion of foods high in starchy carbohydrates begins in the mouth they are chewed and is then completed in the small intestines. This process requires a much less acidic or mildly alkaline environment (pH between 5-10).

Combining protein-rich foods with starchy carbohydrate foods during meals forces your body to attempt to digest the protein foods in a highly acidic environment while simultaneously digesting the starchy carbohydrates in an environment that is mildly alkaline, or at least less acidic. The end result is that both food groups end up partially undigested, causing the undigested elements to build up in the colon, where they will decompose and ferment, creating toxins and mucus.

These food-combining guidelines will make your meal choices easier and healthier.

1. Eat protein-rich foods (meats, fish, poultry, dairy) away from starchy carbohydrate vegetables.

2. Non-starchy carbohydrate vegetables, on the other hand, can be combined with either protein-rich foods or starchy carbohydrates since they won't interfere with the digestion of either proteins or starchy carbohydrates.

3. Fruits are best eaten alone at least 45 minutes prior to other meals, and several hours after a previous meal.

4. Do not combine acid and sweet fruits together. Examples of acid fruits are grapefruit, lemons, and oranges, while sweet fruits include bananas, dates, and raisins.

5. Do not eat more than four or five fruits at a time. In addition, melons are best eaten alone.

It is also best to eat fruits and vegetables when they are in season and, if possible, grown locally. For many people, at least 70 percent of the foods in each meal should be eaten raw or only slightly cooked, while for others cooked foods are the healthier option. This depends in large part on their metabolic type, which is discussed later in this chapter.

Eating To Maintain Your Body's Acid/Alkaline (pH) Balance

Health is all about balance. Inside of your body's cells, tissues, and organs this means having balanced pH levels.

Acid-alkaline balance is determined by measuring pH. pH refers to the relative concentration of hydrogen ions in blood, urine, and saliva. It is a measurement of the acid-alkaline ratio of the body's fluids and tissues. When this ratio is balanced, good health results. When pH levels are imbalanced, proper absorption and utilization of nutrients is interrupted, which impairs cellular energy production, setting the stage for disease.

pH is measured on a scale of 0 to 14. A pH of 7 is considered neutral. A pH reading below 7 is an indication of acidity, and readings above 7 indicate an alkaline condition. In order to thrive, blood chemistry needs to be slightly alkaline, with a pH of 7.365.

Many doctors and health researchers dismiss the importance of eating in a way that supports pH balance, pointing out that the body's own homeostatic mechanisms maintain blood pH levels on their own. This is true. However, what these critics ignore is what the body must do in order to cope with a diet consisting primarily of acid-producing foods and beverages. To neutralize their acidifying effects, your body must call on its stores of the acid-quenching minerals calcium, magnesium, and potassium, all of which play hundreds of other important roles in your body. Eating primarily acidifying foods depletes your body of these vital minerals. Conversely, eating mostly alkalizing foods replenishes your body's supply of these minerals.

The acidifying, alkalizing, or neutral effects produced by foods and beverages are far more significant, in terms of your health, than their pH values prior to their consumption. For example, a number of foods that are acidic in nature, such as certain citrus fruits and vinegars, have an alkalizing effect in the body once they are digested and metabolized. Knowing the effects foods and beverages will have on your pH levels is a key to choosing your foods wisely.

Acidifying foods, beverages, and condiments include alcohol, breads, caffeine products (chocolate, coffee, black tea), fish, most grains, legumes, meats and poultry, milk and dairy products, all refined and processed foods, most seeds and nuts, soda, sugars and artificial sweeteners, tap water, and yeast products.

Alkalizing foods and beverages include all green vegetables, most colored vegetables, cold-pressed oils (flaxseed, olive, coconut, avocado, hemp), sprouts, certain fruits and nuts, herbs and spices, and mineral water. These should make up the biggest portions of every meal you consume. The foundation of every alkalizing meal is plenty of fresh vegetables (ideally organic). Raw vegetables also make an ideal snack food during the day.

Most people do well on a diet consisting of between 60 to 80 percent of foods that are alkalizing. It is also important to eat more alkalizing foods at every meal, rather than eating all your alkalizing foods at one or two meals, and eating acidifying foods the rest of the day. This includes snacks.

The Acid-Alkaline Food Guide by Susan Brown, PhD and Larry Trivieri Jr is an excellent resource to learn about the effect 100s of the most common foods, beverages, and condiments have on the body's pH levels.

Three Other Keys to Improving Digestion and Overall Gut Health

The use of enyzmes, prebiotic, and probiotic supplements, as well as bolstering and supporting hydrochloric acid (HCl) production in the stomach, are other steps you can take to improve and maintain digestion and create better gut health.

Enzymes: Enzymes are specific proteins that are involved in every chemical reaction that occurs in your body. Were it not for enzymes, none of the vitamins, minerals, hormones, and numerous other substances in your body could be activated.

Two enzyme classes—digestive enzymes and pancreatic enzymes—can improve digestion and gut health when taken with meals. Pancreatic enzymes provide additional important benefits when taken away from meals.

Digestive enzymes naturally occur in fruits and vegetables, and are also secreted by the salivary glands, pancreas, and small intestine, as well as by cells in the lining of the stomach. They enable to body to digest and metabolize the proteins, fats, and carbohydrates contained in foods. Enzymes in foods are often depleted due to the use of pesticides and herbicides, pasteurization, genetic engineering, and irradiation. Microwaving and cooking at high temperatures also destroy enzymes in foods.

Digestive enzymes include protease, which digests proteins; amylase, which digests carbohydrates: lipase, which digests fats, and cellulase, which digests soluble fiber. Other types of digestive enzymes include bromelain, papaya leaf or papain, serrapeptase, lumbrokinase, and nattokinase.

Taking digestive enzymes with meals supports proper digestion and improves absorption of the nutrients foods contain. Enzyme supplements also spare the body from having to use its own enzyme supply, resulting in less energy use by the body for digestion. Research has found that the regular use of digestive enzymes with meals both enhances digestion and also helps prevent and reverse a variety of gastrointestinal problems while also boosting immune function.

Pancreatic enzymes are derived from animals, usually pigs. They are also produced by the pancreas and support digestion. However, their greater benefits are derived when they are taken away from meals, as was first shown by the English scientist John Beard.

Beginning in 1902, Beard worked with a surgeon to inject pancreatic extracts directly into cancerous tumors, with considerable success. Dr. William Kelley was influenced by and furthered Beard's research when he developed his Metabolic Typing Diet. Pancreatic enzymes played an important role in helping the patients Dr. Kelley treated recover from cancer.

When taken away from meals, pancreatic enzymes enter directly into the bloodstream and digest undigested protein molecules, foreign particles, viruses, and other harmful microorganisms in the gut. They can also help repair internal scar tissue caused by inflammation and protect against a variety of inflammatory disease conditions, including cancer.

Prebiotics and Probiotics: As discussed earlier, proper functioning of your GI tract depends on the healthy bacteria in your gut, also known as probiotic bacteria. The benefits of probiotic bacteria begin at birth when they first start to colonize the GI tract of newborns after delivery. Human breast milk contains an abundant supply of probiotics known as *bifidobacteria* that support the proper development of babies' digestive and immune systems. Lack of bifidobacteria during early childhood can cause allergies and poor absorption of nutrients.

In addition to supporting digestive function, probiotics sustain gut health by helping produce various substances that kill or deactivate harmful, disease-causing bacteria, viruses, and yeasts. They also enhance the function of natural killer (NK) cells, another reason why they can help prevent and aid in the reversal of cancer.

Many people lack enough probiotic bacteria due to poor diet, modern-day food production techniques, an over-reliance on antibiotics and other pharmaceutical drugs, and other factors. Probiotic deficiencies also occur as we age.

Because they are alive, probiotic bacteria must eat. Foods rich in *prebiotics* provide this nourishment and stimulate their growth and activity. Instead of being digested by the body, prebiotics in food are digested by the bacteria.

Organic yogurt with active probiotic cultures can help replenish friendly bacteria, as can fermented foods such as kimchi, miso, sauerkraut and tempeh. Eating foods rich in prebiotics can also help. Such foods are also good sources of fiber and include asparagus, broccoli, Jerusalem artichokes, sunflower seeds, leeks and onions. Whole grains, such as barley, oats, and wheat, also contain prebiotic compounds, but because of the risk such foods have for triggering fungal overgrowth, they are best avoided, or at least minimized in your diet.

If these dietary measures alone are not enough to boost friendly bacteria levels, consider using inulin. Inulin is a type of fiber found in chicory root and in some of the prebiotic foods mentioned above. Research shows that inulin acts as an excellent aid to digestion because it stimulates the growth of healthy gut bacteria, particularly *Bifidobacteria* and *Lactobacilli*. Inulin also helps to slow overall digestion, thereby enhancing the absorption of nutrients from food. Inulin increases stool bulk and promotes regularity, as well, helping to eliminate waste products from food faster and more efficiently. Inulin supplements are available in both capsule and powder form. Powdered inulin may be preferable for most people because it easily dissolves in water to make a drink you can consume once a day.

Hydrochloric Acid (HCl) Supplments: When you eat, your stomach secretes hydrochloric acid (HCl) to help break down food. This causes the pancreas to secrete bicarbonate, a form of alkalizing salt that neutralizes, or buffers, HCL after it performs its function. If HCl is not neutralized it can interfere with pancreatic enzymes that are also necessary for proper digestion. Poor diet, nutrient deficiencies, and chronic environmental, emotional, and illness-induced stress can interfere with this process. Low stomach acid production disrupts the body's entire digestive system, causing acid-alkaline imbalance and poor absorption of vitamins and minerals.

The most common symptom of this imbalance is heartburn, due to over-acidity. Other symptoms include nausea, cramping, gas, bloating, constipation, diarrhea, undigested food in stool, bad breath, and brittle and dry hair, skin and nails. Low stomach acid can also lead to cancer, diabetes, arthritis, malnutrition, and other conditions.

Research published as early as the 1960s found that in most cases of abnormal HCl production, *too little* HCl is being produced, not too much. This is especially true as we age. When HCl is deficient, certain foods, especially proteins, are only partially digested and begin fermenting in the stomach and intestine, causing inflammation in the small intestine and impairing how well nutrients are absorbed and metabolized.

Supplements that can boost HCl production include de-glycyrrhizinated licorice (DGL), mastic gum, and betaine HCl, all of which stimulate the production of more stomach acid.

Get and Stay Active

In addition to all of the above recommendations, there is one other important step you can take to improve your gut and overall health: exercise. Exercise can significantly improve gut health and function because of how it enhances digestion and promotes healthy and regular bowel movements so that your body easily and efficiently eliminates wastes created after food is digested. In addition, exercise burns calories and helps to maintain healthy metabolism, both of which supply your body with more energy o perform its many tasks, including those that occur within the gastrointestinal system.

You will learn how and why regular exercise is so vital for preventing and helping to reverse cancer in the Chapter 10.

Eating According To Your Metabolic Type

As I noted earlier, there is no such thing as a one-size-fits-all diet that is healthy for everyone because each of us has unique biochemical needs. Knowing and eating according to your biochemical individuality, or metabolic type, makes it easier for your body to digest and assimilate the nutrients foods contain, and also helps maintain proper tissue pH balance.

With regard to diet and cancer, the discoveries of William Donald Kelley, DDS, beginning is the 1960s have played an important role in broadening our understanding of how and why the best diet for each person is based on metabolic type.

Kelley's research began after he was diagnosed with late-stage pancreatic cancer and told that he only had 60 days to live. He rejected his prognosis and began experimenting with his diet in an effort to cure himself. He succeeded and was cancer-free two months later. He attributed his remission to the dietary changes he'd made, along with his intake of high doses of pancreatic enzymes between meals.

Despite having cured himself, Kelley realized that the diet he chose for himself would not necessarily benefit everyone else. As he continued his research, he concluded that diet needs to be tailored to each person's unique metabolism in order to maintain and support the healthy functioning of the autonomic nervous system (ANS) and its two main branches, the sympathetic and parasympathetic nervous systems (see Chapter 7). In Kelley's view, the ANS greatly influences metabolism.

Kelley also found that people metabolize foods differently and have different rates of cellular oxidation, which results in different rates of food conversion into energy from one person to another. As he continued his research, he identified three main metabolic types: sympathetic-vegetarian (carbohydrate type), parasympathetic-carnivore (protein type), and sympathetic-parasympathetic balanced. He then divided each type into four subset categories, resulting in a combined total of 12 metabolic types.

According to Kelley, sympathetic-vegetarian types generally thrive best on a diet that is comprised of 60 percent carbohydrates, 25 percent protein, and 15 percent fat; parasympathetic-carnivore types do best on the diet of comprised of 40 percent protein, 30 percent carbohydrates, and 30 percent fat; and sympathetic-parasympathetic balanced types do best on a diet consisting of 50 percent carbohydrates, 30 percent protein, and 20 percent fat. These ratios vary, however, depending on which metabolic subset a person is in. Some people also do best on a diet comprised mostly of raw, or uncooked, foods compared to people of other metabolic types.

A complete discussion of Kelley's work is beyond the scope of this book. For more information about the metabolic types Kelley identified, visit https://drkelley.info/dr-kelleys-metabolic-typing.

Testing Methods To Help Determine Your Metabolic Type: Despite the success that Kelley achieved helping patients recover from cancer and other serious disease conditions, following his metabolic typing protocols can be difficult because his methods never gained much recognition during his lifetime and, since his passing, few, if any, health practitioners are carrying on his work. Moreover, in addition to specific diets, Kelley's approach also involved nutritional supplement recommendations that were specific for each individual, along with regular coffee enemas, which for most people are impractical.

Today, most practitioners who consider people's metabolic type have reduced Kelley's 12 metabolic categories down to three basic levels: protein type, carbohydrate type, and dual (protein-carbohydrate) type. Protein types typically do well following a diet rich in fats and proteins and low in carbohydrates. Carbohydrate types do better on a plant-based carbohydrate diet that is low in fats and proteins, especially animal fats and proteins. Dual types do best on a diet with a balance of high quality carbohydrates, fats, and proteins.

Fortunately, with the advent of genetic testing, it is now easier to determine the best foods for you to eat, since your genes play a significant role in shaping your metabolic type.

Today, a number of gene testing services are available for consumers to learn more about their genetic predispositions, potential health risks, and the foods and nutrients that best suit their needs. Among them, I recommend The DNA Company's DNA 360 test because of how comprehensive it is compared to other gene testing companies. Instead of simply providing information about genetic predispositions and indicating potential health risks once test results have been analyzed, The DNA Company provides an action plan to help clients most effectively implement the dietary and other lifestyle recommendations the test results indicate are most optimal for restoring and maintaining good health, including recommendations for maximizing healthy sleep, hormone and immune function, cardiovascular health, and the body's detoxification pathways. You can learn more at www.TheDNACompany.com.

Cholesterol and fat (lipid) testing can also be used to help determine your metabolic type. One such company that analyzes cholesterol and lipid profiles is Verisana, which offers a dried blood spot test based on a blood sample you can take from the comfort of your home. The sample is then sent to the company's lab for analysis, with the results then sent back to you, including detailed information about your metabolic type. The company also offers a variety of other tests, including gut and microbiome tests. Visit www.verisana.com/shop/cholesterol-and-lipids-test for more information.

Each of the above tests can be ordered by consumers directly from the companies without the need of a doctor. However, once you obtain your results, discussing them with your physician is highly advisable.

Another type of testing that I recommend is an amino acid profile. This test can be conducted using either a blood plasma or urine sample or, in some cases, both samples. This test screens for potential amino acid imbalances, especially deficiencies. While most often used to screen for health problems in infants and children, the amino acid test is useful for anyone concerned about detecting possible health issues.

Amino acids are used by the body to form proteins. They play important roles in many body functions, including regulating blood flow, blood pressure, food metabolism, growth, liver and lung function, tissue repair, and overall immunity. Various amino acids, such as cysteine, also act as neurotransmitters, supporting cognitive function and helping to protect against mental health issues such as anxiety and depression. An adequate and balanced supply of amino acids is also necessary for healthy sleep.

In addition to evaluating amino acid balance, the plasma amino acid test also looks at detoxification, gastrointestinal, neurological, and magnesium-dependent markers, as well as other providing information about vitamin levels, such as the B vitamins, folate, B6, and B12. Plasma amino acid tests are typically performed after fasting for a minimum of eight hours. The information they provide can be a good indication of whether or not a change in diet is advisable.

The urine amino acid test screens for abnormalities in the kidneys. It can be performed as a spot urine test using morning urine, or as a test of urine samples collected over a 24-hour period. Both amino acid tests can be ordered by your physician.

To restore amino acid balance should testing reveal deficiencies, I recommend the formula Perfect Amino. People with cancer, however, should not supplement with amino acid formulas on their own due to research that indicates certain amino acids, such as arginine, glutamate, and methionine, may act as fuel sources for cancer, promoting cancer cell growth. For this reason, amino acid restrictive diets are now being explored as method of inhibiting the spread of cancer.

Anti-Cancer Diets

Having read this far, you can understand why there is no single diet, regardless of how healthy it may be for others, that is the best choice for all cancer patients. This is why I work with my patients to help them find the diet best suited for their metabolic type, as well as screening for any foods and food ingredients to which they may be sensitive or allergic.

It is also vitally important to assess the current overall health status of cancer patients, including determining how well they are able to eat and metabolize foods to receive the nutrients they contain. In advanced cases of cancer, the first overriding rule is to help patients eat to live. The goal here is to provide them with the nutrients they need to get their strength up, prevent them from "wasting away" (cachexia), and to help restore and maintain their body's homeostasis. Once those goals have been achieved, the next step is to eat to "starve" cancer. This also means eating in a way that supplies patients with all of the nutrients and nutrient co-factors their bodies require, avoiding dietary extremes.

With that in mind, what follow are overviews of the diets that are most worth exploring to prevent and help reverse cancer. Ideally, they are best undertaken under the guidance of a skilled integrative oncologist or other health care specialist who also has training in diet and nutrition.

Plant-Based, Low-Protein Diets: Most of the research into cancer and diet shows that a primarily plant-based diet with low to moderate levels of high quality protein foods is the optimal diet for most people to help prevent and recover from cancer. For some people, this may mean following a vegetarian or even a vegan diet, though I do not recommend them for everyone because of the nutrient deficiencies they can cause, as well as the fact that certain metabolic types cannot thrive on them. Overall, I have found in my practice that plant-based, low-protein diets offer the best benefit for most types of cancer because of the beneficial effects they have on modulating the hormones involved in most cancers, as well as for their antioxidant, anti-inflammatory, and other benefits.

One of the most widely studied diets in this category proven to offer a wide array of health benefits is the **Mediterranean Diet.** It gets its name because it is based on the cultural and lifestyle habits of people from Greece, Crete, southern France, Italy, Morocco, Spain, and other countries in the region. Researchers have found that people from these parts of the world have significantly lower rates of heart disease than their northern European and North American counterparts, as well as an overall lower incidence of most types of cancer, diabetes, and other disease conditions.

The Mediterranean Diet is free of foods high in saturated fats, such as beef and pork, and, with the exception of certain low-fat cheeses, such as feta, and yogurt, is also low on dairy products. Sugar, sweets, and simple (white) carbohydrate foods are also kept to a minimum or eliminated altogether.

In place of such foods, hallmarks of the diet include:

- Eating seven to ten or more servings of fresh fruits and vegetables per day. One way to easily accomplish this is to prepare salads for both lunch and dinner, making sure to include a wide range of vegetables. Walnuts, pine nuts, or other healthy toppings can be added to salads to make them even more nutritious.
- Substituting fish high in omega-3 oils in place of beef and pork. Healthy fish choices include sardines, wild caught salmon, mackerel, trout, and herring. Lean poultry (free-range chicken and turkey) can also be consumed a few times each week, as can lamb, another staple food of a number of Mediterranean countries.
- Eating nuts such as almonds, Brazil nuts, pecans, and walnuts as snacks.
- Eating complex carbohydrate foods such as beans, barley, rich, quinoa, and whole-grain pasta. (Ideally, however, your consumption of carbohydrate foods at each meal should be smaller than your intake of non-starchy vegetables.)
- Cooking with olive oils, and using olive oil in place of butter, margarine, and commercial salad dressings.

The Mediterranean Diet is rich in omega-3 fats. Saturated fat that comes from animal meat and butter is rarely consumed, and hydrogenated fats that come from fried, fast, and processed foods are all absent from the diet.

The healthy non-hydrogenated unsaturated fats consumed in the Mediterranean diet are from food sources like olive oil, nuts, and fish.

Whole grains are also a part of the diet, but refined carbohydrates like flour bread and white rice are eliminated, as is refined sugar. The diet also includes an abundance of fruits and vegetables, with salads often being a part of lunch and dinner meals.

In addition to fish, poultry, and lamb, proteins in the Mediterranean Diet are supplied from various legumes, such as chick peas, kidney and fava beans, and lentils, nuts, and cheeses.

I recommend a modified version of the Mediterranean Diet that increases the amount of fresh, non-starchy vegetables in place of grains and other starchy plant foods in order to avoid the spike in insulin levels that starchy foods can cause. Healthy vegetable substitutes include salad-variety vegetables and root vegetables such as broccoli, asparagus, etc.

Research confirms that the Mediterranean Diet helps protect against both the overall incidence of cancer and cancer deaths. One clinical trial found that the diet reduced the risk for all cancers by 61 percent, and that it is especially effective for reducing the risk of biliary tract, bladder, breast, colorectal, gastric, liver, lung (especially among people who smoke), and prostate cancers, as well as cancers of the head, neck, and gallbladder. The diet has also been shown to reduce the risk of cervical, endometrial, ovarian, and other cancers of the female reproductive tract.

In addition, the Mediterranean Diet helps to prevent and reverse unhealthy weight gain and obesity, both of which increase cancer risk. Moreover, research has confirmed that there is a lower overall incidence of cancer in Mediterranean countries, compared to the cancer rates in northern Europe and the United States, that is directly attributable to the dietary habits in those countries. The widespread use of olive oil in such cultures has also been shown to be a factor, as well as the high nutritional content and overall antioxidant and anti-inflammatory effects of their staple foods.

Studies also confirm that the more closely one follows a Mediterranean Diet, the lower the risk for cancer becomes. One such study involved over 25,000 men and women in Greece who were studied for nearly eight years and evaluated during that time using a 10-point compliance assessment scale. The lowest risk for cancer was found in those who adhered to all 10 points. This was particularly true among the women in the study.

Research also shows that the Mediterranean Diet helps protect healthy cells from DNA damage, supports apoptosis, inhibits cancer cell growth and metastasis, and disrupts angiogenesis. In addition, the full array of nutrients and fiber the diet supplies are known to reduce insulin resistance and support liver function, including its role as a vital organ of detoxification.

Studies also show that the diet modulates hormones and various growth factors in the body that are susceptible to cancer, and reduces the stimulation of hormones and both extra- and intracellular transmitting pathways involved in the onset and growth of cancer. Research also demonstrates that the diet improves and maintains the health of the gut microbiome.

The Ketogenic Diet: This diet, also known as the "keto" diet, has gained in popularity in recent years because of its potential to prevent and reverse cancer.

Ketogenic diets restrict carbohydrate intake to no more than 25 to 50 grams per day (approximately 5 to 10 percent of total food intake). Keto diets are also high in healthy fats, with fats comprising 60 to 75 percent of meals, with high quality protein foods comprising the rest meals.

Breads, cereals, oatmeal, muesli, pasta, rice and other grains and wheat products (including couscous and quinoa), potatoes and yams, most legumes, and snack foods such as chips, bagels, and crackers, are strictly prohibited in keto diets, as are all sugary "sweet" foods and beverages, ice cream, unsweetened yogurt, and fruits with high sugar content, such as bananas, grapes, and mangos. (Berries, coconuts, lemons, and limes are permitted.)

The goal of a ketogenic diet is to shift the body's cells away from using carbohydrate-derived glucose for fuel, to using ketones (fatty acids produced by the liver that are derived from high-fat foods) as the body's primary energy source. The process by which this shift to using ketones as fuel occurs is known as ketosis, or keto-adaptation. The underlying theory of the ketogenic diet for cancer is that the shift to ketones will starve cancer cells because glucose (sugar) acts as cancer cells' primary fuel.

Although its use as an anticancer diet is relatively recent, the ketogenic diet itself has been in use since in the 1920s, when it was first shown to be effective for treating diabetes. The first evidence for this appeared before the discovery of insulin. Since that time, research has shown that ketogenic diets are also effective for treating and reducing epilepsy symptoms, including in childhood epilepsy and in cases for which medications are ineffective.

Because of its long-documented benefits as a treatment for diabetes, today the ketogenic diet is often recommended to control blood glucose levels in both pre-diabetic and diabetic patients. It is also used to help reverse unhealthy weight gain and obesity. In addition to its potential anticancer benefits, researchers are also exploring its possible benefits for helping to reverse and prevent heart disease, as well as Alzheimer's disease and dementia, and other neurological conditions, such as Parkinson's disease.

Research shows that a ketogenic diet may offer benefit in support of an overall cancer treatment plan. However, to date, the benefits that research has found in this regard cannot be considered conclusive because no long-term data on ketogenic diets and cancer exist because all of the studies in this area are recent. In addition, the studies typically only included a small number of test subjects, and in some cases they were also poorly designed.

Still, the research does indicate that a ketogenic diet may be beneficial for some types of cancer. This is especially true for glioblastoma, the most common and aggressive form of brain cancer. Studies also show that the diet may have benefit for cases of endometrial and ovarian cancers. In addition, research indicates that the diet may support and enhance the anticancer effects of chemotherapy and radiation.

A number of possible reasons have been proposed to explain this, including the likelihood that ketogenesis creates a metabolic environment within the body that is unsuitable for cancer cells to thrive within while also inhibiting angiogenesis. Some research also indicates that ketones may have a direct toxic effect on cancer cells and tumors, as was shown in a laboratory experiment when the effects of ketone supplements were studied on cancer cells.

Moreover, research shows that ketones reduce insulin and insulin-like growth factors known to trigger and support the onset and spread of cancer cells and tumors. This effect, as well as the fact that ketones also reduce the production of free radicals while simultaneously boosting antioxidants levels in the body, indicates that a keto diet may also be helpful for preventing cancer. The ketogenic diet's documented weight loss benefits is also a factor, since the majority of people who follow it typically exhibit healthy weight loss.

The diet is not without its shortcomings, however. Common side effects of the diet include constipation, fatigue (especially during exercise or other physical activities), gastrointestinal upsets, muscle cramps, nausea, and poor sleep. Other possible risks include dehydration, hypoglycemia (low blood sugar), gout, and kidney stones. The diet also makes it difficult to obtain a full range of fiber and nutrients, especially the polyphenols and other phytonutrients found in the fruits and vegetables that are off limits when the diet is followed.

For all of these reasons, I do not advise following a ketogenic diet unless you do so under the supervision of a nutritionally-oriented integrative physician familiar with its use.

I hope the information in this chapter encourages you to commit to making healthy eating a key part of your daily lifestyle.

In the next chapter, you will learn how and why you should consider augmenting your diet with nutritional supplements and other anticancer products, and learn which ones I most recommend.

Chapter 9

Cancer-Fighting Supplements

While a shift to a healthier diet is of paramount importance, due to a variety of factors, such as environmental pollutants, the stresses of daily life, and modern farming and food packaging methods, a healthy diet alone, no matter how optimal, is rarely enough to maintain good health. This is particularly true for anyone dealing with cancer. Therefore, I always assess my cancer patient's overall nutritional status and most often recommend the use of various nutritional supplements proven by research to provide anticancer benefits that support their overall treatment program.

Determining Your Nutritional Status

Just as the cancer-screening tests covered in Chapter 1 are essential for knowing whether or not you have cancer or are at risk for developing, so too is knowing your overall nutritional status and whether or not you suffer from any nutritional imbalances. Most often such imbalances are due to nutrient deficiencies, but in some cases excessive levels of a nutrient, such as iron, can be the problem, as you learned in Chapter 2.

Such imbalances can usually and quickly be determined using various blood tests ordered by your physician or, in certain cases, yourself through a number of reputable, high-quality labs that do not require a physician's prescription. (You'll find a list of these labs in the Resources section in the back of this book.)

What follow are a list of blood tests that physicians commonly order for their patients, often as part of an overall annual medical checkup:

- **CBC blood test:** The CBC (complete blood count) test measures the amount of red and white blood cells, plus platelets in your blood.

- **BUN blood test:** BUN stands for "blood urea nitrogen". Elevated BUN levels are an indicator of possible kidney damage or disease.

- **Creatinine blood test:** Creatinine is a waste product produced by your muscles and excreted by your kidneys. The creatinine test is usually ordered in conjunction with the BUN test to compare the ratio level of each substance. Healthy ratios of BUN to creatinine range from 10-1 to 20-1. Ratios above this range indicate a lack of blood flow to the kidneys, which can be an indicator of congestive heart failure, gastrointestinal bleeding, or chronic, low-grade dehydration, while ratios below this range can be signs of malnutrition or liver problems.

- **Glucose blood test:** This test is used to determine your fasting blood sugar (glucose) level.

- **Lipid Panel:** This test measures your HDL, LDL, total cholesterol, and triglyceride levels, all of which are markers for both cardiovascular health and disease.

- **25-hydroxy-vitamin D, or 1,25-dihydroxy vitamin D:** These tests are used to determine vitamin D levels in your bloodstream.

- **Liver blood tests (ALT/AST/ALP/GGT):** These tests measure liver enzymes called *aminotranferases*. Elevated ALT and AST are indications of impaired liver function, liver damage, or disease.

- **Gamma-Glutamyl-Transferase (GGT):** GGT is an enzyme produced in the liver bile ducts, kidneys and a few other organs. This test measures the amount of GGT in the blood to screen for inflammation in the liver and/or the bile ducts.

- **Prothrombin Test:** In addition to analyzing the body's blood clotting performance and detecting bleeding or clotting disorders, this test can help detect liver problems, vitamin K deficiencies, immune diseases, and certain types of cancer, such as leukemia.

- **Uric Acid Test:** The uric acid test is a blood test measures uric acid levels. Elevated uric acid levels can be an indication of gout, risk of kidney stones and other types of kidney disease, and cancer.

- **Comprehensive Metabolic Panel (CMP):** This test includes blood measurements of BUN, creatinine, glucose, ALP (alkaline phosphatase), ALT and AST. It also measures blood levels of albumin, calcium, carbon dioxide (bicarbonate), chloride, sodium, potassium, total bilirubin, and protein. The CMP test is very useful for assessing your body's overall health metabolism, chemical balance, and kidney and liver function.

- **Comprehensive Vitamin and Mineral Panel Tests:** These tests measure vitamin and mineral levels in the bloodstream to determine both vitamin and mineral deficiencies and excesses. (**Note:** Both of these tests can be measured with urine as well as blood.)

- **Thyroid Panel:** The thyroid panel test measures three thyroid hormones—T3, T4, and TSH. It helps doctors determine how well the thyroid is functioning and screens for symptoms of both an overactive and underactive thyroid (hyperthyroidism and hypothyroidism, respectively), and Hashimoto's disease, an autoimmune disease that is the primary cause of hypothyroidism if it persists.

- **B12 and Folic Acid (Folate) Tests:** This test screens for B vitamin deficiencies, especially deficiencies of B12 and folic acid.

- **Homocysteine:** This test is useful for diagnosing malnutrition, folate and vitamin B12 deficiencies, and genetic defects in intracellular methylation enzymes. It can also help detect cardiovascular disease risk.

- **hs-C-reactive Protein (CRP) and Fibrinogen:** These inexpensive tests measure the amount of the pro-inflammatory markers high sensitivity C-reactive protein, or hs-CRP, and fibrinogen in the bloodstream, and can be used to detect chronic inflammation and to monitor your progress as you work to reduce inflammation levels in your body.

- **Hemoglobin A1C (A1C):** The hemoglobin A1C test measures the average amount of glucose in the bloodstream over an 8 to 12 week time period. It is a more accurate marker for diabetes (both type I and type II) and prediabetes than the blood glucose test. In addition, it can be used to screen for other serious health conditions, including heart disease, stroke, nerve damage, kidney disease, and eye damage.

- **Ferritin Test:** This test screens for iron overload and excess free iron (unbound iron in the blood).

- **Mg RBC:** The Mg RBC test measures the amount of magnesium inside the red blood cells and is a far more accurate measurement of your body's overall magnesium status than a standard serum (blood) test.

- **MTHFR:** MTHFR is an abbreviation for a gene that codes for an enzyme called *methylenetetrahydrofolate reductase*. People with a mutation of MTHFR may have difficulty eliminating toxins from the body. In addition, mutations in the *MTHFR* gene have been linked to thrombosis and heart disease, and can lead to blood clots, stroke, embolism, and/or heart attacks. MTHFR mutations can also be a factor in elevated homocysteine levels. The risk of birth defects and difficult pregnancies can also be increased when MTHFR mutations are present.

- **Comprehensive Female or Male Hormone Panel:** This test is available either as a single blood draw or a spit test in which saliva is collected multiple times over a 24-hour period. Hormone panel tests on saliva or blood typically measure the cycling and production of cortisol, DHEA, estradiol, pregnenolone, progesterone, and testosterone. Blood only is used to test thyroid hormones and sex hormone binding globulin (SHBG).
- **DHEA:** This test measures DHEA in the form of DHEA-sulfate (DHEA-s). Low DHEA levels can be indications of a range of diseases, ranging from anxiety and depression, autoimmune and immune disease, cancer, chronic fatigue, dementia, diabetes, heart disease, high blood pressure, low libido, and obesity.

Two other types of testing for nutritional imbalances are the SpectraCell Micronutrient Test (MNT) and autonomic response testing (ART).

SpectraCell Micronutrient Test (MNT): The MNT is a proprietary screening test developed by and only available from SpectraCell Laboratories. What makes it unique is its ability to measure the functional level and capability of micronutrients within white blood cells, which is where metabolism occurs. Unlike standard serum (blood) tests, which only measure and assess the concentration of nutrients in the bloodstream outside of cells, and only provide a snapshot of your health, the MNT provides a longer (4 to 6 months) assessment of a person's nutrient status that addresses the functional impact (performance) of micronutrients, while also taking a person's biochemical individuality into account.

Included in the MNT assessment is information about vitamins A, B1, B2, B3, B5, B6, B12, C, D, E, K2, biotin, folate, and inositol, as well as calcium, chromium, copper, magnesium, manganese, selenium, zinc, various amino acids, fatty acids, plus the antioxidants alpha lipoic acid, coenzyme Q10 (CoQ10), and glutathione. In addition, MNT provides an assessment of a person's carbohydrate metabolism, fructose sensitivity, total antioxidant function, and immune response score.

Among its other clinical applications, MNT can be used to screen for indications of cancer, as well as Alzheimer's and other neurological conditions, autism and other spectrum disorders, cardiovascular disease, diabetes, cellular fatigue, and other conditions.

The MNT can only be ordered by a physician. As of this writing, is not available for residents of New York State.

For more information about SpectraCell Laboratories and MNT, visit www.spectracell.com.

Autonomic Response Testing (ART): ART, sometimes referred to as autonomic reflex screening, is a highly accurate form of muscle testing (kinesiology) developed by Dietrich Klinghardt, MD. My clinical experience has proven it to be a valuable aid for assessing my patients' dietary and nutritional needs, as well as for determining many other aspects of their health.

I refer to ART as a biofeedback enhanced physical exam that uses changes in muscle tone as a primary indicator of my patients' health status. ART assesses the body through the autonomic nervous system (ANS) by observing how it responds to introduced stressors. Since the ANS is in direct contact with every cell, organ, tissue, muscle, and system in the body, the amount of information that can be gained through ART goes beyond that provided by blood tests. ART practitioners use it to not only find out which organ or system of the body may be struggling, but also to determine what nutritional interventions may be needed and why.

In my experience, Autonomic Response Testing is often effective even when other conventional and alternative testing methods fail, and is an effective tool for screening for and helping to treat both acute and chronic illnesses, including cancer. It is also an excellent tool for developing the most effective and restorative nutritional strategies for patients based on their unique needs. This includes helping to determine the best diet for each patient's metabolic type (see Chapter 8).

Dr. Klinghardt has trained a growing number of physicians and other health care practitioners in ART. To locate an ART practitioner near you, visit https://klinghardtinstitute.com/contact-us.

Proven Anticancer Supplements

What follow are overviews of the supplements I most commonly instruct my patients to consider.

Apigenin: Apigenin is a bioflavonoid compound found in a wide variety of fruits and vegetables, as well as in chamomile tea, where it acts as an anti-anxiety agent. It has been used for centuries in various cultures around the world because of the antibacterial and antiviral benefits it provides

Research shows that apigenin also has potent anticancer, anti-inflammatory, and antioxidant properties. Moreover, studies found that its ability to help protect against cancer has to do with how it selectively targets cancer cells, as opposed to normal cells, as well as its ability to help prevent healthy cells from mutating, or devolving, into cancer cells. Studies have also shown that apigenin can induce apoptosis, stimulate immune function, and support the body's detoxification enzymes.

Among the cancers for which apigenin potentially has benefit are adrenal, breast, cervical, colon, liver, lung, ovarian, pancreatic, prostate, skin, stomach, throat, and thyroid cancer, as well as neuroblastoma and blood cancers (leukemia, lymphoma and myeloma).

Apigenin is available as a supplement (primarily as a standardized chamomile extract). It is also available in high quantities in parsley.

Artemesinin: Artemisinin, also known as wormwood, is derived from the *Artemisia* plant and has been a staple herbal remedy for treating malaria for centuries. It is also use to balance certain hormones, especially excess estrogen and prolactin levels. Research shows it is also beneficial for protecting against and fighting more than 50 different types of cancer.

One of the main ways that artemisinin acts as an effective anticancer agent has to do with how it interacts with iron. Excess and unbound levels of iron, as you learned in Chapter 2, are a risk factor for cancer and research proves that cancer cells and tumors need large amount of iron in order to grow. As a result, as cancer takes hold in the body, iron is stored by cancer cells and tumors. When artemesinin comes in contact with iron, it generates free radicals which kill cancer cells. This fact has been confirmed by research, which has also shown that cancer cells are approximately 100 times more susceptible to this cytotoxic effect of artemisinin than normal cells are.

Research also shows that artemesinin disrupts the blood supply to tumors (angiogeneis), triggers apoptosis, and regulates and repairs various genes that protect against cancer, while also inhibiting the activity of various enzymes that are involved in cancer growth.

Artemesinin is available as a fat-soluble supplement. Researchers into its use advise taking it once a day in conjunction with a low-carbohydrate diet, along with vitamin D, organic coconut or extra virgin olive oil, or omega-3 fatty acids, in order to enhance its absorption in the body. It should always be taken at least 3 hours away from meals. Because the body can become used to artemesinin's effects, researcher also advise taking it for 5 to 8 days, then not taking it for 3 days, then repeating this cycle.

Note: Artemesinin should not be used by anyone undergoing radiation therapy, people who smoke, and people taking glutathione supplements.

Coenzyme Q10 (CoQ10): CoQ10 is a fat-soluble antioxidant that is present in most tissues, with the highest concentrations found in the heart, kidneys, liver, and pancreas. CoQ10 is important for cellular energy production because of how it transports protons and electrons into the inner membrane of the mitochondria, where energy is produced. It also supports and boosts immune function, plays key roles in healthy cell growth, and helps repair damaged cells, tissues, and organs. Research has found that cancer patients typically have low levels of CoQ10.

According to the National Cancer Institute (NCI), coenzyme Q10 has been shown to stimulate the immune system of patients with cancer, and to protect the heart from damage caused by a class of chemotherapy drugs called anthracyclines that are known to have the potential to damage the heart.

The NCI adds that while CoQ10 "may show indirect anticancer activity through its effect(s) on the immune system, there is evidence to suggest that analogs of this compound can suppress cancer growth directly.

Analogs of coenzyme Q10 have been shown to inhibit the proliferation of cancer cells *in vitro* and the growth of cancer cells transplanted into rats and mice."

Additional research has found that CoQ10 has the ability to cause cancer cells to self-destruct before they can multiply and grow by inducing apoptosis, thereby preventing metastasis.

To enhance absorption, CoQ10 supplements should be taken with a high-fat meal. It should not be taken during radiation therapy, however, as it reduces the effectiveness of radiation treatments.

Curcumin: Curcumin is the primary active ingredient in turmeric and is available in capsule form as a supplement. More than 50 years of research has confirmed that curcumin supplements provide numerous anticancer benefits that are far greater than those provided by turmeric itself.

Curcumin's benefits are primarily due to its ability to protect against free radical damage and inflammation, increase cellular glutathione levels, induce normal cell death (apoptosis), inhibit tumor growth, inhibit cancer cells from developing their own network of blood vessels that supply nutrient fuel for cancer cells and tumors (angiogenesis), increase the activity of enzymes that help eliminate carcinogens, and block estrogen-mimicking chemicals. Research has also found that curcumin helps prevent and stop the spread of bacterial, fungal, and viral infections that can trigger cancer.

As a potent anti-inflammatory, curcumin inhibits the activation of nuclear factor-kappaB (NF-kB), which, as you learned in Chapter 2, can trigger the expression of pro-inflammatory genes. Curcumin also inhibits the expression of cyclooxygenase-2 (COX-2) and 5-lypoxygenase (5-LOX), two enzymes involved in inflammation. Additionally, curcumin binds to 5-LOX to directly inhibit its activity. These genes and enzymes, when unchecked, play a role in the development and spread of cancer.

Research also shows that curcumin inhibits the expression of various cell surface adhesion molecules, cytokines, and chemokines, all of which are directly related to inflammation, and all of which can cause healthy, normal cells in the body to become cancerous.

Studies also show that curcumin inhibits the effects of tumor-causing reactive oxygen species (ROS), including in white blood cells (leukocytes) within the body's immune system. Additional research shows that curcumin is an effective scavenger of reactive nitrogen species (RNS), which can also cause cancer. Other studies have demonstrated curcumin's protective effects against oxidative damage to the skin, and its ability to protect against cellular DNA damage caused by oxidation, and the oxidation of healthy fats (lipid peroxidation), both of which can cause the formation of cancer cells.

Curcumin's ability to increase cellular glutathione levels is another important health benefit. Glutathione is an important antioxidant that plays a critical role in supporting cellular adaptation to stress. The better cells are able to resist such stress, the more resistant they are to cancer. Research has shown that curcumin elevates cellular glutathione levels through its ability to enhance the gene expression of glutamate cysteine ligase (GCL), an enzyme involved in glutathione synthesis.

Curcumin also blocks health-damaging chemicals from entering inside cells, something that sets it apart from most other natural anticancer compounds. Curcumin is especially effective for preventing estrogen-mimicking chemicals, such as DDT, dioxin, chlordane, and endosulfane, from penetrating inside cells. It does this by its ability to pass through a cell receptor called aryl hydrocarbon, which acts as a cellular doorway. Both estrogen and the chemicals that mimic it also enter cells through aryl hydrocarbon receptors. Because curcumin can compete with them for the receptor, it has the ability to block their access into cells, thus preventing the cells from becoming damaged and turning cancerous.

Like estrogen itself, estrogen-mimicking chemicals promote the growth and spread of breast cancer. One study of human breast cancer cells showed that curcumin reversed the growth of breast cancer cells caused by 17b-estradiol by 98 percent. The same study also found that curcumin reversed breast cancer cell growth caused by DDT by 75 percent. Additional research showed that curcumin reversed the growth of breast cancer cell growth caused by chlordane and endosulfane, both of which also mimic estrogen, by 90 percent. When combined with the soy-derived compound genistein, curcumin resulted in a 100 percent halt to cancer cell growth. Curcumin also has the ability to block other carcinogenic chemicals from entering inside cells. Studies have also found that curcumin's mechanisms of actions in the body are in many ways similar to various classes of anti-cancer drugs, including recently discovered tumor necrosis factor blocking drugs such as Humira, Remicade, and Enbrel, vascular endothelial cell growth factor blocking drugs such as Avastin, human epidermal growth factor receptor blocking drugs such as Erbitux, Erlotinib, and Geftinib, and HER2 blocking drugs such as Herceptin. Cancer researchers and physicians today increasingly employ multi-targeted therapies that combine these different classes of drugs to improve cancer outcomes. Curcumin offers many of these same multi-targeted benefits.

Among the cancers that curcumin has been shown to protect against include bladder, brain, breast, colon, liver, pancreatic, prostate, and skin cancers. It has also been found to offer protection against leukemia, myeloma, and non-Hodgkin's lymphoma.

When choosing a curcumin supplement, look for brands that contain BCM-95®. One of the challenges associated with curcumin supplements is the relatively low bio-availabilty of curcumin once it is isolated from turmeric. Curcumin products with BCM-95 combine curcumin with the essential oils turmeric contains, using a patented process that has been shown to increase absorption by as much as 700 percent, compared to other curcumin and tumeric extract supplements.

EGCG: EGCG stands for epigallocatechin-3-gallate. It belongs to a class of compounds called catechins. EGCG is the most abundant catechin in green tea and considered the primary reason why, as you learned in the last chapter, green tea has been shown to help protect against cancer. The advantage of using EGCG as a nutritional supplement, as opposed to drinking green tea, is that its beneficial anticancer effects can be achieved more easily, since it would require drinking many cups of green tea in order to gain similar benefits as those provided by an EGCG supplement.

According to the NCI, EGCG has "substantial free radical scavenging activity and may protect cells from DNA damage caused by reactive oxygen species." Studies show that EGCG also promotes apoptosis, inhibits angiogenesis and tumor cell invasiveness, and can protect against damage caused by ultraviolet (UV) radiation, thus helping to protect against skin cancer. EGCG has also been shown to support immune function and to activate detoxification enzymes in the body that help prevent the formation of tumors. It also helps prevent tumor formation because of its anti-inflammatory properties, and by inhibiting the expression of oncogenes (genes known to increase the risk of cancer), as well as other cancer-promoting biochemicals in the body. Taken in high doses (over 1,000 mg), EGCG acts as a pro-oxidant, creating oxidative stress in cancer cells, making it an useful aid for enhancing the effects of certain chemotherapy treatments.

In addition to skin cancer (including melanoma), other cancers that EGCG has been shown to protect against include cancers of the bladder and urinary tract, breast, colon, esophageal, lung, pancreas, prostate, and stomach.

Note: Because EGCG can deplete vitamin E stores in the body, taking 400 IU of mixed tocopherol vitamin E containing at least 10 percent gamma tocopherol once a day is also advised.

Ellagic Acid: Ellagic acid (EA) is a compound known to have potent antioxidant properties. It is found in many fruits and nuts, with apples, grapes, pomegranates, blackberries, cranberries, raspberries, and strawberries being among its richest food sources, along with cashews, pecans, pistachios, and walnuts.

Research has established that EA offers strong protection against various cancers. Studies show that EA is able to prevent the formation of cancer cells in part because of its anti-inflammatory effects and its ability to bind to and neutralize free radicals and cancer-causing chemicals.

EA has also been shown to positively influence the expression of genes involved in apoptosis, as well as inhibiting the activity of genes, proteins, and various cellular signaling pathways associated with cancer formation and proliferation. Moreover, studies confirm that EA can inhibit the spread of cancer cells, prevent angiogenesis, and prevent cancer cells from invading the extra-cellular matrix surrounding healthy cells. This matrix is a network consisting of various enzymes, minerals, proteins, and other compounds that provide structural and biochemical support to cells. Other studies indicate that EA may also increase the effectiveness of chemotherapy and radiation therapy to fight tumors.

In addition to its direct anticancer properties, studies show that EA can indirectly protect against cancer because of its ability to regulate lipid (fat) metabolism, thus reducing the risk of insulin resistance, nonalcoholic fatty liver disease, type II diabetes, and unhealthy weight gain and obesity, all of which increase cancer risk.

Cancers for which EA has shown benefit include bladder, blood, breast, cervical, colorectal, liver, non-small cell lung cancer, pancreas, prostate, and ovarian cancers, as well as melanoma.

While ellagic acid can be obtained by eating the fruits and nuts mentioned above, even a diet high in such foods will not supply the dosage levels of EA that were used in studies examining its anticancer benefits, which is why the use of ellagic acid supplements are advisable. Pomegranate extract is the primary ingredient in most brands of EA supplements.

Fermented Wheat Germ Extract (FWGE): Wheat germ is the embryo portion of wheat kernals and is a rich source of vitamins, minerals, and proteins. In studies published in the 1980s, Hungarian scientist and Nobel laureate Abert Szent-Gyorgyi, who, in 1928, became the first person to isolate vitamin C, noted that compounds wheat germ could help restore healthy cell metabolic function. This led his fellow Hungarian scientist Dr. Mate Hidvegi to research FWGE, leading to his invention in the 1990s of a new, fermented wheat germ extract suitable for human consumption. It was originally named as Avermar under the brand names Ave'[R] and Oncomar[R] and sold as a powdered supplement that could be mixed in water or other beverages.

Since that time, Avemar has been extensively researched in both animal and human studies and clinical trials, as well as in vitro with human cell lines, including research carried out to determine Avemar's potential benefits for cancer patients struggling with both the effects of their disease and the side-effects of chemotherapy and radiation therapy.

The studies demonstrated that FWGE offers a number of anticancer benefits, including helping to regulate cell metabolism, inhibiting non-oxidative glucose metabolism, enhancing oxidative glucose metabolism, and supporting many mechanisms of immune system regulation. In addition, research has found that FWGE also restores healthy mitochondrial function and helps prevent tumors growth.

Based on the results of this research, Avemar is approved as a dietary food supplement for cancer patients by the National Institute of Food Safety and Nutrition of Hungary. (**Note:** Because the proprietary extraction and fermentation process used to produce Avemar substantially changes the original composition of wheat germ, Avemar's benefits cannot be achieved by using wheat germ, germinated wheat, or any other wheat germ extract or derivative.)

Since 2006, Dr. Hidvegi has collaborated with the company America BioSciences, Inc to distribute Avermar is the US and to invest in new manufacturing technology to produce a more potent version of this supplement. This resulted in the creation of a gluten-free fermented wheat germ extract super-concentrate sold under the brand names Metatrol(R) and Metatrol PRO(R). For more information about these FGWE products, visit www.americanbiosciences.com. For a full list of studies about FGWE, visit fwgeresearch.org.

Honokiol: Honokiol is a highly active compound extracted from the bark of Magnolia trees. It has been a staple remedy in both traditional medicine systems of China and Japan for centuries. Because of the numerous health benefits it provides, Dr. Isaac Eliaz refers to honokiol as nature's "smart drug".

"Thousands of published studies and extensive clinical use show that pure honokiol delivers a remarkable array of powerful therapeutic actions," he says. "Because of its broad-spectrum of benefits and excellent safety profile, pure honokiol has become an essential strategy for protecting and enhancing numerous key areas of health. It's rare that one single ingredient can exert so many powerful actions. Pure honokiol is one of these unique compounds. It supports the treatment and prevention of numerous health conditions, targeting a diverse range of pathways with potent bioactivity."

Research has established that honokiol acts as a powerful antioxidant, anti-inflammatory, and antimicrobial agent. It has also been shown to promote calm, relaxation, and restful sleep because of its ability to enhance the effects of the amino acid GABA (gamma amino butyric acid).

"It also supports neurological and cognitive health," Dr. Eilaz says "because of its unique ability to cross the blood-brain and blood-cerebral-spinal fluid barriers, delivering powerful protection and support for neurological health. Research shows it promotes the growth of healthy nerve cells, inhibits neuroinflammation, and addresses amyloid plaque buildup in the brain associated with Alzheimer's. Pure honokiol is also shown to support against other neurological conditions such as Parkinson's disease."

Studies also show that honokiol protects against and fights cancer through multiple mechanisms of action. "Extensive published research shows pure honokiol works on critical cell signaling and genetic pathways to halt cancer growth, promote apoptosis in cancer cells, and disable the metastatic process," Dr. Eliaz explains. "It is also shown to enhance certain conventional cancer protocols —including synergy with chemotherapy and radiation— and prevent multi-drug resistance."

Honokiol has also been shown to inhibit angiogenesis and regulate gene expression. In addition, studies show that it can enhance the effects of specific chemotherapy drugs and cause cancer cells to become more susceptible to radiation therapy. Significantly, honokiol has also been shown to help prevent the spread of cancer cells through the lymphatic system.

This is important because circulating tumor cells (CTCs) and cancer stem cells (CSCs) can not only spread via the bloodstream but also through the lymph, which is why lymph nodes are often biopsied when cancer is detected in the breast and other organs.

Honokiol also helps prevent and fight cancer because of its effectiveness for scavenging free radicals, addressing oxidative stress, and supporting mitochondrial function. It also helps destroy harmful bacteria, fungi, viruses, and parasites, all of which can act as triggers for cancer because of the infections they cause.

"When it comes to honokiol's efficacy, purity matters," Dr. Eliaz says. "Research continues to show that the important benefits of honokiol are achieved with a purified extract versus a lower-grade combination of honokiol and other compounds."

Inodole-3-Carbinol (I3C): As you learned in Chapter 8, idole-3-carbinol is found in cruciferous vegetables, including Brussels sprouts, broccoli, cabbage, cauliflower, collard greens and mustard greens, kale, radishes, and turnips. Foods in the cruciferous family offer broad cancer protection. But eating such foods is often not enough to obtain the same level of benefit that I3C supplements provide.

I3C has been studied since the 1960s when researchers first began investigating for its ability to protect against various carcinogens. Since then, studies show that I3C has multiple anticancer mechanisms of action. Among these actions, I3C induces apoptosis, blocks estrogen excess and inhibits the growth of estrogen receptor positive and negative breast cancer cells, protects against DNA damage, and inhibits the growth of prostate cancer cells. It has also been shown to protect against dioxin, a highly toxic carcinogen. In addition, research shows I3C enhances the effectiveness of Tamoxifen, a drug commonly used to treat breast cancer. Animal studies also indicate that I3C may protect against cervical and other uterine-related cancers.

In addition, studies show that, besides helping to regulate estrogen levels, I3C modulates other hormones, including androsterone, androstenedione and testosterone, indicating that it may provide benefit for people undergoing hormone replacement therapy.

Though there are many supplements containing ingredients derived from the cruciferous vegetable family, I3C is the compound that has been most extensively researched.

Melatonin: Melatonin is a hormone that is secreted by the pineal gland in the brain over a 24-hour cycle. It is also produced in bone marrow, the gastrointestinal tract, the retinas of the eyes, and the skin.

The highest levels of melatonin are produced during nighttime sleep. For this reason, melatonin is commonly considered to be a sleep hormone, and over-the-counter melatonin supplements, usually in a dosage range of between 1 to 3 mg, are often used as a sleep aid and for helping to prevent and recover from jet lag.

However, melatonin provides many other health benefits, as well. It acts as a powerful antioxidant, protecting against oxidative stress and inflammation (including neuroinflammation in the brain), and also helps regulate and support immune function, including enhancing natural killer (NK) cell function. Research shows that it also regulates antioxidant enzymes in the body, enhancing their activity. In addition, melatonin helps to improve mood and protect against anxiety and depression because it increases serotonin production in the body. Moreover, it helps regulate body temperature and maintain energy levels in the body, supports bone health, and helps to maintain healthy blood pressure and blood sugar levels. It also plays a role in lipid metabolism, and helps regulate cortisol activity, thus reducing cortisol's negative effects on immune function.

Research shows that melatonin not only helps to prevent cancer, but can be effective as a treatment for most types of cancer, both on its own and in conjunction with other cancer therapies. Among its mechanism of actions in this regard, studies show that melatonin stimulates apoptosis, inhibits the growth and spread of tumor cells, disrupts angiogenesis, and enhances pro-survival signaling in cells. It also has been shown to maintain the genomic integrity of cells, protecting against the genomic instability that is one of the risk factors for the onset and spread of cancer.

In low doses, melatonin's antioxidant properties have been found to protect cellular DNA, RNA, and cellular membranes against damage. In high doses, melatonin acts as a pro-oxidant cytotoxic agent capable of killing cancer cells. It has also been found to block the effects of hormones and growth factors related to cancer growth, and to modulate estrogen, testosterone, and other hormones in ways that make tumors more hormone-dependent and therefore more responsive to cancer treatments.

In addition, melatonin has also been shown to enhance the therapeutic benefits of chemotherapy and radiation, while reducing their side effects. Melatonin supplementation by itself has also been shown to improve survival time in cases of terminal cancer, and to double the survival time and response rate to conventional cancer treatments for hormone-sensitive cancers.

Note: Melatonin should not be used in cases of leukemia, lymphoma, and multiple myeloma, however, unless it is prescribed by a physician experienced in integrative oncology. Even then, it typically should only be used short-term in conjunction with chemotherapy or radiation treatments.

Many people today are unable to produce enough melatonin due to the use of cell phones, tablets, computers, and other devices that emit blue light, which is known to impair the body's melatonin production, as well as because of the widespread exposure to electromagnetic fields (EMFs), including WiFi, both in the home and elsewhere.

You can assist your body's production of melatonin by getting at least 20 minutes exposure to outdoor sunlight early in the morning, and by sleeping in a completely dark room at night, using an eye mask if necessary. I also recommend turning off WiFi before going to bed, and, if possible, keeping your head at least three feet away from any electrical outlets in your bedroom.

For basic health maintenance, a daily supplement dose of between 1 to 3 mg may be suitable for some people, but higher doses may be advisable, especially to help prevent cancer. Even at high doses (20 mg or higher), melatonin has a very good safety profile. Any sides effects that may arise are typically mild and not long-lasting.

Modified Citrus Pectin (Pecta-Sol⁽ᴿ⁾): Modified citrus pectin (MCP) is another supplement product that can be effective for preventing and helping to reverse cancer, as well as other diseases, especially those caused by chronic inflammation.

MCP is derived from the peels of citrus fruits (grapefruit, lemons, limes, and oranges). "It is called modified citrus pectin (MCP) because the pectin has been changed so that it's easier for the body to absorb it in the gut," explains Dr. Eliaz. "This change involves taking regular pectin and making the molecules smaller, with a special enzyme- and pH-controlled process to break them up."

Dr. Eliaz is one of the foremost experts in MCP's use, and the developer of Pecto-Sol⁽ᴿ⁾, the most studied form of MCP. "Ongoing research has shown that MCP can prevent cancer cells from growing and metastasizing," he says. "It is also shown to benefit the immune system, reduce inflammation and fibrosis (uncontrolled scar tissue build up inside the body), remove toxins and heavy metals, and support numerous other key areas of health.

MCP's cancer-fighting properties are in large part due to its ability to block the effects of galectin-3. As I discussed in Chapter 2, galectin-3 is a naturally occurring protein in the body that is beneficial inside, and in small amounts outside, cells, but which in larger, unchecked amounts can cause and worsen inflammation and impair immune function, triggering cancer formation and metastasis. "MCP is able to circulate throughout the body, find galectin-3 molecules, and bind to them, blocking and often reversing their devastating effects in the body," Eliaz says. "When MCP ties up galectin-3 on cancer cells' surfaces, it can disable their ability to communicate, feed themselves, or grow. MCP's ability to bind to galectin-3 makes it a powerful weapon in blocking the spread of cancer."

Among the cancers for which MCP has been shown to have benefit are breast, colon cancer, leukemia, melanoma, ovarian cancer, and prostate cancer, including in cases where these cancers are advanced. This is particularly true of Pecta-Sol, the most researched MCP product for these types of cancer.

"Furthermore, MCP can also enhance the effects of other treatments," Eliaz points out. "For example, when MCP is combined with cefotaxime, an antibiotic, it is shown to strengthen cefotaxamine's effects against six methicillin-resistant *Staphylococcus aureus* (MRSA) strains that were analyzed. And MCP complements and enhances the benefits of some chemotherapy drugs, radiation therapy, and even botanical treatments for cancer. This can allow for better outcomes from conventional treatments, with potentially fewer side effects.»

For more information about MCP and Pecta-Sol, visit dreliaz.org.

Poly-MVA: Poly-MVA is a proprietary dietary supplement consisting of a unique formula of lipoic acid mineral complexes known as nucleotide reductases that have been shown to protect RNA and DNA. The unique combination of these molecules are bound with Vitamin B1 and palladium (a mineral) through an exclusive patent that uses the distinct characteristics of these elements to effectively address cancer promoting patterns.

Poly-MVA was developed by Dr. Merrill Garnett, a biochemist and researcher, who devoted nearly forty years of his life probing the secrets of cellular and molecular biology. During the course of his research, he recognized that cellular dysfunction is the failure of cells to mature and regenerate themselves normally, repeatedly reproducing themselves in an abnormal unhealthy state instead. He theorized that this failure of some cells to mature and reproduce properly was caused by a problem with how energy is used in the cells. With regard to cancer, Garnett also knew that cancer cells rely on simple sugars and the presence of an anaerobic (low-oxygen) environment for metabolic growth and cell replication.

After testing approximately 20,000 compounds, Garnett discovered that the combination of compounds in the Poly-MVA product disrupted the metabolic development of cancer cells while also supporting the conversion of cancer-causing free radicals into water and energy. He patented this formula in 1991. Subsequent testing has confirmed that Poly-MVA is completely safe, nontoxic, and effective.

Additional research has found that Poly-MVA helps to promote health and homeostasis in the body, as well as enhancing detoxification because its ability to improve energy production, protect against cellular oxidative stress, improve and support immune function, and generate adenosine-triphosphate (ATP) and water within cells to produce energy and to fuel other cellular processes.

Poly-MVA also detoxifies the liver, helps maintain proper pH levels, and provides essential minerals that maintain various other organ systems and cellular functions in the body.

Studies have also confirmed Poly-MVA's anticancer benefits, including its ability to reduce damage caused by radiation treatments. In one study, for example, administration of Poly-MVA showed a reduction of radiation-induced DNA damage when given to laboratory animals exposed to lethal doses of whole-body gamma-radiation. The use of Poly-MVA provided a significant decrease in mortality caused by gamma-radiation exposure and also aided in recovery from body weight reduction due to radiation use in surviving mice post-gamma-radiation exposure.

In another study, when administered beforehand, the use of Poly-MVA with and without radiation was shown to enhance the anti-tumor effects of radiation. When Poly-MVA was administered once daily for two weeks following radiation therapy, DNA protection was achieved in peripheral blood, as was protection against radiation-caused reduction of platelet counts.

All of these reasons explain why a growing number of integrative oncologists, as well as myself, now often include Poly-MVA as part of an overall cancer treatment plan. (For more information about Poly-MVA, visit PolyMVA.com and www.polymvasurvivors.com/scientific_research.html.

Onkobel Pro®: Onkobel Pro® is a dietary supplement developed by Mirko Beljanski, Ph.D., Inspired by Dr. Beljanski's pioneering observations on the nature of inflamed and cancerous cells, Onkobel Pro harnesses the unique properties of three distinct botanical extracts— *Pao pereira, Rauwolfia vomitoria,* and *Golden Leaf* of *Ginkgo biloba*—to deliver multiple health benefits, especially in the domain of cancer care.

Central to understanding the effectiveness of Onkobel Pro is Dr. Beljanski's finding that destabilized DNA, characterized by open loops between the DNA strands, is indicative of inflamed and potentially cancerous cells. Both *Pao pereira* and *Rauwolfia vomitoria* extracts selectively recognize the destabilized DNA of damaged cells and support the natural process of their elimination from the body. Research has shown that the two extracts work by different mechanisms of action and combining the two yields a synergistic effect.

Research has shown that both extracts provide substantial support for prostate health, pancreatic health, and ovarian health, among other benefits. These studies are available on the Beljanski Foundation's website Beljanski.org.

Pao Pereira extract has also been shown to induce apoptosis in destabilized cells, helping the body rid itself of cells that have gone astray. In addition, Pao pereira provides substantial antiviral and anti-inflammatory benefits, adding another layer of defense to the body.

Rauwolfia Vomitoria extract also induces the arrest of destabilized cells, thereby acting as a checkpoint against the proliferation of such cells. Beyond its cellular actions, this extract also offers the added advantage of hormone regulation, restoring balance to the male and female reproductive systems.

Unlike more common green leaf extracts, Onkobel Pro's Golden Leaf of Ginkgo biloba extract offers a variety of unique benefits. Because of the rich supply of antioxidants it contains, this extract is particularly useful in safeguarding tissues from various forms of electromagnetic radiation. In addition, Dr. Beljanski's research documented the golden leaf extract's potential to significantly curtail radiation-induced fibrosis. Furthermore, this extract ensures a healthy regulation of ribonucleases enzymes, which often see imbalances under cellular stress. By doing so, it also plays a role in liver functions and general cellular health.

While each extract within Onkobel Pro's proprietary formula offers its own set of benefits, their combination results in a synergistic effect, enhancing the body's ability to target and remove destabilized cells.

Helpful Vitamins and Other Nutrients: A number of nutrients are also well-known for their anticancer benefits. Among them are vitamin B6, inositol, and vitamins C, D, and K.

Vitamin B6, also known as pyridoxine, plays an essential role in immune function and has been shown to help prevent bladder, breast, cervical, and non-small lung ovarian cancer, as well as colorectal adenocarcinoma. In addition, studies show that supplementing with B6 during chemotherapy can reduce chemo's side effects while increasing its effectiveness, including when ovarian cancer is treated with chemotherapy. B6 is also important for maintaining the health of mucous membranes lining the body's respiratory tract, helping them to prevent the entry of potential cancer-causing infections and environmental toxins into the sinus cavity and lungs.

Inositol, another B vitamin, is found in nearly all of the body's cells, and naturally occurs in fiber-rich foods, which is likely one of the reasons a diet high in fiber-rich foods protects against cancer. In addition to its antioxidant properties, inositol plays an important role in the transmission of signals between cells and their environment, and is essential for healthy immune function and for proper cell growth and differentiation.

Studies show that inositol, especially in the supplement form of inositol hexaphosphate, or IP6, is effective for inhibiting tumor growth, cancer progression, and metastasis. In addition to reducing cancer cell growth, IP6 also causes cancer cells to differentiate. This, combined with IP6's immune-enhancing and antioxidant properties, also enable it to destroy tumor cells. Studies have also demonstrated that IP6 and other forms of inositol can boost the effectiveness of chemotherapy and improve cancer patients' quality of life.

Vitamin C is one of the most potent antioxidants and anti-inflammatory nutrients, and is essential for healthy immune function. Research has shown that vitamin C can help protect against a variety of cancers, and is also effective as part of an overall cancer treatment plan. One reason for this is because of the role vitamin C plays in the functioning of the immune systems natural killer (NK) cells. Research has established that NK cells can only be activated by adequate amounts of vitamin C. Studies show that vitamin C also boosts the body's production of interferon, another anticancer compound.

For many cancer patients, vitamin C in the form of ascorbic acid, when administered intravenously (IV vitamin C therapy) at high doses (typically between 50 to 100 grams or more), may offer the most significant benefits. IV vitamin C bypasses normal gut metabolism and excretion pathways to create blood levels that are 100 to 500 times higher than levels than levels achieved when vitamin C is taken orally. At these high doses, ascorbic acid shifts from acting as an antioxidant (as it is in lower, oral doses) to become a pro-oxidant, generating hydrogen peroxide ($H2O2$). The production of $H2O2$ is able to damage and kill cancer tumor cells because such cells have low levels of catalase enzyme activity compared to normal, healthy cells, and are therefore much less capable of removing $H2O2$ than normal cells are. (Normal cells are able to remove $H2O2$ in several ways, keeping it at very low levels so it does not damage them.)

I discuss IV vitamin C treatments in more detail in Chapter 12.

Vitamin D actually acts more like a hormone than a vitamin in the body. All of the body's cells contain receptors for vitamin D, which indicate how important vitamin D is to overall health.

Research has demonstrated that vitamin D deficiencies can increase the risk for certain types of cancer, while increasing the body's vitamin D levels can reduce the risk for developing these same cancers. This is especially true for the protection vitamin D offers for breast and colon cancers, two of the most common types of cancer today.

The risk for bladder, bone, lung, and ovarian cancer, as well as melanoma, may also be reduced by vitamin D, according to research. Research has also linked vitamin D deficiency to an increased risk of infection (including COVID-19), as well as a greater risk for asthma, diabetes (both type 1 and 2), cardiovascular disease, inflammatory bowel disease (IBS), and various neurological conditions.

Vitamin D's anticancer benefits are due in large part to its ability to maintain healthy cell differentiation, while preventing abnormal cell growth and mutations. In addition, vitamin D has also been shown to maintain natural cell death (apoptosis).

While the research into vitamin D as a preventive and therapeutic aid against cancer is still ongoing, many oncologists and other physicians today now prescribe vitamin D3 supplementation to their patients to aid in the fight against cancer.

While the use of vitamin D supplements has become more popular in recent decades, sunlight exposure remains the best way of providing your body with vitamin D. In grade school you likely learned how plants convert sunlight into food through a process called photosynthesis. The human body converts sunlight, specifically its ultraviolet B (UVB) rays, into vitamin D in much the same way.

However, various factors make sunlight exposure alone an insufficient method for ensuring adequate vitamin D levels. While sunlight exposure is still encouraged, vitamin D supplements are also advisable. One of the best supplement forms is cod liver oil. When supplementing with vitamin D in capsule form, it is always advisable to also take a vitamin K supplement, since vitamin D supplements, especially in high doses, can displace calcium in the body, sending it into the arteries and kidneys. Vitamin K helps prevent such displacement.

Vitamin K, especially in the form of K2, which is synthesized in the gut by bacteria, has been shown by research to protect against colorectal, liver, lung, prostate, stomach, and other types of cancer in multiple ways. Among its anticancer mechanisms is vitamin K's ability to suppress the growth and spread of tumor cells. It does this by modifying various growth factors and their receptor molecules (molecules on the surface of cells that receive chemical signals), making them less apt to trigger tumor growth. Vitamin K has also been shown to block replication of tumor cells, and to initiate apoptosis. Additionally, vitamin K stimulates the release of proteins that cancer cells typically suppress in order to repair themselves. By triggering these proteins, vitamin K helps to prevent this repair process, inhibiting tumor cells' ability to survive.

Other research has found that vitamin K causes oxidation among cancer cells without harming healthy, normal cells. Cancer cells are highly vulnerable to oxygen, compared to normal cells, and thus more likely to die when exposed to oxidative stress.

Vitamin K has also been shown to block the formation of new blood vessels that cancer cells use to support their rapid spread and growth. Researchers continue to discover other ways in which vitamin K helps to protect against cancer, both by itself, and in combination with other cancer-fighting nutrients, especially vitamins C and D and magnesium.

A variety of other nutritional supplements also provide anticancer properties, including calcium, glutathione, iodine, magnesium, MSM (methylsulfonylmethane), omega-3 fatty acids, quercetin, selenium, taurine, and zinc.

Other natural anticancer agents include astragalus, berberine, black cumin seed (nigella sativa), boswellia, grapeseed extract, Korean ginseng, and the mushrooms coriolus, reishi and skullcap. Some of these are discussed in Chapter 11.

To discuss all natural anticancer compounds and products, as well as providing recommended dosages, is beyond the scope of this book. When using such products, it is always best to do so under the guidance of a physician trained in their use, especially a nutritionally-oriented integrative oncologist when dealing with cancer.

For more information about the full range of anticancer nutrients, herbs, and other supplements, I recommend the book *Beating Cancer With*

Nutrition by Patrick Quillin, PhD, an internationally recognized expert in the area of nutrition and cancer.

Guidelines for Using Nutritional Supplements

The following guidelines can help ensure that you receive the fullest benefits when using nutritional supplements.

Read the label. Since not all brands of nutritional supplements are the same in terms of quality, efficacy and price, it is important to know the quality of the brand you are buying. By reading the label of the supplements you purchase, you can determine their dosage range and whether or not the supplements also contain fillers, binders, and other additives of no nutritional value, and to which you might be allergic or sensitive, such as sugars or gluten. (Generally safe additives include alginic acid, cellulose, calcium or magnesium stearate, dicalcium phosphate, gum accacia, and silica.) Reputable companies typically list all ingredients in their nutritional formulas and, upon request, are usually willing to also provide further information regarding their efficacy.

Know when and how to take your supplements. As a general rule, vitamin and mineral supplements are best taken during meals or 15 minutes before or after eating, in order to enhance their assimilation. This is especially true of fat-soluble vitamins, which ideally should also be taken during the meal of the day with the highest fat content. Overall, however, most vitamin and mineral supplements are best taken with the first meal of the day. In addition, single B vitamins are best consumed along with a total B-complex supplement.

Beware of "megadosing." Certain nutrients, including all fat-soluble vitamins and certain minerals and B-complex vitamins, can be toxic in high doses. To avoid the risk of toxicity, avoid taking high doses of nutrients unless you do so under the guidance of physician trained in their use.

Pay attention to any reactions following supplementation. Nutritional supplements, if properly used, rarely cause adverse reactions. However, if you experience nausea or other side effects after taking supplements, immediately discontinue their use. In many cases, such reactions are due to excessive dosages or symptoms of detoxification provoked by supplementation and will cease once supplementation is discontinued. But if symptoms persist, seek medical attention.

Consult with your physician before using supplements with medication. While most supplements taken in moderate doses are generally safe, certain nutrients can be contraindicated when used with prescribed medications, and can also interfere with chemotherapy and radiation treatments. To ensure safety, always consult with a nutritionally-oriented physician prior to beginning any nutritional supplementation program.

Be consistent. Irregular use of nutritional supplements provides little or no benefit, since the benefits of diet and proper nutrition are cumulative and accrue over time. By following a daily supplement routine, you can ensure that your body regularly receives the nutritional support it requires to properly perform its many functions.

While the therapeutic use of diet and nutritional supplements is generally safe, and in many cases can be adapted as part of an overall self-care regimen, for best results it is advisable to seek the professional assistance of an integrative physician or nutritional therapist to ensure that your nutrient needs are optimally met.

Chapter 10

The Importance of Regular Exercise

Your body is designed for daily physical activity. Numerous studies show that sedentary people, on average, don't live as long and do not enjoy good health to the same degree as people who exercise regularly. The reason for this is simple: Movement is LIFE.

To be blunt, the moment we stop moving, we start dying. Your body is designed in a very specific way in order to preserve its resources and will actually shut down the areas not being used. In fact, many studies show that people who exercise and keep moving increase their chance of beating cancer by more than 30 percent.

When we move we continually cleanse the fluid around our cells, which leads to the cells being bathed in a nutrient-rich, toxic-free fluid. Much like the water of a stagnant pond versus a continually flowing river; where there is stagnation, toxins begin to build up, pathogens proliferate, and the nutritional resources are quickly used. The same can be said for the body. A cell living in that type of environment cannot remain healthy. So the key here is to do whatever you can to stay active and keep moving.

We all have cancer cells floating around our bodies every single day, and it's our immune system that is patrolling the body to identify and eliminate them. So we need to do all we can to help keep the immune system functioning the way that it needs to. This includes exercising regularly because exercise stimulates the proliferation and activity of the various components of the immune system.

Overall Benefits of Exercise

In addition to helping prevent cancer and improving the odds of recovering from it, regular exercise and physical activity provides many other health benefits, including:

- Increased longevity
- Prevention of other serious, degenerative diseases
- Improved recovery from heart disease and reduced risk of repeat heart conditions
- Prevention of and relief from tension
- Decreased "fight or flight" response, and therefore less stress
- Prevention of and relief from stress, anxiety, and depression
- Reduced risk of alcoholism and drug addiction
- Increased muscle to fat ratio, making dieting and weight loss easier
- Increased muscular strength, increased flexibility, and improved balance, especially among older people
- Better quality of sleep
- Improved cognitive function
- Increased stamina and energy
- Increased aerobic capacity
- Improved self-esteem and greater confidence
- Increased incidence of positive attitudes and emotions, including joy.

Regular exercise also aids digestion, increases circulation, stimulates the lymphatic system (your body's filtration and purification system), and promotes enhanced levels of positive emotions and a balanced mood. (Regular exercise of an aerobic nature has been shown to increase serotonin levels in the brain. Serotonin levels are associated with feelings of calm and well-being, improved brain function and enhanced sleep.) Given all of the above benefits, you can see why you need to make regular exercise a priority in your life.

Exercise and Cancer

One of the biggest myths about receiving a diagnosis of cancer is the mistaken belief that people with cancer need to rest and "take it easy," curtailing exercise and other physical activities as much as possible. Not only is this belief false, if its advice is accepted, it can significantly reduce the likelihood of a full recovery from cancer. The truth is that people with cancer who engage in regular exercise typically achieve better and longer-lasting results from their cancer treatments, compared to cancer patients who do not. Moreover, regular exercise has been shown by research to improve and enhance one's mindset, leading to more positive attitudes and emotions, the importance of which we discussed in Chapter 7.

Similarly, engaging in regular exercise is one of the most important self-care steps you can take to prevent cancer, as well as disease in general.

A growing body of research confirms how an inactive, sedentary lifestyle is a contributing cause of cancer. For example, one study of men and women aged 30 and older found that over a three-year period (2013 to 2016), lack of exercise was responsible for over 46,000 cases of cancer in the U.S. This was particularly true of sedentary women, who accounted for over 32,000 of those cases.

Additional research shows that lack of exercise is a known risk factor for colon cancer, endometrial cancer, esophageal cancer, female breast cancer, kidney cancer, stomach cancer and urinary bladder cancer.

Conversely, according to the National Cancer Institute (NCI), "There is strong evidence that higher levels of physical activity are linked to lower risk of several types of cancer."

What follow are study findings summarized by the NCI:

- "Bladder cancer: In a 2014 meta-analysis of 11 cohort studies and 4 case-control studies, the risk of bladder cancer was 15% lower for individuals with the highest level of recreational or occupational physical activity than in those with the lowest level. A pooled analysis of over 1 million individuals found that leisure-time physical activity was linked to a 13% reduced risk of bladder cancer.

- "Breast cancer: Many studies have shown that physically active women have a lower risk of breast cancer than inactive women. In a 2016 meta-analysis that included 38 cohort studies, the most physically active women had a 12–21% lower risk of breast cancer than those who were least physically active. Physical activity has been associated with similar reductions in risk of breast cancer among both premenopausal and postmenopausal women. Women who increase their physical activity after menopause may also have a lower risk of breast cancer than women who do not.

- "Colon cancer: In a 2016 meta-analysis of 126 studies, individuals who engaged in the highest level of physical activity had a 19% lower risk of colon cancer than those who were the least physically active.

- "Endometrial cancer: Several meta-analyses and cohort studies have examined the relationship between physical activity and the risk of endometrial cancer (cancer of the lining of the uterus). In a meta-analysis of 33 studies, highly physically active women had a 20% lower risk of endometrial cancer than women with low levels of physical activity. There is some evidence that the association is indirect, in that physical activity would have to reduce obesity for the benefits to be observed. Obesity is a strong risk factor for endometrial cancer.

- "Esophageal cancer: A 2014 meta-analysis of nine cohort and 15 case–control studies found that the individuals who were most physically active had a 21% lower risk of esophageal adenocarcinoma than those who were least physically active.

- "Kidney (renal cell) cancer: In a 2013 meta-analysis of 11 cohort studies and 8 case–control studies, individuals who were the most physically active had a 12% lower risk of renal cancer than those who were the least active. A pooled analysis of over 1 million individuals found that leisure-time physical activity was linked to a 23% reduced risk of kidney cancer."Stomach (gastric) cancer: A 2016 meta-analysis of 10 cohort studies and 12 case–control studies reported that individuals who were the most physically active had a 19% lower risk of stomach cancer than those who were least active."

The NCI adds, "There is some evidence that physical activity is associated with a reduced risk of lung cancer...In a 2016 meta-analysis of 25 observational studies, physical activity was associated with reduced risk of lung cancer among former and current smokers but was not associated with risk of lung cancer among never smokers.

"For several other cancers, there is more limited evidence of an association. These include certain cancers of the blood, as well as cancers of the pancreas, prostate, ovaries, thyroid, liver, and rectum."

These findings are supported by a meta-analysis of hundreds of epidemiologic studies with a combined several million study participants. The analysis "found strong evidence for an association between highest versus lowest physical activity levels and reduced risks of bladder, breast, colon, endometrial, esophageal adenocarcinoma, renal, and gastric cancers. Relative risk reductions ranged from approximately 10% to 20%. Based on 18 systematic reviews and meta-analyses, the report also found moderate or limited associations between greater amounts of physical activity and decreased all-cause and cancer-specific mortality in individuals with a diagnosis of breast, colorectal, or prostate cancer, with relative risk reductions ranging almost up to 40% to 50%. The updated search, with five meta-analyses and 25 source articles reviewed, confirmed these findings."

These and other studies proving the effectiveness of exercise for cancer has led to a new medical field called exercise oncology.

One of the leading experts and researchers in this field is Kathryn H. Schmitz, PhD, MPH, who has spent decades researching the benefits of exercise for cancer patients. Dr. Schmitz is professor in the University of Pittsburgh Department of Medicine, Division of Hematology/Oncology and the UPMC Hillman Cancer Center, an NCI-designated Comprehensive Cancer Center. In addition to having published approximately 300 peer-reviewed scientific papers, she was the lead author of the First American College of Sports Medicine Roundtable on Exercise for Cancer Survivors. I consider her book, *Moving Through Cancer: An Exercise and Strength-Training Program for the Fight of Your Life*, essential reading for anyone with cancer, as well as for their loved ones and caregivers.

I've had the privilege of interviewing Dr. Schmitz on my podcast. During our conversation, she noted that society hasn't really caught up to the reality of what cancer patients look like today. Instead, when they think of cancer patients, what they envision is similar to how cancer patients are portrayed in movies and on television.

"They're generally shown with a blanket over their knees, and an IV in their arm," she says. "They look a little waxy. They might have a scarf on their head, they're in bed, and they look sick. The average cancer patient doesn't look like that anymore. Most people are being diagnosed with early stage cancer, and they're still working. There are people in the grocery store right now walking around buying their groceries who have cancer."

One of the challenges for medical doctors , Dr. Schmitz points out, is that educating patients about exercise takes time. "They're used to their prescription pad and prescribing drugs and instructions on when to take them, for how long, and at what dose. You have a direct correlation between this pill for that illness. Exercise is not as defined when it comes to cancer and other illnesses. People need to know what type of exercise they need for their health condition, how often they need it, how long they should exercise each time, and in what intensity. Exercise oncology is evolving towards having answers to such questions.

"The American College of Sports Medicine most recent round table on the topic of exercise and cancer reviewed 16 different cancer health related outcomes to see whether there was sufficient evidence for us to make a fit prescription, meaning frequency, intensity, time, and type of exercise. We don't tell people with cancer to just go get some chemotherapy, right? We give them a very specific chemotherapy for a very specific cancer at a very specific dose, at a very specific frequency, for a very specific number of times. We want to make sure that we are prescribing exercise with that kind of precision.

"What we were able to conclude on the basis of that systematic review was that there were eight different cancer health-related outcomes for which we could make a fit prescription. The outcomes are fatigue, anxiety, depression, physical function, breast cancer-related lymphedema, sleep, bone health, and overall quality of life. For all of these, it was interesting that the dose actually coalesced during treatment. Three times a week of aerobic exercise for 30 minutes each time, and twice weekly strength training was beneficial for all of these outcomes."

One point that's important for cancer patients to understand is that just because a doctor does not prescribe exercise does not mean that it is not vital. Dr. Schmitz points out, for example, that, "There actually is peer-reviewed evidence in oncology, in particular with lung cancer patients, that if physicians do not say anything about exercise, patients walk away with the impression the doctors do not want them to exercise. That the absence of saying anything translates for many patients into 'Rest. Take it easy. Don't push yourself.' That's why it's so crucial for us to get physicians into the habit of telling their patients, 'I do want you to exercise.'"

How Exercise Boosts Resistance To and Aids In the Recovery From Cancer

While there is still more to discover in the field of exercise oncology, research has clearly established some of the ways that exercise acts as a powerful anticancer self-care strategy. It is well-known, for example, that regular exercise and other physical activities improves mood and an overall sense of well-being, while simultaneously improving overall physical function, aerobic capacity, and muscle strength. Regular exercise also prevents and can help reduce excess weight gain and obesity, a major risk factor for many types of cancer.

Research also demonstrates that regular exercise:

- Lowers levels of sex hormones, including estrogen, as well as various growth factors associated with the development and progression of certain cancers, especially breast and colon cancer.

- Prevents insulin spikes and insulin resistance, which also contribute to cancer development and progression.

- Alters the metabolism of bile acids in the gastrointestinal tract, which in turn decreases exposures to various carcinogens found in nonorganic foods and beverages.

- Reduces the transit time of food moving through the GI tract, which also decreases exposures to carcinogens.

But perhaps the most important anticancer benefits of exercise are its ability to boost immune function, reduce inflammation, and enhance metabolic function, including "starving" cancer by depriving tumors of glucose, their primary fuel.

Immune Function: One of the most notable immune-enhancing benefits of exercise is its ability to alter the metabolism of immune white blood cells known as cytotoxic T cells (also known as CB8+ T cells). These cells play an essential role in targeting and eliminating cancer cells in the body, and exercise improves their ability to do so.

Research involving both mice and humans confirm this. In one study, conducted by researchers at the prestigious Karolinska Institutet in Sweden, mice with cancer were separated into two groups. One group was trained to exercise regularly on a spinning wheel, while the other group was kept inactive. Compared to the sedentary mice, tumor growth in the exercise group slowed down, and the incidence of death was reduced.

The researchers then injected antibodies to remove the cytotoxic T cells in both groups. Once this was done, the exercise mice exhibited no positive differences in tumor growth and survival compared to the other mice.

To further examine their findings, the researchers then transferred cytotoxic T cells from the both groups of mice to other mice with cancerous tumors. The mice that received cytotoxic T cells taken from the exercise mice group had better outcomes than those that received the same T cells taken from the sedentary mice.

Finally, the researchers isolated T cells, along with blood and tissue samples, from mice after they finished a session on the spinning wheels in order to measure various metabolites produced in muscle and excreted into blood at high levels during exercise. Among these metabolites was lactate, which is known to alter T cell metabolism and increase their immune function activity. The researchers found that the cytotoxic T cells isolated from the mice after exercise positively altered the cells' metabolism compared to T cells taken from the mice that did not exercise.

The researchers then examined how these same metabolites are altered after humans exercise. During that part of the study, blood samples were isolated and examined from eight healthy men after they completed 30 minutes of intense exercise. The examination revealed that exercise released the same metabolites.

Helene Rundqvist, one of the study's authors, stated, "Our research shows that exercise affects the production of several molecules and metabolites that activate cancer-fighting immune cells and thereby inhibit cancer growth. We hope these results may contribute to a deeper understanding of how our lifestyle impacts our immune system and inform the development of new immunotherapies against cancer."

Dr. Schmitz points out that numerous other animal studies have shown similar results. "We have shown over and over again that exercising animals with cancer will reduce both tumor size and tumor burden," she says. "When we do these studies, we show that exercise while the animal has a tumor makes a very large difference. The animals are able to live longer, and their tumors shrink.

"Animal models show that exercise changes the effectiveness of chemotherapy, as well. The likelihood of a complete response or the shrinkage of the tumor is much greater in animals that exercise with chemotherapy as opposed to just the chemotherapy. Generally speaking, most animal studies are divided into four groups. All the animals have cancer. One group receive no intervention, one group is trained to exercise, the third group receives chemotherapy, and the fourth group is trained to exercise in combination with chemotherapy. The group that always does best is the group with the combination of exercise and chemotherapy."

Inflammation: Exercise has a tremendous positive impact on inflammation in the body, which is one more reason why regular exercise is so important for helping to prevent and reverse cancer.

These anti-inflammatory benefits can be gained in as little as 20 minutes of brisk yet non-strenuous walking. This fact was confirmed in a study of 47 men and women who walked on a treadmill for 20 minutes. Blood samples were taken from the participants before and immediately after they finished exercising. The study found that after a single treadmill session inflammation markers in the bodies of all of the participants were reduced. This included a five percent reduction in the production of tumor necrosis factor (TNF), which, as you learned in Chapter 2, not only plays a role in the body's inflammation response, but can also damage DNA and inhibit DNA repair, as well as contributing to the growth, proliferation, angiogenesis, and metastasis of cancer cells and tumors.

According to Suzi Hong, the study's lead researcher, "Our study shows a workout session does not have to be intense to have anti-inflammatory effects. Twenty minutes to half an hour of moderate exercise, including fast walking, appears to be sufficient. Feeling like a workout needs to be at a peak exertion level for long duration can intimidate those who suffer from chronic inflammatory diseases and [who] could greatly benefit from physical activity." Remember, among other things, cancer is also a chronic inflammatory disease.

Exercise also causes muscle cells to release interleukin-6 (IL-6), a protein that reduces inflammation in several ways, including lowering TNF levels. IL-6 also inhibits the signaling effects of another protein called interleukin-1 beta (IL-1β). IL-1β signaling triggers inflammation capable of damaging cells in the pancreas that produce insulin.

One study demonstrating IL-6's ability to reduce inflammation involved human volunteers who received injections of a molecule from *E. coli* bacteria known to trigger an inflammatory response. During the study, participants experienced a 200 to 300 percent increase in levels of TNF alpha. But when the participants engaged in three hours of exercise on stationary bikes prior to receiving the injection, they experienced an increase in their IL-6 levels, but not a corresponding rise in TNF alpha.

While three hours of exercise at one time may be beyond the capability of many cancer patients, even a 30 minute workout has been shown to increase IL-6 levels by as much as 500 percent.

Animal studies show that regular exercise also increases the production of interleukin-15 (IL-15) in muscle cells. This protein helps prevent the accumulation of excess abdominal fat, a known trigger of inflammation and a serious risk factor for various cancers.

Another important way in which exercise benefits cancer patients has to do with its effects on shear stress, the force that is exerted within the inner lining (endothelium) of the arteries, affecting the production of nitric oxide (NO).

As you learned in Chapter 8, adequate NO production is needed to ensure that the arteries remain open wide enough to ensure proper blood flow throughout the body. According to Abigail L. Cook, PhD, "Shear stress can be characterized in different ways, with each form resulting in different responses from the inner lining of the vessels. High levels of unidirectional shear stress occur in the straight sections of blood vessels. This is associated with the production of molecules that *fight* inflammation, which protect the cell from abnormal growth and proliferation, and even cell death. Low levels of bidirectional shear stress are most often found at curvatures and at branches of blood vessels. This type of shear stress generates molecules that are associated with inflammation."

Research shows that a sedentary lifestyle results in low levels of healthy, unidirectional shear stress, and that exercise is an excellent way to increase this type of shear stress. Moreover, both in vitro research and studies with both animals and humans show that fluid [blood and plasma] shear stress can destroy circulating tumor cells (CTCs).

"Exercise changes sheer stress in a way that alters how the vasculature attaches to tumors," Dr. Schmitz explains. "It probably also alters how chemotherapy is delivered to the tumor. If you look at the vasculature around a tumor, it's generally very tortured because it's being built to support tumor growth in a way that the body is trying to fight. If you open up the vasculature to the tumors, the tumors are better able to receive the chemotherapy. That is one of the hottest issues among researchers trying to understand why exercise would have an effect on improving the likelihood of chemotherapy to do its job."

Metabolic Function: Healthy metabolic function is also vital for preventing cancer. Restoring impaired metabolic function is also a key component of a comprehensive cancer treatment program. Exercise can help in this regard in a number of ways.

First, it helps starve cancer cells and tumors by depriving them of the glucose (sugar) cancer feeds upon in order to survive. Glucose stored in the body is known as glycogen, which the body draws upon in order to produce energy. When we exercise, glycogen storage is depleted because of the increased energy expenditure that exercising requires. In cancer patients, this exercise-induced glycogen depletion cuts off the supply of glucose to cancer cells. This, in turn, makes cancer less resistant to cancer chemotherapy and other cancer treatments.

"We are able to diagnose cancer in part because of the amount of glucose that is going to cancer cells," Dr. Schmitz points out. "If we are regularly exercising, then that glucose is needed elsewhere. This is one of the ways that we believe that exercise is likely involved in prevention of cancer. It pulls the glucose away from the metabolic processes that are developing tumors and sends it towards a more functional place in the body where it's needed."

In addition, regular exercise improves levels of A1c, a marker of blood sugar levels, and also causes hemoglobin in the blood to release more oxygen. Increased oxygen in the body is known to protect against and help reverse cancer. Exercise also lowers blood pressure and offers many other cardiovascular benefits, which is also important, since chemotherapy is known to weaken the heart in many cases.

"All of these factors are difficult to regulate and manage in the setting of a growing tumor," Dr. Schmitz says. "The body becomes less and less able to regulate metabolism while it's dealing with a tumor, as well as with the onslaught of chemotherapy or radiation therapy. Because exercise helps to regulate the body's metabolic processes, it can help keep things from going awry while patients are receiving chemotherapy. We also know that cancer patients who have diabetes, hyperlipidemia, or hypertension are much more likely to be hospitalized while they're going through their chemotherapy. Exercise can be quite helpful for reducing that likelihood in such patients."

Exercise also helps maintain overall metabolism, as well as the microenvironment of the cells and their mitochondria (discussed in more detail in the next chapter). "We know that exercise has a tremendous impact on the metabolic microenvironment in general, but there is evidence to show that exercise has an effect on the tumor microenvironment, as well," says Dr. Schmitz. "As I mentioned, the vessels around a tumor are really tortured and growing in a way that the body is trying to fight at the same time. The entire tumor microenvironment is inflamed and resistant to cancer-fighting immune cells trying to enter it to do their job. These strange metabolic processes in the tumor are not at all consistent with a healthy body. But when we are exercising on a regular basis, then all systems in the body will lead towards the regulation of that tumor microenvironment in a way that helps kill the tumor. Moreover, by reducing the inflammation through exercise, you're reducing cancer signaling, which will also reduce the risk for metastases."

Components of A Healthy Exercise Routine

A healthy exercise routine geared towards preventing disease, including cancer, will ideally incorporate a blend of strength training and aerobic exercises that work in conjunction with each other.

Strength Training: Building and maintaining muscle strength is an essential component of an overall exercise program. This is particularly true as we age. Research shows that strength training helps to maintain healthy hormone levels, improve metabolism, reduce the risk of bone loss, and improve the body's ability to efficiently burn calories.

Weight training (weight lifting and training on weight machines) is perhaps the most popular form of strength training, but you can get many of the same strength-building benefits without the use of such equipment. Moreover, not having to rely on weights and weight machines makes it far likelier that you will commit to your training routine.

Aerobic Exercise: The word *aerobic* means "with oxygen". Aerobic exercise is exercise that requires extra oxygen to supply energy to the muscles. In general, aerobic exercise causes moderate shortness of breath, perspiration, and an increase in resting pulse rate. The heart in particular benefits from aerobic exercise due to the increased oxygen that such exercise provides to it, as well as the rest of your body.

Jogging, bicycling, running on treadmills, and using stair climbers are all popular forms of aerobic exercise, as are swimming and sports such as tennis, racquetball, and basketball. However, the easiest form of aerobic exercise is walking.

Making Your Exercise Routine Work For You: To get the best results from your exercise program follow these guidelines to avoid injury or over-exertion.

Avoid exercising during times of emotional crises or when you are angry. Exercise under such conditions is counterproductive and can put a dangerous strain on your heart.

Wait at least two hours after eating before exercising. Additionally, when exercising before meals, wait at least 30 minutes after your exercise session ends before eating. Also drink plenty of water at least half an hour before you begin. You can also drink water during the exercise session, if you are thirsty, but do so sparingly.

When performing any type of exercise, be sure to breathe in a relaxed, deep manner. Doing so will enhance the benefits of the exercise itself by increasing the amount of oxygen that is available for your body's cells, tissues, and organs.

Start off exercise sessions with proper warm-up and stretching exercises. This will help to avoid post-exercise soreness or injury.

Wear the proper attire when exercising, including athletic shoes with the proper support for the activity. Tight clothing and shoes can restrict your circulation and dissipation of heat during exercise. Avoid them.

If possible, exercise outdoors, dressing appropriately for the weather. The combination of fresh air and bright sunshine will make exercising more enjoyable.

When exercising indoors, make sure your room is well ventilated. Open windows or turn on the fan or the air-conditioner during summer months to avoid exercising in a room that is too hot.

Just as warming-up and stretching is important as you begin each exercise session, so is a cool-down period at the end of your exercise activity. This should include at least several minutes of gentle stretching or walking.

The key to long-term success is to find exercise activities you enjoy and commit to them on a regular basis.

Exercise Guidelines for People with Cancer

The first key to exercise for cancer patients is to start slow and then gradually building up to more exercise as strength and endurance improves. Going slow is especially important for cancer patients who are unused to exercising and have lived a sedentary lifestyle. Cancer patients should also inform their physicians before beginning any exercise program.

An effective exercise routine does not need to be complicated. Doing any activity is better than none, and the best exercise is the one you actually do, even if in the beginning that means only a few minutes of daily movement. Over time, commitment and persistence will lead to consistent gains and better results.

Dr. Schmitz, along with many health associations, including the American Cancer Society, the National Cancer Institute, the CDC, the American College of Sports Medicine, and the National Comprehensive Cancer Network, endorse following exercise recommendations for cancer patients.

Aerobic Activity (Movement): The recommendations for the amount of aerobic activity varies according to where patients are with regard to their cancer treatments.

Ideally, before patients begin their treatments, they should try to build up to 150 to 300 minutes of aerobic activity per week. This equates to 30 to 60 minutes of movement exercise per day, five days a week. One of the easiest and most enjoyable methods for achieving this is by taking a daily walk.

Once treatment begins, especially if treatment includes chemotherapy or radiation, or a combination of the two, 30 minutes of moderately intense aerobic activity three times a week is advised, or a daily 30-minute walk of low intensity if symptoms make more intense aerobic activity inadvisable.

Following surgery, if it is necessary, patients should try to get out of bed as soon as their physicians deem it safe to do so to take short walks or engage in other light aerobic activity. Over the course of the next two months, aerobic activity can gradually be increased to 150 to 300 minutes of aerobic activity each week. "The focus post surgery is on duration, not intensity," Dr. Schmitz says.

Hormonal therapy is sometimes used to treat cancer. Patients who undergo hormone therapy should also aim for 150 to 300 minutes of aerobic activity each week, as should patients who have completed their cancer treatments.

Over time, as strength improves, patients can engage in more vigorous aerobic activities. For most patients, 75 to 150 minutes of more intense aerobic exercise per week offers optimal benefits.

Strength Training (Resistance) Exercises: In addition to regular aerobic exercise before, during, and after their treatments, cancer patients should also engage in strength training exercise at least twice a week in order to maintain their muscle strength.

"Cancer patients and survivors need to pay attention to maintaining their muscle mass," Dr. Schmitz says. "It is common for muscle mass to decrease during and after cancer treatment. This contributes to the feeling expressed by many patients and survivors that they have aged more than would be expected during the time they went through treatment. I strongly recommend that cancer patients develop and maintain a program of progressive resistance training before, during, and after treatment to address the expected loss of muscle, function, and increased fatigue.

"Activities should work all the major muscle groups of your body—legs, hips, back, chest, abdomen, shoulders, and arms. To gain health benefits, you need to do muscle-strengthening activities to the point where it's hard for you to do another repetition without help. A repetition is one complete movement of an activity like lifting a weight or doing a sit-up. Try to do eight to 12 repetitions per activity, which counts as one set. Try to do at least one set. To gain even more benefits, do two or three sets. You can do activities that strengthen your muscles on the same or different days that you do aerobic activity. Do whatever works best for you."

There are many ways you can strengthen your muscles. You can lift weights (even five-pound weights are enough to get started) or work with resistance bands. Body weight exercises, such as push-ups, chin-ups, sit-ups, and squats, are also excellent ways to build and strengthen muscles.

"If exercise was a pill that we could bottle, it would be prescribed by every physician," Dr. Schmitz sums up. I wholeheartedly agree.

To find out more about the benefits of exercise for cancer, as well as the latest research and exercise guidelines, visit www.movingthroughcancer.com, the companion site to Dr. Schmitz's book of the same name.

Chapter 11

Optimizing Immune and Mitochondrial Function to Fight Cancer

This chapter will provide you with a deeper understanding of your immune system and your body's mitochondria, the cellular "energy factories" that we first discussed in Chapter 1. It will also explain more about why optimal immune and mitochondria function is so vital for both preventing and helping to fight cancer, and reveal specific action steps you can begin today on your own to improve both functions. These action steps will also help your body to produce new, healthy mitochondria for better overall health.

Let's begin by taking a closer look at your immune system and how it protects against cancer.

Your Body's First Line of Defense

You may have been surprised when you read in Chapter 1 that your body produces cancer cells each and every day. In many respects, this production occurs because each of us is constantly being exposed to carcinogens in our food, air and water supply. In a state of health, your immune system is constantly on the alert for such abnormal cells and is quick to destroy them before they can grow and spread once it detects them. This inactivation and elimination of cancer cells is known as "spontaneous regression." But in reality it occurs because of the immune system as part of the overall protective role it performs to help maintain your overall health.

Based on these facts, here are three key things to remember:

1. The health of immune system is one of the most important factors that determine cancer patients' survival.

2. The presence of cancer cells in the body is far less important than the immune system's ability to properly identify and eliminate such cells.

3. Cancer takes hold in the body largely as a result of a functional breakdown in the immune system. This can occur as a result of many factors, including poor diet, nutritional deficiencies, chronic exposure to toxins, unhealthy lifestyle choices (smoking, alcohol or drug abuse, etc), chronic stress, unresolved emotional issues, and other factors that impair and overwhelm immune function over time.

Your immune system protects against cancer in a number of important ways. First, it assesses whether normal cells have been transformed into cancer cells. This task is performed by specialized white blood cells known as T lymphocytes, or T cells. T cells are produced by the thymus gland and travel throughout the body where they seek out abnormal cells and foreign proteins known as tumor-associated antigens that are released by tumor cells.

If cancer cells are present, certain types of T cells signal other types of white blood cells to spring into action. These include B cells that produce antibodies that neutralize foreign matter in both blood and tissues, as well as other lymphocytes that produce anticancer chemicals known as cytokines. Cytokines act like a natural form of chemotherapy and include tumor necrosis factor, interleukin, and interferon. When the immune system is functioning properly, cytokines do their work without harming healthy cells.

Other cancer fighters in your immune system's arsenal include natural killer (NK) cells and macrophages. NK cells are one of your body's most immediate and powerful agents for protecting against cancer. A specialized class of lymphocytes, NK cells lock onto cancer cell sites to destroy malignant cells before they can multiply and spread. NK cells are especially important in the early stages of cancer, when they descend directly upon tiny tumors to devour them or cause them to disintegrate before the tumors can grow and cause harm. NK cells have little effect against large tumors, however.

Like NK cells, macrophages also destroy cancer cells by ingesting them. They also support your body's detoxification system by scavenging for waste and debris and help to regulate cell reproduction as well as the activity of other immune cells. Research has shown a direct correlation between increased macrophage activity and a decreased incidence of tumors and tumor growth. For this reason, macrophage function by itself can often accurately determine whether tumors will thrive or die.

What follows is a closer look at the primary classes of immune cells, along with their respective roles in battling cancer:

Th1 Cells (T-helper 1 Cells): These cells are a subset of CD4+ T cells. They release pro-inflammatory cytokines, such as IFN-gamma and TNF-alpha, that activate macrophages and cytotoxic T cells, leading to enhanced tumor cell killing and inhibition of tumor growth.

Natural Killer (NK) Cells: NK cells are part of the innate immune system and have the ability to recognize and eliminate cancer cells without prior sensitization. They release cytotoxic substances that cause target cell destruction and apoptosis.

Dendritic Cells: These cells are antigen-presenting cells that play a vital role in initiating and shaping the adaptive immune response against cancer. They capture, process, and present tumor antigens to T cells, leading to the activation of specific cytotoxic T cells and the generation of a robust antitumor response.

Macrophages: These cells are part of the innate immune system and can exhibit both pro- and anti-tumor activities. M1 macrophages promote antitumor responses by releasing pro-inflammatory cytokines and exhibiting direct cytotoxicity against tumor cells, while M2 macrophages can suppress antitumor immune responses and promote tumor growth.

Neutrophils: These cells are the most abundant class of white blood cells and play a complex role in cancer. They can both promote and inhibit tumor growth, depending on factors such as the tumor microenvironment and the presence of specific cytokines.

T-Suppressors (Tregs): These cells are a subset of CD4+ T cells that express the transcription factor FoxP3. When immune function is impaired, they can suppress antitumor immune responses by inhibiting the activation and function of effector T cells and other immune cells, thereby promoting tumor growth and immune evasion.

T-Effectors (Cytotoxic T cells, or CTLs): These cells are a subset of CD8+ T cells that help detect and kill cancer cells by releasing cytotoxic substances. They play a critical role in antitumor immune responses.

T-Regulators (Tregs, mentioned above as T-Suppressors): These cells help maintain immune tolerance and prevent autoimmunity, but in the context of cancer and weakened immunity, they can suppress antitumor immune responses and facilitate immune evasion by the tumor.

Plasma Cells: These cells are responsible for producing and secreting antibodies that help eliminate tumor cells through mechanisms such as antibody-dependent cellular cytotoxicity (ADCC) and complement-dependent cytotoxicity (CDC).

All of these immune cell types interact in a complex and dynamic manner within the tumor microenvironment, and their balance and activity can influence the outcome of cancer progression and the response to therapy.

Cytokines and signaling pathways also play critical roles in regulating the immune system's response to cancer, either promoting or suppressing cancer development and progression. Key cytokines and signaling pathways involved in these processes include:

CD47 Protein Signal: CD47 is a cell surface protein that acts as a "do not eat me" signal when bound to its receptor, SIRPα, on macrophages. Cancer cells can over express CD47 to escape detection by immune cells and avoid phagocytosis (the engulfing and destruction of cancer and infectious microorganism by macrophahes and neutrophils).

WNT Pathway: The WNT signaling pathway is involved in various cellular processes, including cell proliferation, differentiation, and migration. Abnormal activation of the WNT pathway can promote cancer development and progression by enhancing cancer cell growth, survival, and invasion.

TGF-β Signaling Pathway: Transforming growth factor-beta (TGF-β) is a cytokine with multiple effects. In early-stage cancer, TGF-β helps suppress tumor growth by inhibiting cell proliferation and promoting apoptosis. However, in advanced stages, TGF-β can suppress immune function and promote tumor progression, invasion, and metastasis.

TNF-α: Tumor necrosis factor-alpha (TNF-α) is a pro-inflammatory cytokine that can have both pro- and anti-tumor effects. TNF-α can promote cancer cell death and inhibit angiogenesis, but it can also contribute to chronic inflammation and stimulate cancer cell proliferation and survival.

Interleukin-6 (IL-6): This cytokine is involved in various immune responses. It can promote tumor growth and survival by activating various signaling pathways, inducing angiogenesis, and suppressing antitumor immunity.

Interleukin-10 (IL-10): This anti-inflammatory cytokine that can suppress antitumor immunity by inhibiting the activation and function of T cells, NK cells, and macrophages. It can also promote tumor growth and metastasis by stimulating angiogenesis in tumors and suppressing detection of cancer cells.

Interleukin-12 (IL-12): IL-12 is a pro-inflammatory cytokine that promotes antitumor immunity by activating Th1 cells, cytotoxic T cells, and NK cells. It enhances the production of IFN-γ and other pro-inflammatory cytokines, leading to increased tumor cell killing.

Interferon-Gamma (IFN-γ): IFN-γ is a cytokine produced by Th1 cells, cytotoxic T cells, and NK cells. It plays a crucial role in antitumor immunity by promoting the activation and function of immune cells, enhancing antigen presentation (a vital immune system process essential for T cell immune response triggering), and inhibiting angiogenesis.

PD-1/PD-L1 Pathway: Programmed cell death protein 1 (PD-1) is an inhibitory receptor expressed on T cells, and its ligand, PD-L1, can be expressed on cancer cells. When PD-1 binds to PD-L1, it inhibits T cell activation and function, allowing cancer cells to evade immune system detection.

CTLA-4 Pathway: Cytotoxic T-lymphocyte-associated protein 4 (CTLA-4) is an inhibitory receptor expressed on T cells that can cause T cell inhibition and immune system evasion by cancer cells.

Notch Signaling Pathway: The Notch signaling pathway is involved in cell differentiation, proliferation, and survival. Dysregulation of Notch signaling can contribute to cancer development by promoting cancer cell survival, angiogenesis, and metastasis. Notch signaling can also modulate the tumor immune microenvironment, influencing immune cell function and promoting immune evasion.

JAK/STAT Pathway: This pathway plays a crucial role in regulating cytokine signaling and immune responses. Abnormal activation of the JAK/STAT pathway can contribute to cancer development and progression by promoting cancer cell survival, proliferation, and immune evasion.

PI3K/AKT/mTOR Pathway: This pathway is involved in regulating cell growth, survival, and metabolism. Deregulation of this pathway is common in cancer and can contribute to tumor development, progression, and resistance to therapy. This pathway can also modulate immune cell function and impact the antitumor immune response.

These cytokines and signaling pathways contribute to the complex interplay between the immune system and cancer cells, shaping the tumor microenvironment, and determining the outcome of cancer progression and therapy. Targeting these pathways and modulating the immune response has become a promising strategy for cancer treatment. Immunotherapies such as immune checkpoint inhibitors, cytokine therapies, and adoptive T cell transfer are already showing great promise in treating various types of cancer and improving patient outcomes. For example, immune checkpoint inhibitors such as anti-PD-1/PD-L1 and anti-CTLA-4 antibodies have shown remarkable success in treating various types of cancer by reinvigorating antitumor immune responses.

Naturopathic oncologists such as myself, along with other integrative cancer physicians, have long recognized the importance of the immune system when it comes to treating cancer effectively. For this reason, we emphasize immune-boosting therapies as part of our overall strategies for addressing cancer. This produces better and long-lasting results compared to simply focusing on killing cancer cells and tumors through the use of chemotherapy and/or radiation, both of which wreck havoc on cancer and healthy cells alike, especially immune cells. This difference in approach helps to explain why integrative approaches for cancer are often far more effective than conventional cancer treatments, both in the short-term and in the long-term.

Bolstering immune function can be accomplished in a variety of ways, starting with improving patients' diets so that the foods they eat enhance all of the body's functions, rather than impede them. One of the biggest impediments to healthy immune function is the nutritionally deficient standard American diet (SAD). The healthiest dietary approaches were covered in Chapter 8 and will be revisited later in this chapter.

Other therapies that can support the immune system include specific nutritional supplements (see Chapter 9 and more below), detoxification therapies and hyperthermia (heat-based therapies), both of which are covered in Chapter 12, regular exercise (see Chapter 10), and mind/body medicine for stress relief and to heal painful emotions (see Chapters 6 and 7).

In addition, should chemotherapy be necessary, I recommend that patients discuss with their oncologist the lab tests I covered in Chapter 5 in order to determine the most appropriate chemo drugs that are most specific to each patient's needs. By tailor-making chemotherapy treatments to match each patient's unique needs the effectiveness of chemotherapy can usually be improved, while also reducing the side effects chemotherapy is noted for, thus minimizing harm to the immune system.

Mitochondria and Your Health

None of the functions carried out by the body's immune system—or, indeed, any of the other functions performed by the body's other systems—can be performed without an sufficient supply of energy. As you learned in Chapter 1, it is the cells' mitochondria that produce nearly all (90 percent) of the body's energy supply. Ensuring that mitochondria stay healthy is therefore a major key to maintaining optimal health.

Here are just a few reasons why healthy mitochondria are so important:

1. As mentioned, mitochondria produce most of the body's energy. If they are not functioning correctly you will feel tired.

2. Mitochondria play a pivotal role in immunity. Impaired mitochondrial function increases the risk of infections and disease, including cancer.

3. Mitochondria are involved in programmed cell death (apoptosis), a process that helps to eliminate old and damaged cells, and support the body's creation of new, healthy cells. When mitochondria become damaged this process is also impaired, making it easier for cells to turn cancerous.

4. Mitochondria help to regulate metabolism. If your mitochondria are not healthy you may find it difficult to maintain a healthy weight, thus increasing your risk of unhealthy weight gain and obesity.

5. Mitochondria help regulate the cellular response to oxidative stress by producing antioxidants.

6. Mitochondria are essential for the development and function of many organs in the body, including the brain, heart, and muscles.

7. Researchers now recognize that impaired mitochondrial function is a primary cause of not only cancer but also many other diseases, including diabetes, heart disease, and neurodegenerative diseases.

8. Mitochondria also play key roles in the aging process, with damage to mitochondria over time resulting in premature aging due to declining cellular function.

These and other functions of mitochondria are why their healthy function is essential for preventing cancer, as well as why impaired mitochondrial function is a major risk factor for the onset and spread of cancer.

Here are some other facts about mitochondria:

- Mitochondria are believed to have originated from ancient bacteria that were engulfed by larger cells, leading to a symbiotic, or "win-win", relationship between the host cells and the mitochondria.

- The mitochondria in your body were inherited from your mother.

- Each cell in the body contains between 1,000 to 2,500 mitochondria, and mitochondria comprise as much as 25 percent of total cell volume. (The only exception to this is red blood cells, which do not contain any mitochondria.)

- As you learned in Chapter 1, mitochondria produce energy in the body by converting adenosine diphosphate (ADP) into adenosine triphoshate (ATP). This is accomplished through a process called cellular respiration.

- Your body at rest produces your body weight in ATP every day, and this production level increases during intense periods of exercise and other physical activities.

- ATP cannot be stored in the body. Instead, it must be produced by mitochondria every second of every day.

- The greatest number of mitochondria are found in the brain, heart, liver, and muscles, all of which use the most energy in the body.

- Mitochondria have their own DNA that is separate from the DNA found in the cell's nucleus. This DNA is used to help produce some of the proteins found in the mitochondria.

- When cells require more energy, the mitochondria reproduce to make more of themselves so they can meet that need.

- Many commonly prescribed pharmaceutical drugs can damage mitochondria and impair their function, especially if such drugs are used over long periods of time. Among the most common classes of drugs known to damage mitochondria are antibiotics, statins and other cholesterol-lowering drugs, and nonsteroidal anti-inflammatory drugs (NSAIDs) and other painkillers, including acetaminophen and aspirin.

Mitochondria and Cancer

The role of mitochondria in the initiation and progression of cancer has long been debated, but it is now generally accepted that mitochondria do play an important role in cancer through replication and energy production. Identifying the important roles that mitochondria play in cancer development and progression can help identify ways in which repairing mitochondrial function may be used for therapeutic benefit. That's because **cancer is a metabolic disease caused by dysfunction in how energy is produced within the cell.**

Many cancer researchers tend to adopt a reductionist approach in their research, seeking to condense complex biological processes down into their many parts in order to find and understand a single cause and devise a cure. It is this approach that has long spurred the hope of finding a "magic bullet" cure for cancer. With cancer, seeking out a single cure is an over-simplification, as is claiming cancer to be one disease, or that it has only one cause. In addition, cancer types differ broadly in such ways as the primary site, anatomical changes in cells, the genes involved, staging criteria, level of evidence, and, perhaps, at what point the mitochondria become involved.

As you learned in Chapter 1, despite inconsistencies in the understanding of biochemical processes, cancer has long been considered by many researchers and oncologists to be caused by genes gone awry. In science, this is called the somatic mutation theory (SMT), which posits that the initiating disease process is the result of nuclear mutations in oncogenes and tumor suppressor genes. This view is responsible for the ongoing development of cancer drugs that block specific genetic mutations, with some promise that one day a single drug could potentially treat all tumor types that share the same mutation.

Newer research, however, continues to demonstrate that such a hope is likely unfounded. My own clinical experience confirms this, as well. A more comprehensive, holistic approach is what is needed, both for preventing cancer and for effectively treating it. A better understanding of the mitochondria may be the gateway for this alternative approach.

The Mitochondria and the Krebs Cycle: The mitochondria are the home of the Krebs cycle, which you may remember learning about in school. The Krebs cycle is also known as the tricarboxylic acid cycle (TCA). It is through this cycle that mitochondria produce chemical energy in the form of adenosine triphosphate (ATP). Through the cycle's processes of oxidizing (losing an electron) the fat, protein, and carbohydrates we consume through food and drink energy-abundant molecules are created for cells. These processes are known as cellular respiration. Within the TCA, substrates such as oxygen and glucose are converted through enzymatic processes, first into pyruvate, then into acetyl-CoA, ultimately leading to the production of an ATP molecule, water, and carbon dioxide.

Researchers at the United Mitochondrial Disease Foundation have reported that only three percent of genetic material per mitochondrion (one hundred in every three thousand) is required to produce up to 90 percent of the body's ATP, and thus its energy. This efficiency enables 97 percent of the mitochondria to perform other roles in regulating the body's metabolic pathways.

The mitochondria are also genetically independent from the nucleus of the cell and communicate via nuclear transport and messenger proteins. In addition to producing ATP, mitochondria are responsible for building and encoding the nucleic acids and proteins responsible for cellular respiration, communicating with the nucleus, causing cells to grow, function, and recycle their molecular building blocks through regulation of apoptosis pathways.

Mitochondria and the Warburg Effect: Normal cells produce energy through a process known as mitochondrial oxidative phosphorylation (OXPHOS). When oxygen is not available, they produce energy via the less efficient route of anaerobic glycolysis (the extraction of energy from glucose in a low oxygen environment). In the 1920s, Nobel laureate Otto Warburg observed that cancer cells do not produce energy in the efficient way that normal cells do. Rather, they produce most of their energy through an inefficient, high rate of anaerobic glycolysis and glutaminolysis (the process by which cells convert glucose and glutamine into TCA cycle metabolites, the substances used for metabolism) through the activity of multiple enzymes. This then followed by fermentation of lactate into lactic acid.

Glutamine is the most abundant amino acid circulating in blood and muscle. It is critical for many healthy cellular functions, including maintaining mitochondrial metabolism, the production of antioxidants to remove reactive oxygen species (ROS), the activation of cell signaling, and the synthesis of nonessential amino acids, fatty acids, and other substances needed for cellular replication. Altered or unhealthy glutaminolysis results in these same benefits being provided to cancer cells.

In an anaerobic environment, as cancer occurs and spreads, glucose and glutamine metabolites are then diverted from producing ATP to a process to promote unchecked cell growth. Warburg described this process as aerobic fermentation. Today, it is known as aerobic glycolysis, or the *Warburg Effect*.

Since lactate production is considered an indicator of respiratory insufficiency in biological systems, Warburg regarded aerobic production of lactate in cancer cells to be a sign and gauge of respiratory insufficiency. (Differentiated cells produce large amounts of lactate only under anaerobic conditions.) This observation remains a controversial one, not so much as to the involvement of the mitochondria in cancer, but as to what point mitochondria become involved in the cancer process and whether they are still functioning within cancer cells.

Cancer researcher Thomas Seyfried, PhD, professor of biology at Boston College, is a leading proponent of cancer as a mitochondrial metabolic disease. He outlines the key points of Warburg's research and theories about cancer very well when he states that 1) insufficient respiration initiates tumorigenesis and ultimately cancer, 2) energy through glycolysis gradually compensates for insufficient energy through respiration, 3) cancer cells continue to ferment glucose, creating lactate as an end-product both with and without the presence of oxygen, and 4) respiratory insufficiency eventually becomes irreversible.

The view that cancer is a metabolic mitochondrial disease appears to be the only cancer initiation theory that relates to all cancers, in contrast to the somatic mutation theory. This is because all evidence supports the Warburg effect – whether causal or not – as being constant in the initiation and/or progression of cancer. Seyfried's model regards somatic mutation as an event that follows mitochondrial disruption. He and other researchers have concluded that respiratory insufficiency is the origin of cancer, and that the other theories about what causes cancer, including the SMT, also arise either directly or indirectly from insufficient respiration.

Disruptions in any of the cellular processes controlled by mitochondria can initiate cancer. This includes disruptions in how mitochondria regulate cellular energy production and oxidation–reduction (redox) status, generate reactive oxygen species (ROS), and initiate apoptosis through the activation of the mitochondrial permeability transition pore and Cytochrome C. Changes in any of these mechanisms of action can shift cells towards a cancerous state. Other disruptors of mitochondria function are genetic mutations, enzyme defects, and acid buildup in the cellular microenvironment caused by the conversion of glucose to lactic acid.

When mutations in mitochondrial genes are present, as they often are in cancer cells, they alter the mitochondria's oxygen rate, extracellular acidification rate, and cell proliferation. Cancer cells have been shown to display genetic and epigenetic mutations that activate irregular programs that optimize the cancer cell environment by reprogramming adjacent cells for their benefit, using retrograde signaling. Mutated mitochondrial genes regulate the transcription factor hypoxia-inducible factor 1 (HIF-1), which induces glycolysis under anaerobic conditions, allowing cancer cells to thrive. HIF-1 is increasingly being studied because it allows for the survival and proliferation of cancerous cells due to its angiogenic properties. Thus, inhibition of HIF-1 potentially could prevent the spread of cancer.

Enzyme defects also play a role because cancer cells require altered metabolism to efficiently divert and incorporate nutrients into tumors and to support abnormal proliferation. In addition, the survival of tumor cells outside of normal tissue requires adaptation of metabolism to different microenvironments. Warburg theorized that, in order to treat cancer effectively, targeting the enzymes that cancer cells depend upon more than normal cells for tumor cell growth, survival and proliferation was more important that targeting mutated genes. These defective enzymes are present in virtually all cancers.

There are several metabolic enzyme defects that are susceptible to certain treatments that target these enzymes. However, long-term success with this approach depends on understanding why specific metabolic pathways are important for cancer cells and being able to determine which patients are likely to respond to such treatments.

Reactions involving electron transfers are known as oxidation-reduction, or redox, reactions for which OXPHOS is the metabolic pathway. A redox reaction occurs as a result of two smaller reactions; one molecule loses one or more electrons and simultaneously gains an oxygen atom to become oxidized, and another molecule gains an electron and loses an oxygen atom to become reduced. Cancer cells have an amazing tendency to reprogram their metabolic capability by inhibiting OXPHOS to elevate glucose metabolism. Inhibiting glycolysis to shift cellular metabolism back to normal OXPHOS pathway activity is another element of integrative cancer treatments.

The increase of reactive oxygen species (ROS) in cancer cells is linked to many irregularities in cellular functions, such as cell proliferation, migration, differentiation and apoptosis. The increased promotion of ROS in tumor cells with mitochondrial dysfunction makes them more prone to further oxidative stress, compared to normal cells with lower levels of ROS. When mitochondrial ROS production is too high it is toxic to healthy cells and can cause abnormal tissue growth.

Understanding the role that lactic acid buildup in the cellular microenvironment plays in cancer, and to what degree, is another important area of cancer research. Whether cancer cells opt for fermentation to proliferate, or if they must choose this path over cellular respiration due to mitochondrial damage, continues to be debated by researchers. However, there is growing agreement that the Warburg effect is common to all cancers and that, regardless of the availability of oxygen, cancer cells convert most glucose to lactic acid.

Studies have shown that lactic acid is not merely a byproduct but that it informs a predictive role in the proliferation of cancerous cells, metastasis of cancer, and patient survival. Acidosis generated from lactic acid impedes the function of normal immune cells, including loss of T-cell function, thereby suppressing the anticancer immune response and enhancing tumor cell survival.

Cytochrome C function and apoptosis must also be examined in order to treat cancer. Cytochrome C is a small, water-soluble protein found within mitochondrial membranes. In normal cells and in the presence of oxygen Cytochrome C acts like a shuttle to move electrons from glucose to ATP production. Cytochrome C also has an opposite function, signaling cells to begin the process of apoptosis. While apoptosis is part of healthy growth and development, if the apoptosis system is malfunctioning it can trigger the growth and spread of cancer cells and tumors.

All of the above factors demonstrate that, even given the role that ongogenes and tumor suppression genes play in cancer, the underlying common denominator of cancer's onset and progression is controlled by mitochondria function. Since the mitochondria have so few parts to them and play such a major role in tumorigenesis, they are an obvious target for cancer therapies. To this end, new drugs are being developed to inhibit mitochondrial respiration of cancer cells and induce mitochondrial structural damage within them. The additional nontoxic cancer treatments you will learn about in Part Three also offer significant benefit in this regard.

Self-Care Steps To Support Immunity and Mitochondrial Function

The self-care measures I shared with you in Chapters 8, 9, and 10 all help to boost immunity, support healthy mitochondrial function, and prevent cancer. What follows is more information about them, as well as other proven self-care tips you can use to help keep your immune system and mitochondria healthy.

Diet

Your diet is especially important when it comes to maintaining the health of your immune system and mitochondria. Following the healthy eating guidelines I shared with you in Chapter 8 will go a long way to helping you achieve this goal.

As I discussed in that chapter, in recent years the ketogenic, or keto, diet has gained in popularity for the benefits it may provide for cancer patients and as a possible means of preventing cancer. According to research, much of the diet's value in this regard has to do with its effects on mitochondrial metabolism.

To recap what you learned in Chapter 8, the ketogenic diet involves replacing one's intake of carbohydrates with healthy fats, so that fats become the main source of fuel in the body. This, in turn, pushes the body's metabolism into a state of ketosis, which prevents cancer cells from deriving energy from the glucose in carbohydrate foods. Some research takes a broader view, suggesting that cancer growth and progression can be managed by following an individualized nutritional protocol so that the TCA (Krebs) cycle will shift the whole body from fermentable end-products of metabolism (primarily glucose and glutamine) to respiratory metabolic end-products (primarily ketones). A pilot study has shown that the ketogenic diet is safe even for late stage cancer patients.

Research also suggests that the diet may support first line cancer treatments via two different mechanisms, both of which increase oxidative stress inside cancer cells. First, lipid (fat) metabolism obliges the cells to generate energy from mitochondrial metabolism instead of anaerobic glycolysis as the glucose is not available for that process. This reduction in the availability of glucose limits glycolysis, depriving cancer cells of energy. In addition, because dysfunctional mitochondria lead to reactive oxygen species (ROS) production, cancer cells are more likely to experience and be damaged by oxidative stress, compared to normal cells, when glucose metabolism is restricted.

In 2017, a systematic review was done on the ketogenic diet in animal models. All 13 articles included in the review indicated that the diet was shown to inhibit tumor growth and nine articles stated that the diet could enhance survival time. Multiple research trials have also assessed ketogenic diets as an aid to primary cancer therapies. In the University of Würzburg, Germany, patients who failed traditional cancer therapy but who were able to continue the ketogenic diet therapy for over three months showed improvement, including a stable physical condition, tumor shrinkage, or slowed cancer growth.

I recommend including broccoli and other cruciferous vegetables when following the ketogenic diet, not only because they are low in carbohydrate value, but because of the proven anticancer benefits they provide (see Chapter 8). This includes the fact that they contain a compound called phenethyl isothiocyanate (PI), which has been shown to exhibit a potent anticancer ability to disable the glutathione antioxidant system, which results in severe ROS accumulation in cancer cells. Consequently, the oxidative damage initiates death of the cancer cells.

Based on current research, I agree that ketogenic diets can be useful for correcting inherent oxidative metabolic differences between cancer cells and normal cells, and for improving standard therapeutic outcomes by selectively enhancing oxidative stress and ROS in cancer cells and tumors. I especially recommend such a diet for patients suffering from brain cancer and other cancers that are not primarily being driven by hormonal imbalances and abnormalities. Overall, however, I find that the plant-based diets discussed in Chapter 8 offer equal, and perhaps greater value, for most cases of cancer, and are more advisable for most noncancer patients because of the greater array of nutrients they provide, and also because they are much easier to implement and abide by, especially long-term. Moreover, studies show that such diets also strongly support immune and mitochondrial function and overall health to at least the same degree that ketogenic diets do.

This is especially true of plant-based diets low in starchy carbohydrate foods and rich in organic fruits and vegetables because of the abundance of polyphenols and other nutrients they contain. Other immune- and mitochondrial-supporting food groups include non-farm-raised fish, grass-fed meats (including organ meats such as liver) and poultry, and certain nuts and seeds, such as Brazil nuts and pumpkin seeds.

Nutritional and Herbal Supplement Aids

An extensive body of research proves that certain types of supplements are also effective for boosting immune and mitochondrial function, thereby helping to both prevent and reverse cancer. Of particular value in this regard are the following:

Astragalus, a traditional Chinese medicine (TCM) herb with immune-enhancing and antitumor effects that has been shown to enhance the cytotoxic activity of immune cells, such as NK cells and T cells. Some clinical studies have reported that Astragalus may improve immune function and survival in cancer patients when used as an adjunct to conventional therapies but more research is needed.

Cat's claw is another herbal remedy that supports the immune system and has anti-inflammatory effects. It has been shown to stimulate the immune system and inhibit the production of inflammatory agents like TNF-α, COX-2, and PGE2. However, the evidence for its effectiveness in cancer treatment is limited and more research is needed to establish its clinical effectiveness in fighting cancer.

Curcumin, the active compound in turmeric, has been extensively studied for its anti-inflammatory, antioxidant, and anticancer properties. It has been shown to regulate the activity of various immune cells and inhibit signaling pathways like NF-κB and STAT3 that are involved in inflammation and tumor progression.

Echinacea is a popular herbal remedy with proven immune stimulation effects. Echinacea has been shown to enhance the activity of immune cells, such as NK cells, macrophages, and T-cells. However, the research on echinacea's effectiveness in cancer treatment is limited and more research is needed to determine its clinical usefulness in cancer patients.

Fermented wheat germ extract (FWGE) has been shown in more than two dozen in vitro and in vivo studies to have strong anticancer, anti-metastatic, and immune-enhancing effects, including tumor-inhibiting effects in human breast adenocarcinoma cells equal to or better than tamoxifen. In addition, several human clinical studies indicate that FWGE may help improve quality of life as well as having a further beneficial role in patients with various forms of cancer.

FWGE promotes apoptosis directly by increasing levels of Cytochrome C as well as indirectly by cleaving PARP, a family of proteins, which prevent cancer cells from repairing DNA. FWGE inhibits glycolysis, helping to curtail cancer cell proliferation.

FWGE also inhibits the enzyme glucose-6-phosphate dehydrogenase, a metabolic enzyme essential for using glucose carbons to make ribose. FWGE may virtually eliminate cancer cell proliferation through inhibition of both major and minor pathways of cancer cell synthesis of ribose. Lastly, FWGE rescues mitochondria via apoptosis and induces cancer cells to engage in mitochondrial OXPHOS so that they produce energy like a normal cell.

Green tea extract (EGCG), the polyphenol found in green tea, also provides antioxidant, anti-inflammatory, and anticancer benefits. It has also been shown to support the immune response and inhibit tumor growth by targeting various signaling pathways and enzymes, such as NF-κB, STAT3, and COX-2.

Ginseng, especially Panax ginseng, has been used in TCM for centuries and is known for its adaptogenic and immune-enhancing properties because of the ginsenosides and other bioactive compounds it contains.

Medicinal mushrooms and mushroom extracts such as reishi, turkey tail, and shiitake, also provide immunomodulatory and antitumor properties. They also contain bioactive compounds, including beta-glucans, that can stimulate immune cells, including NK cells, dendritic cells, and T cells. Some clinical trials indicate that mushroom extracts may improve immune function and survival in cancer patients when used alongside conventional therapies.

Milk thistle is an herb that contains a group of bioactive compounds called silymarin which have antioxidant, anti-inflammatory, and anticancer properties. Silymarin has been shown to regulate the immune response and inhibit various signaling pathways like NF-κB that are involved in tumor progression. Some studies have reported potential benefits of milk thistle in cancer patients, such as reduced liver toxicity from chemotherapy, but more research is needed to confirm these findings.

Mistletoe extracts contain various bioactive compounds that can stimulate immune cells and induce cancer cell death. Some clinical trials have reported that mistletoe extracts may also improve quality of life and survival in cancer patients, but more research is needed to establish its effectiveness in this area.

Omega-3 fatty acids are found in fish, fish oils, and certain plant sources. Omega-3s have anti-inflammatory effects and can help modulate the immune response in cancer by affecting the function of immune cells, such as T cells and macrophages, and by inhibiting the production of inflammatory mediators like PGE2 and COX-2. Some clinical studies have suggested that omega-3 fatty acids may improve the effectiveness of chemotherapy and reduce treatment-related side effects.

Quercetin, a plant-derived flavonoid commonly found in fruits, vegetables, and certain beverages like tea and wine, possesses antioxidant, anti-inflammatory, and anticancer properties. One of the mechanisms by which quercetin exerts its anti-inflammatory effects is by blocking the inflammatory cascades caused by tumor necrosis factor-alpha (TNFα). As you learned in Chapter 2, TNFα plays a significant role in inflammation and can promote tumor growth, angiogenesis, and metastasis. Quercetin's interference with TNFα signaling has several downstream effects that further contribute to its anti-inflammatory and anticancer properties. However, more research is needed to fully understand its mechanisms and to establish its safety and effectiveness as a cancer-fighting supplement.

A variety of other nutritional and other supplements known to support immune and mitochondrial function include:

- Alpha-Lipoic Acid (ALA)
- Apigenin
- Coenzyme Q10 (CoQ10)

- D-Ribose
- Glutathione
- L-Carnitine
- Magnesium
- Melatonin
- N-Acetyl Cysteine (NAC)
- Resveratrol
- Selenium
- Taurine
- Vitamin C
- Vitamin D
- Vitamin E
- Yerba mate
- Zinc.

It's important to emphasize, however, that the value of these supplements can vary greatly from person to person depending on each person's unique biochemical individuality. This is especially true for cancer patients and the type and stage of cancer they are dealing with. This is why I always recommend that my patients ideally take supplements under the guidance of physician or other health care practitioner experienced in their use and properties.

Time-Restricted Eating (TRE) and Fasting

Time restricted eating, also known as intermittent fasting, means consuming all of the foods you eat each day within an eight to 12-hour period. By doing so you allow your body 12 to 16 hours to rest and repair itself through a process known as autophagy.

Autophagy is a natural process of cellular cleansing in which the body essentially "eats" parts of itself by breaking down and then eliminating old, worn down proteins, cell membranes, and other parts of cells which can no longer be sustained by the body's energy. This enables the body to replace these cellular components with new, healthier versions, thereby helping the body to better maintain itself.

Autophagy can only occur during times of fasting, which TRE mimics to some extent. TRE is not the same thing as dieting or calorie restriction. You can eat as you normally do as long as you limit the window of time each day in which you do so.

Research suggests that TRE can also increase mitochondrial energy production in the body. That's because TRE has been shown to increase levels of a metabolite called nicotinamide adenine dinucleotide (NAD). Research by Otto Warburg, among others, demonstrated that NAD is an essential cofactor of many of the body's biochemical reactions, either in its oxidized (NAD+) or reduced (NADH) form. NAD+, in addition to helping the body metabolize fats and glucose, helps to improve mitochondrial function and increases the ability of mitochondria to produce ATP, resulting in increased levels of cellular energy.

If you are new to TRE and want to explore it, I suggest starting out slowly, eating all of your meals within a 12-hour window. As you become more used to TRE, you can move on to eating all of your meals, as well as snacks, within an eight-hour window.

As a substitute for or enhancement to TRE, you can increase the benefits autophagy provides by periodically fasting. A 24-hour water fast done weekly or every other week is safe for most people to undergo. In addition to its autophagy benefits, fasting has been shown to stimulate the body's production of growth hormones, which typically decline as we age. You may also wish to explore periodic longer fasts of three to five days, although these should initially be undertaken under the supervision of a doctor or other health practitioner familiar with fasting's therapeutic benefits.

Exercise

Research confirms that regular exercise also boosts immunity and mitochondria function. When you exercise, your body's energy supply is temporarily reduced. This depletion causes an increase in NAD+ molecules, thereby improving mitochondrial function and increasing the production of ATP in much the same way that time-restricted eating does. Mitochondrial enzymes necessary for proper mitochondrial function are also increased during exercise.

Research also shows that regular exercise increases the amount of mitochondria and therefore ATP in muscles cells to meet the energy demands that occur while exercising, and helping to slow muscle loss associated with aging. This includes skeletal muscles, as was confirmed in a small study of eight healthy elderly test subjects who engaged in high intensity interval training (HIIT). After only two weeks of HIIT, all of the test members were found to have significantly improved mitochondrial function in their skeletal muscles.

See Chapter 10 for more on the health benefits of exercise and how to incorporate exercise into your daily life.

Regular Sunlight Exposure

It's well-established that sunlight exposure enables to body to produce vitamin D, and that vitamin D provides many important immune function benefits. What is less known is that vitamin D is also vital for mitochondrial health.

This fact was confirmed by researchers who explored what happened when they "silenced" the vitamin D receptor (VDR) in a study of both healthy and cancer cells. VDR is responsible for regulating the various effects of vitamin D. Without it, vitamin D cannot perform its functions. In their published study, the researchers wrote, "We demonstrated that, in silenced cells, the increased respiratory activity was associated with elevated reactive oxygen species (ROS) production. In the long run, the absence of the receptor caused impairment of mitochondrial integrity and, finally, cell death. Our data reveal that VDR plays a central role in protecting cells from excessive respiration and production of ROS that leads to cell damage. Because we confirmed our observations in different models of both normal and cancer cells, we conclude that VDR is essential for the health of human tissues."

Regular sunlight exposure is also important because it increases an antioxidant gene in the body called Nrf2 (nuclear factor erythroid 2 p45-related factor 2). Nrf2 is known to increase mitochondrial function and signaling, and also to protect against cancer. Its production is increased by sunlight's infrared ultraviolet-B (UVB) rays.

Nrf2 is the master regulator of cellular redox homeostasis, and targets genes in an extensive network of antioxidant enzymes and proteins involved in the body's various detoxification processes. It is also involved in the repair and removal of damaged proteins and inhibits inflammation. According to researchers, "Studies using isolated mitochondria and cultured cells have demonstrated that Nrf2 deficiency leads to impaired mitochondrial fatty acid oxidation, respiration, and ATP production."

Finally, mitochondria themselves also have the ability to convert sunlight into energy via a process of photosynthesis that is similar to photosynthesis in plants. This better enables mitochondria to increase ATP, as well as cellular respiration to supply cells with more energy.

Fortunately, you can obtain all of sunlight's health benefits in as little as 20 to 30 minutes of daily sunlight exposure, ideally in the early morning hours.

In addition to the above measures, it is vitally important that you obtain at least seven hours of deep, restorative sleep each night, and that you do your best to reduce your exposures to environmental toxins both in your home and work environments in order to achieve and maintain optimum immune and mitochondrial function,.

By applying the information in this chapter on a consistent basis, as well as implementing the many other self-care measures you learned about in the preceding chapters of this book, you will soon discover how much control you actually have over your health and begin to experience improvements throughout your whole person—body, mind, and spirit.

Chapter 12

Why An Integrative Medicine Approach Is Crucial For Treating Cancer

Learning that you or a loved one has cancer can be devastating. Even worse, navigating the cancer treatment process can be scary and confusing. In fact, one of the primary obstacles cancer patients face is not knowing the full range of options that are available to them. These options, when properly used, can significantly improve the likelihood that they will not only recover from cancer, but also that they will avoid a recurrence of cancer in the future. That's why it is crucial that cancer patients and their oncologists first do all they can to determine the best course of action.

Unfortunately, the primary approaches used by oncologists for treating cancer today continue to be surgery, chemotherapy, and/or radiation therapies. While each of these procedures certainly has value on their own and when they are used in combination with each other, their long-term success rates overall continue to be suboptimal. This is why I advocate for a far more comprehensive and integrative approach for treating cancer.

In this chapter, you will learn what such an approach entails, as well as what therapies my staff and I employ at The Karlfeldt Center, both on their own, and to support and improve the effectiveness of surgery, chemo, and radiation should they be needed. Many of these therapies may be unfamiliar to you, yet, as you will learn, research supports their use, as does the clinical results my staff and I are achieving with our cancer patients. Other integrative oncologists are, as well.

It is my hope that the information in this chapter will educate cancer patients and oncologists alike about how and why the use of such therapies within an integrative medicine framework can achieve greater rates of successful remission and longer lasting recovery than what is typically achieved by conventional treatments alone.

In the remainder of this chapter, you will learn about the benefits, limitations, and side effect risks of these conventional cancer treatments, the steps needed to most effectively diagnose cancer and develop an individualized treatment plan, and additional treatment options that are proven to be effective for treating cancer.

The Pros and Cons of Conventional Cancer Treatments

I want to emphasize that I do not oppose the use of surgery, chemotherapy, and radiation. All three of these treatments have great value and, indeed, can be life-savers. Moreover, I often recommend such treatments to my cancer patients and work with them in tandem with their oncologists. However, I also make sure to advise my patients of the limitations and side effects each of these therapies can have, as well as what can be done to reduce these risks.

The biggest limitation of these conventional therapies is their poor long-term survival rates despite the fact that the number of cancer survivors continues to increase in the United States due to advances in early detection and treatment.

According to the most recent (September/October 2022) data reported by the American Cancer Society (ACS), only a combined 31 percent of male and female cancer patients who received conventional cancer treatments, whether separately or in combination, were still alive five years later (33 percent of men and 29 percent of women). And after five years, this percentage dropped to a combined 22 percent (23 percent of men and 21 percent of women), and then continued to drop precipitously in each successive five-year period. This means that nearly 70 percent of all cancer patients who receive conventional cancer treatments alone will not be alive five years later.

The five-year survival time among cancer patients whose cancer has spread into other organs (stage-4 cancer) can be significantly less. For example, the five-year survival rate of patients with colon cancer that has metastasized into other organs is only 13 percent, according to the ACS. It's worth noting that colon cancer is one of the most common types of cancer in the US, with over 40 percent of all American men and women likely to develop it at some point in their lives.

Moreover, even among those who do survive whichever type of cancer they develop, many of them suffer long-standing diminished quality of life issues that are caused by the treatments' side effects, including functional and cognitive impairments, as well as other psychological and economic challenges.

What follow are overviews of the most common of these side effects for each type of conventional cancer treatment.

Surgery: Surgery is often advisable as a cancer treatment. It works best for solid, localized tumors in one area of the body. It is not used for leukemia (a type of blood cancer) or for cancers that have metastasized. In some cases, surgery alone may be the only treatment needed, but most often other treatments are also required.

Depending on the type of cancer and how advanced it is, surgery can be used to remove an entire localized tumor or to debulk a tumor. Debulking removes part, but not all of a tumor, and is used when the removal of an entire tumor is likely to damage an organ. Debulking is also often used to improve the effectiveness of other cancer treatments. In some cases, surgery is also used to ease pain and other cancer symptoms caused by pressure exerted by tumors.

Surgery often requires cutting through skin, muscles, and sometimes bone. These cuts can be painful and take some time to heal. Before they are made, patients receive either local or general anesthesia to prevent feelings of pain as the surgery is performed.

There are many types of surgery, which differ based on the purpose of the surgery, the part of the body that requires surgery, the amount of tissue to be removed, and, in some cases, what the patient prefers. Surgery can be open or minimally invasive.

In open surgery, the surgeon makes one large cut to remove the tumor, some healthy tissue, and possibly some nearby lymph nodes. In minimally invasive, or laparoscopic, surgery, the surgeon makes a few small cuts instead of one large one. A long, thin tube called a laparoscope to which a tiny camera is attached is inserted into one of the small cuts. The camera projects images from the inside of the body onto a monitor, which allows surgeons to see what they are doing. Special surgery tools that are inserted through the other small cuts remove the tumor and some healthy tissue. Because minimally invasive surgery requires smaller cuts, it takes less time to recover from than open surgery. Biopsy, which involves the removal of tissue samples for diagnostic purposes, is another commonly used surgery that is minimally invasive.

Two other surgical procedures sometimes used to treat cancer are cryosurgery, also known as cryotherapy, and laser surgery. Cryosurgery is a procedure that uses extreme cold produced by liquid nitrogen or argon gas to destroy abnormal tissue. Among the cancers it can treat are early-stage skin cancer, precancerous growths on the skin and cervix, and retinoblastoma, a rare form of cancer of the retina that is most common in young children.

Laser surgery employs laser tools that emit powerful beams of light to cut through tissue. Since lasers can focus very accurately on tiny areas, they can be used for precise surgeries. Lasers can also be used to shrink or destroy tumors or growths that might turn cancerous. Laser surgery is most often used to treat tumors on the surface of the body or on the inside lining of internal organs. Cancers for which laser surgery can be useful include basal cell carcinoma, cervical changes that might turn into cancer, and cervical, vaginal, esophageal, and non-small cell lung cancers.

The most common side effect of cancer surgery is pain in the part of the body that was operated on. The degree of pain depends on how extensive the surgery was, as well as on the part of the body where surgery was performed. Doctors and their staff educate patients on how to best manage pain after surgery, as well as providing them with pain medications.

Other risks of surgery include bleeding, damage to nearby tissues, infections, and reactions to the anesthesia, all of which can weaken immune function, which is already affected by surgery itself. Prior to having surgery, patients should always talk with their doctors about possible risks for the type of surgery they will have.

While the above risks are well known to and monitored by cancer surgeons and oncologists following surgical procedures, less attention is paid to the circulating tumor cells (CTCs) that invariably break apart from tumors as they are surgically removed or debulked. Even biopsy procedures can cause CTCs to dislodge from tumor samples. As you learned in Chapter 4, unless CTCs are properly screened for and dealt with, they can cause a recurrence of cancer that is often more deadly and more difficult to treat than the original cancer was.

Finally, another serious, yet unfortunately not rare, risk factor of surgery is the removal of more parts of the body than are necessary when tumors are removed. Examples of this include radical mastectomy of the breast when a far less invasive lumpectomy may be all that was required, or the unnecessary removal of the prostate gland in cases of prostate cancer, which can leave men with multiple side effects, including urinary incontinence, erectile dysfunction, and impotence.

For all of these reasons, anyone considering surgery for cancer should first learn all they can about the potential risks and complications that are involved, and also do all they can to prepare themselves prior to the procedure, including bolstering their bodies with appropriate dietary and other nutritional measures. These education and preparation measures are a standard part of integrative oncology. Surgery suppresses the immune system and leaves the body more vulnerable to potential CTCs that are breaking off or that are already in other areas of the body. It is essential to support the immune system both before and after surgery. I frequently have my patients do a series of vitamin C IVs to support the activity of the immune system.

Chemotherapy: Chemotherapy, or chemo, is the most common conventional care treatment for cancer. In many cases, it is introduced after surgery is used to either biopsy or remove a malignant tumor since surgery alone cannot ensure that malignancy does not still exist or that cancer may recur later. In such cases, chemo is used to try to eliminate any remaining cancer cells and reduce the risk of recurrence.

In many other cases, chemo is the conventional treatment of choice when oncologists determine that surgery is not advisable due to cancer having moved beyond its early stage. Even if chemo is not effective in reversing cancer, it can often used to help prolong life and manage cancer pain and other symptoms.

Chemo can sometimes also be used prior to surgery in order to shrink tumors before they are surgically removed.

The types of chemo treatment that patients receive depends on the type of cancer they have developed, its stage, where in the body it is located, and whether or not it has spread. Patients' overall health status is also a determining factor, especially if they are dealing with other health conditions, such as diabetes or heart disease. Any additional medications patients may be taking are also considered.

Once a treatment plan is devised, chemotherapy can be administered in one of many ways. The most common forms of administration are:

- Orally, via capsules, pills, or liquids.
- Intravenously directly into a vein.

- Via injection into a muscle in the arm, hip, or thigh, or right under the skin in the fatty part of the arm, leg, or belly.
- Intra-arterially, with chemo injected directly into the artery that leads to the tumor site.
- Intraperitoneally, meaning directly into the peritoneal cavity, the area in the body that contains organs such as the intestines, stomach, and liver.
- Intrathecally, meaning injected into the space between the layers of tissue that cover the brain and spinal cord.
- And topically, as a cream applied to the skin.

Of all the methods mentioned above, chemotherapy is most often given via an IV, through a thin needle that is placed in a vein at the start of each treatment, which is then removed when treatment is over. IV chemotherapy may also be administered via a catheter or port, sometimes with the help of a pump.

A catheter is a thin, soft tube. For chemotherapy, one end of the catheter is inserted into a large vein, most often in the chest area, with the other end remaining outside the body. Most catheters stay in place until patients finish all of their chemotherapy treatments. Catheters can also be used to administer other drugs and to draw blood.

A port is a small, round disc that is placed under the skin during minor surgery. Like a catheter, it is put in place before treatment begins, and remains there until all treatments are finished. A catheter connects the port to a large vein, typically in the chest. A needle can be inserted into a port to administer chemotherapy or to draw blood. This needle can remain in place for chemotherapy treatments that are given for longer than one day.

Cancer patients who receive a catheter and/or port need to watch for signs of infection that can sometimes occur around them. Should infection occur, patients' oncologists should be informed immediately.

Pumps are often attached to catheters or ports in order to control how much and how fast chemotherapy goes into a catheter or port. The use of a pump allows cancer patients to receive chemotherapy outside of the hospital. Pumps can be internal or external. External pumps remain outside the body. Internal pumps are placed under the skin during surgery.

A more recent delivery method for chemotherapy drugs is the use of nanotechnology in which chemo drugs are encapsulated within nanoparticle carriers. Although still in the early stages of research and development, nanotechnology shows promise because of its ability to inject chemo drugs directly into cancerous cells and tumors, enhancing the drugs' effectiveness while reducing the risk of debilitating side effects, thereby potentially improving the likelihood of survival.

Treatment schedules for chemotherapy vary widely. How often and how long patients receive chemotherapy depends on their type of cancer and how advanced it is, the type of chemo drug or drugs (chemo drugs are often given as a combination cocktail) being used, and the purpose for which chemo is used (to cure cancer, control its growth, or ease patient symptoms). Another important determining fact is how well patients respond to chemotherapy.

Chemotherapy is typically administered in cycles. A cycle is a period of chemotherapy treatment followed by a period of rest. For example, a patient might receive chemotherapy every day for one week followed by three weeks for rest and recuperation. This total of four weeks comprise one cycle.

Chemotherapy affects cancer patients in different ways. How patients respond to chemo depends on the type and stage of cancer they have, their state of overall health prior to beginning treatment, the type of chemo they are receiving, and the dosage. Because patients respond differently, prior to treatment it is not possible for oncologists to predict with certainty how each individual patient will be affected by chemotherapy. Even so, prior to beginning chemotherapy, patients should be sure to educate themselves about the benefits, limitations, and risks associated with chemotherapy, including having discussions with their oncologists.

During the course of treatment, patients are regularly monitored by their oncologists to assess how well chemo is working and to address any potential side effects. During office visits, patients will be asked how they feel, receive physical exams, and may undergo tumor marker and other blood test, as well as MRI, CT, and/or PET scans.

The primary purpose of chemotherapy is to kill rapidly growing cancer cells and halt tumor growth. But because of their high toxicity, chemo drugs can also damage the body's healthy cells and tissues, resulting in a wide range of harmful side effects, including reducing and impairing the production of both red and white blood cells in bone marrow. Although this effect is temporary and will usually resolve over time once the cycle of chemo treatments ends, when it happens, it can suppress immune function, increase the risk of infection, and cause ongoing fatigue, which can often be severe.

Chemo can also damage cells within the gastrointestinal tract, including in the mouth and stomach, resulting in mouth sores, loss of appetite and impaired digestion, constipation and/or diarrhea, nausea, and vomiting.

Other common side effects of chemotherapy include hair loss, and memory and cognition problems (sometimes referred to as "chemo brain"). Pain and discomfort are also common, as are sleep problems. During treatment, chemo can also interfere with any other medications patients may be prescribed, complicating other pre-existing conditions they may have. In most cases, these side-effects are temporary.

Another side effect, which can often be long-lasting, is peripheral neuropathy that causes numbness, tingling, and pain in fingers and/or toes.

Chemo can also cause long-term damage to the heart, liver, and lungs.

Many chemo drugs, because of their toxicity, are known to carry a higher risk of heart issues which, collectively, are known as cardiotoxicity. Cardiotoxicity risks include cardiomyopathy, myocardial infarction (heart attack), coronary heart disease, arrhythmia (irregular heartbeat rhythm), heart valve disease, and heart failure. Blood pressure problems (both high and low), fluid buildup around the heart, constrictive pericarditis (thinning of the heart's lining), and a slower than normal heart rate can also be caused by chemo drugs.

Warning signs and symptoms of cardiotoxicity include abdominal distension, chest pain, dizziness, edema (swelling and fluid retention in the legs), heart palpitations, and shortness of breath.

Because there is no way to prevent cardiotoxicity during chemotherapy, during and following chemo treatments, patients should be regularly monitored with electrocardiograms (EKG or ECG), echocardiograms, and/or cardiac CT and MRI scans.

Liver damage can also be caused by chemotherapy due to the fact that it is the liver that breaks down both oral and intravenous chemo drugs (as well as all drugs in general) to help the body clear their toxic residues. Liver damage can be a direct result of chemotherapy drugs alone, or a compounded reaction to chemo and various drugs such as analgesics (painkillers), antibiotics, anti-emetics (drugs used to relieve nausea and vomiting), and other medications that may be used to lessen the severity of other side effects that chemo can cause.

Common side effects and damage to the liver caused by chemotherapy include liver inflammation due to elevated liver enzyme levels, jaundice due to elevated bilirubin levels, hepatitis, damage to and destruction of hepatocytes (the liver's main functional cells), liver fibrosis and scar tissue formation, impaired or completely stalled bile flow (hepatic cholestasis), obstruction of the small veins in the liver (hepatic veno-occlusive disease, which can be life-threatening), and outright liver failure.

Researchers have also found that up to 85 percent of patients who receive chemotherapy develop a condition known as fatty liver disease, and that many patients also develop a chronic liver disease known as steatosis hepatitis, especially if chemo drugs cause an increase in bilirubin levels.

Lung damage is another potential serious and long-term side effect of chemotherapy. It is more common in patients who smoke or who have pre-existing lung conditions, and can be worsened when chemo is used with radiation therapy. But lung damage can potentially affect anyone receiving chemo.

One of the most common lung issues caused by chemotherapy is inflammation and/or scarring of lung tissues, which can reduce the amount of air patients can breathe. Lung inflammation often presents as pneumonitis, a condition that affects the cells that line small sacs in the lungs called the alveoli. The alveoli are responsible for exchanging oxygen from the air with carbon dioxide in the blood. Inflammation in the alveoli impairs this oxygen and carbon dioxide exchange, reducing the amount of oxygen that is delivered to the body.

Pulmonary fibrosis is another lung condition that chemotherapy can cause. This condition is characterized by fibrous, or stiff, scar tissue in the lungs. In healthy lungs, lung tissue is elastic and easily expands when we inhale, allowing proper intake of air. Pulmonary fibrosis reduces this elasticity and thus the amount of air patients can breathe in. Pulmonary fibrosis can occur even if lung inflammation is not present and often worsens over time, causing long-term complications.

Chronic dry cough, shortness of breath, fatigue caused by impaired oxygen intake, and chest pain due to lung damage are other risk factors of chemotherapy.

Patients receiving chemotherapy should be regularly monitored to screen for signs of chemo-induced lung issues. Screening methods include bronchoscopy (the insertion of thin, flexible tube called a bronchoscope into the lungs), chest x-ray or CT scan, and a pulmonary function test.

Radiation Therapy: Radiation at low doses is used diagnostically to screen for issues inside the body, including bone and teeth screening. Diagnostic techniques that employ radiation include x-rays, CT and MRI scans, fluoroscopy, and PET and SPECT scans, among others. The radiation emitted from such procedures is generally harmless. On the other hand, high-dose radiation therapy, also called radiotherapy, is harmful, which is why it is often used to kill cancer cells and shrink tumors. Radiation therapy achieves these goals by damaging the DNA of cancer cells.

If this damage to cancer cell DNA is beyond repair, the cancer cells stop dividing or die, and ideally are removed by the body.

Radiation therapy does not kill cancer cells immediately, however. Typically, days or weeks of treatment are required before enough damage is caused to DNA for cancer cells to die. Once radiation-induced cancer cell death begins, cancer cells will usually continue to die off for weeks, and even months, after radiation therapy is completed.

Like chemotherapy drugs, the type of radiation therapy that is used depends on multiple factors, especially the type of cancer one has, the size and location of the tumor in the body, and how close the tumor is to healthy tissues that are likely to be damaged by radiation. Other factors include the patient's age, overall health and medical history, and what, if any, other types of cancer treatments the patient may be undergoing.

There are two main types of radiation therapy—external beam and internal.

External beam radiation is the most common type of radiation therapy. It is a localized treatment in which radiation is emitted by machines called linear accelerators and directed at the area of the body where cancer is located.

Internal radiation therapy is also a localized treatment. It involves placing a source of radiation inside the body. The radiation source can be either solid or liquid. Internal radiation therapy that uses a solid source of radiation is known as brachytherapy. In this procedure, capsules containing a protected radiation source are inserted into the body, inside or in close proximity to a tumor so that the radiation can kill it. The capsule may be removed later, or be kept in place, depending on the patient's treatment plan.

Internal radiation therapy using a liquid source is called systemic therapy. In this procedure, the irradiated liquid moves through the bloodstream to tissues throughout the body, seeking out and killing cancer cells as it does so. The liquid source of radiation can be swallowed, directly injected into a vein, or be administered intravenously.

Regardless of which type of radiation therapy is used, there is a limit to how much radiation treated areas of the body can safely receive. In addition, patients who receive radiation therapy need to be closely monitored by their oncologist to address any side effects that can arise as a result of treatment.

Many people who undergo radiation therapy experience fatigue, which in some cases can be debilitating. Fatigue can occur suddenly or slowly over time. Other common side effects are hair loss and abnormal skin changes in the areas of the body targeted by radiation. Side effects of radiation therapy also depend on the part of the body that is treated.

Additional side effects for the brain include blurred vision, headache, memory and cognition problems, and nausea and vomiting. Other side effects in the breast include edema and tenderness in and around the breasts, while radiation directed at the chest can cause cough, shortness of breath, and throat problems, such as difficulty swallowing.

Radiation directed at the head or neck can damage the thyroid gland and impair thyroid function, and cause mouth and throat problems, and changes in taste, whereas radiation directed at the pelvis and to the area of the rectum can cause bladder and urinary problems, diarrhea, infertility, and sexual problems in both men and women. Many of these same symptoms can also occur as a result of radiation therapy directed at the stomach and abdomen.

Healthy cells and tissues can also be damaged as a result of radiation treatments. Although this damage will often heal within a few months once treatment is over, in some cases the damage may be permanent.

Late Effects of Chemotherapy and Radiation Therapy: Sometimes the side effects of both chemo and radiation therapy may not occur until months or even years after these treatments end. Delayed side effects are called late effects. Such effects are specific to the types of treatments and the dosages patients received and can differ greatly from patient to patient.

One potential late effect that can be caused by both chemo and radiation therapy is bone loss. With radiation therapy, bone loss, should it occur, will only do so in the area of the body that was treated, whereas chemotherapy can cause bone loss in multiple areas of the body.

In addition to bone loss, both chemo and radiation can cause scar tissue to form in the joints, which can lead to loss of motion in joints and overall impaired mobility.

Unhealthy brain changes and behaviors can also occur months or years after chemo or radiation treatments. They include memory loss, problems concentrating, cognitive impairment (including difficulties doing simple mathematic calculations and impaired ability to process information), and changes in personality. According to the National Cancer Institute (NCI), "In rare cases, radiation to the brain can cause radiation necrosis. This problem may happen when an area of dead tissue forms at the site of the brain tumor. Radiation necrosis can cause movement problems, problems concentrating, slow processing of information, and headaches."

Delayed vision, hearing, and mouth problems are other late effects. The most common late effect vision problems are cataracts and dry eye syndrome. Common hearing late effects are tinnitus and hearing loss. Late effects in the mouth include dry mouth, cavities, and/or bone loss in the jaw.

Late effect damage and unhealthy changes to the organs of the endocrine system can also occur, particularly to the thyroid gland, ovaries, and testes. This can lead to hypo- or hyperthyroidism, infertility (in both men and women), premature (early) menopause, and unhealthy weight gain, as well as sleep issues and impaired metabolism of food.

Other common late side effects are the heart and lung problems discussed earlier in this chapter, lymphedema, and ongoing feelings of stress and fear. In addition, according to the NCI, both chemo and radiation "can sometimes cause a new cancer many years after you have finished treatment. When a new primary cancer occurs in a person with a history of cancer, it is known as a second primary cancer. Second primary cancer is not the same thing as metastatic cancer, which is when cancer spreads from where it started."

The risk for all of the above side effects associated with surgery, chemo, and radiation can be significantly reduced when those therapies are supported by the additional integrative therapies covered in the remainder of this chapter. In fact, these integrative therapies that I employ for cancer patients at The Karlfeldt Center are so effective that physicians at the hospital near my clinic not only approve of them, but in many cases recommend that local cancer patients work with my staff and me while they receive their conventional cancer treatments. My staff and I are well-versed in this process and provide a wide variety of therapies that, either by themselves or integrated with conventional cancer treatments, help to maximize patients' health and well-being to not only defeat cancer, but to create an internal environment that is unfriendly to cancer, thereby reducing the risk of recurrence.

Immunotherapy

Immunotherapy is a groundbreaking form of cancer treatment that leverages the body's immune system to target and destroy cancer cells. Unlike conventional chemotherapy, which attacks all rapidly dividing cells, immunotherapy is a targeted therapy, meaning it precisely homes in on specific attributes of cancer cells.

There are different types of immunotherapy. The major types include:

- **Monoclonal Antibodies:** These are laboratory-made molecules that bind to specific parts of cancer cells, enabling the immune system to better recognize and attack them.

- **Checkpoint Inhibitors:** These drugs block certain proteins that can help cancer cells evade the immune system, thus boosting the immune response against the cancer cells.

- **T-cell Transfer Therapy:** In this therapy, T-cells are genetically modified to enhance their ability to detect and kill cancer cells. **CAR-T cells (Chimeric Antigen Receptor T-cells)** is an increasingly used type of this immunotherapy.

- **Cancer Vaccines:** These types of vaccines are comprised of substances that are introduced into the body to stimulate an immune response against certain types of cancer.

Immunotherapy's roots can be traced back to the late 19th century when the first cancer vaccines were experimented with. The real acceleration in the field, however, began in the late 20th and early 21st centuries with the development of more sophisticated targeted therapies like monoclonal antibodies. This evolving field has transformed cancer treatment and holds great promise for the future of medical oncology. Its targeted approach aligns well with the growing emphasis on personalized medicine and the shift away from traditional, more toxic, chemotherapy.

The advent of immunotherapy marks not just an advance in treatment strategies, but also a paradigm shift in understanding the very nature of cancer and the body's relationship to it. As a result, immunotherapy is often heralded as the future of oncology. It's the bridge between conventional medicine and the body's innate healing power, opening doors to novel collaboration between oncologists and integrative medicine practitioners such as naturopathic physicians.

The emergence of immunotherapy demonstrates the continuing evolution of cancer care, blending scientific innovation with a renewed appreciation for the body's natural defenses. This field's potential is vast, and as more is uncovered about the complexities of the immune system, immunotherapy is poised to play an ever-increasing role in the fight against cancer.

How Immunotherapy Works: Immunotherapy focuses on enhancing the immune system's ability to combat cancer. Unlike traditional treatments that attack cancer directly, immunotherapy modulates the immune system, improving its natural ability to detect and destroy cancer cells.

In the case of monoclonal antibodies, these laboratory-engineered molecules latch onto specific proteins on the surface of cancer cells. By binding to these markers, the monoclonal antibodies flag the cancer cells for destruction by the immune system. By contrast, CAR-T and other types of T-cell transfer therapies involve removing T-cells (a class of immune system cells) from the patient, genetically modifying them to target specific cancer cells, and then infusing them back into the patient. This supercharges the T-cells' ability to find and kill the targeted cancer cells. These and other types of immunotherapy provide a strategic advantage by enhancing the body's inherent defense mechanisms, offering a more precise and often less toxic means of battling cancer.

Unlike traditional chemotherapy, which can harm health cells along with cancerous ones, immunotherapy's true potential lies in its precision as a targeted therapy aimed directly at cancer cells and tumors. By focusing on specific targets found on cancer cells, immunotherapy minimizes collateral damage to healthy tissues. For instance, certain monclonal antibodies are designed to attach themselves to particular proteins expressed only by specific types of cancer. This means that the immune system's attack is directed more accurately at the cancer, reducing harm to normal cells. This represents a significant advancement over more indiscriminate conventional treatment methods, prioritizing accuracy and effectiveness without the broad harmful impact that can be caused by both chemotherapy and radiation therapy.

Integration With Conventional Treatments: While immunotherapy can be administered as a standalone therapy, it often provides its most promising benefits when combined with other treatments. Whether integrated with chemotherapy, radiation, or other targeted drugs, immunotherapy can complement these methods, often improving their effectiveness or mitigating some of their side effects. For example, combining immunotherapy with traditional chemotherapy might enable a reduction in chemotherapy dosage, potentially minimizing its toxicity while still attacking cancer aggressively.

This collaborative potential expands the toolkit available to oncologists and offers patients a more nuanced, personalized approach to treatment. By aligning itself both with the body's natural defenses and conventional medical wisdom, immunotherapy shows promise as a more effective and humane way to fight cancer, integrating science's cutting-edge capabilities with the timeless wisdom of the body's intrinsic healing powers.

The Pros and Cons of Immunotherapy: Although immunotherapy has shwon significant benefit in treating various types of cancer, its response rate can vary widely depending on the types of cancer it is used to treat.It has been most effective in treating malignancies like melanoma, lung cancer, and certain types of lumphomas. CAR-T and other T-cell transfer therapies, in particular, have shown substantial success in treating some leukemia and lymphoma cases. Overall, the variation in response rates is influenced by the type of immunotherapy that is used, the specific type of cancer, the stage of the disease, and individual patient factors.

While immunotherapy represents an important and substantial advancement in cancer care, it is essential to recognize that immunotherapy does not work for everyone. Its effectiveness is often linked to the unique biological characteristics of the patient's cancer. In addition, while immunotherapy's targeted approach often reduces the collateral damage to healthy cells, it is not entirely without the risks of side effects.

Common side effects include fatigue, fever, inflammation, and more serious issues such as autoimmune reactions that cause the immune system to mistakenly attack healthy tissues. Moreover, although immunotherapy often results in fewer toxic side effects than traditional chemotherapy, it may cause unique and sometimes severe immune-related side effects, also known as "immune -related adverse events," which can affect various organs in the body. The toxicities associated with immunotherapy are generally different from those seen with chemotherapy, requiring careful management and monitoring.

Balancing the Pros and Cons: As with all other cancer treatments, both conventional and integrative, immunotherapy is not a one-size-fits-all solution. Its varying success rates and potential toxicities necessitate a tailored approach to patient care. Comprehensive understanding, patient selection, and continuous monitoring are vital in maximizing the benefits and minimizing the risks of immunotherapy. The balancing act between success and safety emphasizes the need for personalized medicine and highlights the critical role of both oncologists and integrative practitioners in navigating this intricate landscape.

Combining Immunotherapy with Integrative Therapies: The combination of immunotherapy with with natural and integrative therapies holds immense potential in cancer treatment. The integrative therapies discussed later in this chapter can enhance immunotherapy's effectiveness by supporting the immune system and overall well-being, while also helping to alleviate and reduce the risk of harmful side effects. Research and clinical observation support the potential benefits of combining immunotherapy with these integrative approaches, although more extensive studies are required.

Diagnosis and Testing

An accurate and comprehensive diagnosis is essential for effectively dealing with cancer. Such a diagnosis needs to include testing to not only determine what type of cancer patients have, and at what stage, but also a thorough exploration of all potential factors that are contributing to each patient's cancer. This is vital, because cancer is a complex multifactorial disease and the causes and behavior of cancer is unique to each patient. This is why no "magic bullet, cookie-cutter solution" for cancer exists.

Each cancer patient is unique and every cancer type must be treated in accordance with each patient's specific needs and challenges. Determining how to best do so is not something that the conventional cancer tests and markers that I covered in Part One are capable of providing complete information about. This is why, in addition to the use of such tests and markers, I also employ the nonconventional diagnostic and testing methods discussed in Chapter 5, while also screening for all of the cancer drivers discussed in Chapter 3. In addition, I evaluate my patients' diet, lifestyle, exercise and sleep habits, and their individual internal terrain and how it may be contributing to cancer growth. This evaluation includes screening them for dietary and nutritional deficiencies or imbalances, food sensitivities and allergies, chronic infections, chemical and other environmental exposures, and organ weaknesses, as well as measuring their bodies' level of inflammation and assessing the status of their immune system, mitochondrial function, and microbiome. (For more about the importance of all of these factors, refer back to Chapters 8-11.)

Perhaps most importantly, I also discuss their spiritual mindset and share how and why a connection to God or Spirit is so important (see Chapter 6). In addition, I also take time to address any toxic emotions and limited belief systems patients may be dealing with (see Chapter 7). I also make it a point to listen to any concerns my patients have, including answering their questions about their prognosis and the risk/reward ratio of the treatments they may choose to undergo, including the benefits and risks of surgery, chemotherapy, and radiation.

In order to defeat cancer, the body must be supported at every level and with every method necessary to reverse cancer's multi-pronged assault. All this must be done while maintaining the maximum possible well-being of the patient. Proper diagnosis and testing helps ensure that this happens with all of the patients I treat. I encourage cancer patients and their loved ones who are working with other physicians and oncologists to ask their doctors to follow a similar comprehensive diagnostic approach. Since the diagnostic approach of most oncologists, as of yet, does not employ all of the screening and testing methods I recommend, I advise seeking out integrative naturopathic and other integrative physicians who do make use of them, as well as working with spiritual and psychological counselors to further support patients' journey through cancer.

Treatment

Although attacking cancer with chemotherapy or radiation will kill a great number of the fast-growing cancer cells, neither of these therapies, alone or together, will kill all of them. There will always be a certain percentage that will survive. Focusing only on tumor shrinkage can leave patients handicapped in fighting the long-term battle. Treatment cannot just focus on the cancer. It needs to take into account the individual with cancer, and address all of the factors that allowed cancer to develop and continue. In my experience, this can best be done by taking a comprehensive, integrative approach.

Such an approach can, and often will, include surgery, chemo, and/or radiation, but in many cases, patients may elect to forgo such treatments to avoid their unwanted side effects. The choice belongs to each patient to make for her or himself.

With or without the inclusion of conventional cancer treatments, a truly integrative approach will also include a range of nontoxic treatments to boost immune function, potentially halt and reverse the progression of cancer cells and tumors, support and enhance the body's detoxification system, and provide all of the necessary nutrition, including potential nutritional and other supplements and products that patients may need that directly impact cancer cells, along with the most appropriate diet tailor-made for each patient's individual genetic and metabolic requirements. Proper support for patients' spiritual and psychological needs is also essential.

When cancer patients first come to me, in addition to conducting an extensive evaluation of their situation using the diagnostic and testing methods I've shared in this book, I take time to inform them about all of their treatment options to ensure they have a better understanding of the treatment choices available to them, the benefits and limitations of each treatment, and what they can expect once their treatments begin. I also inform them of other resources that are available to them, including cancer support groups, both locally and online, as well as putting them in touch with spiritual and psychological counselors with experience in helping patients dealing with cancer and related health challenges.

For patients that I see at The Karlfeldt Center, I often recommend the services of a minister, priest, rabbi, or other spiritual counselors to provide spiritual encouragement to our patients, as well as their families and friends who assist them as they undergo their treatments. In many cases, they offer personal in-home visits, as well as at my clinic, providing patients and their families with prayers and counseling.

As I explained in Chapter 6, I consider helping patients to cultivate or deepen their connection with God to be of paramount importance because of the positive and significant influence doing so can have on patient outcomes. During our darkest times, we sometimes need a guide to assist us in reconnecting with that ever-present healing power. My goal is to equip patients and their support team with tools they can use to bring God's healing into their lives.

Once my staff and I obtain the results of the various tests I order for each patient, we then create a customized cancer treatment plan for that patient that is designed to attack cancer cells, inhibit their ability to spread, eliminate any underlying cancer-causing factors, and boost overall health to defeat the disease.

I firmly believe that patients should have the final say regarding the choices they make about their treatment plan once they have been informed about and understand what their options are. Many patients will choose to follow a combination of conventional cancer treatments (surgery, chemo, and/or radiation) and integrative therapies. I often recommend this approach, as well, particularly if removal or debulking of tumors is advisable.

Other patients may opt to pursue integrative, naturopathic cancer treatments alone, often because they have witnessed successful outcomes other patients have experienced with integrative medicine, or because they want to avoid the toxic and unwanted side effects of chemotherapy and radiation. With so much at stake in the cancer treatment process, at The Karlfeldt Center we use our extensive knowledge of naturopathic oncology and integrative medicine to create the most advisable treatment plan for each patient that offers them the greatest chance of regaining their health and wellness.

At the core of all of the treatment plans I employ is a two-week intensive round of treatments that take a multi-pronged approach in order to jump-start and fast track patient recovery. This approach includes addressing a multitude of cancer drivers while boosting each patient's immune system and mitochondrial function, as well as stimulating apoptosis, shifting the body's internal terrain (microbiome) to create an anticancer environment, improving oxygenation so that cancer cells and tumors are unable to continue thriving in a low-oxygen state (hypoxia), and targeting cancer stem cells (CSCs) and circulating tumor cells (CTCs).

Cancer drivers: As you learned in Chapters 1-3, the survival and progression of cancer depends on a number of cancer drivers. These drivers can be targeted using various nutritional interventions such as curcumin, quercetin, melatonin, and medicinal mushrooms. The pharmaceutical industry has spent billions of dollars trying to duplicate what some of these substances, including curcumin, do naturally without the toxic side effects that many pharmaceutical drugs can cause.

Immune and mitochondrial function: It is the body's immune system that does most of the work to kill cancer cells and tumors. Supporting immune function is therefore vitally important. This is especially true in patients who chose to undergo surgery, chemotherapy, and/or radiation. None of these therapies get rid of all of the cancer, which is why we need to rely on the immune system to clear out whatever cancer remains. A weakened immune system will do a very poor job of this, particularly if it is subjected to chemo or radiation.

Working hand in hand with the immune system are the mitochondria, which not only produce most of the body's energy, but also control the cancer death switch (apoptosis). Cancer cells become immortal by bypassing normal mitochondria to produce their own energy supply via a fermentation cycle. Repairing and activating the mitochondria in cancer cells turns on the cell death switch to kill cancer cells. In addition, supporting mitochondrial health of normal cells prevents them from becoming cancerous, which inhibits the growth of cancer and metastasis.

Apoptosis: As we've previously discussed, apoptosis is the process of programmed cell death that rids the body of cells that have aged or been damaged beyond repair. When this process is impaired or interrupted, it leads to uncontrolled cell division and the subsequent development of cancer cells and tumors. In addition to supporting apoptosis by improving immune system and mitochondrial function, apoptosis can also be triggered by oxidative therapies, and by starving cancer cells of sugar (glucose). This starvation reduces the ability of cancer cells to maintain themselves, making them more vulnerable to oxidative and photodynamic therapies, as well as to chemotherapy and radiation.

Changing the body's internal terrain: Rather than being an isolated event that "just happens," cancer is actually a process that can only develop in an environment that promotes its existence. Changing this environment changes the behavior of the tumor and arrests the ability of cancer cells and tumors to grow and spread. Toxins, infections, and nutritional deficiencies, all of which can be exacerbated by emotional stressors and traumas, are known factors that create a pro-cancerous environment. Eliminating them through dietary, nutritional, and detoxification therapies, along with various emotional healing and other mind/body therapies if needed, helps to restore a healthy terrain, enabling the immune system to more efficiently attack and kill cancer cells and tumors.

Hypoxia: When cells become hypoxic, or oxygen-deficient, they shift how they produce energy from an aerobic (oxygenated) process within the mitochondria to an anaerobic process using fermentation (the Warburg effect discussed in Chapter 11). Fermentation produces byproducts that support the survival of cancer cells and tumors and promote metastasis. Using various therapies that promote healthy cell and tissue oxygenation counteracts this fermentation process, depriving cancer cells and tumor of energy. This, in turns, weakens and helps to kill them and makes them more susceptible to other cancer therapies.

Cancer stem cells (CSCs) and circulating tumor cells (CTCs): While conventional cancer therapies can be effective at shrinking and debulking tumors, they are incapable of protecting the body from CSCs and CTCs. All too often, oncologists focus on initial tumor shrinking while failing to place similar attention on preventing metastatic tumors, which cause more than 90 percent of all cancer-related deaths. Cancer stem cells are the engine of tumor evolution and drive the colonization of cancer cells to distant organs and tissue. Studies show that CSCs are enriched after chemotherapy because a small subpopulation of them remain in tumor tissue where they can survive and expand even though most chemotherapeutic agents kill the bulk of tumors. Therefore, we need to incorporate strategies to reduce the activity of CSCs while patients undergo traditional care, and support the immune system's ability to keep them in check.

We also need to recognize that biopsies and cancer surgeries to remove tumors cause microscopic tumor cells to break off from tumors to circulate in the bloodstream and eventually lodge in other tissues and organs away from the primary tumor site. Locating and eliminating these CTCs is also imperative in order to prevent metastasis and later recurrences of cancer.

For patients who elect to undergo surgery and receive chemo or radiation, this two-week protocol is ideally followed at the same time, or immediately following their conventional treatments, in order to best support the effectiveness of those treatments while minimizing the risk of their harmful side effects.

An Overview of the Two-Week Protocol

An example of therapies that I incorporate into this two weeks of treatment, along with their timing, follows below, beginning with the IV (intravenous) protocol. (An explanation of each of the therapies is provided later in this chapter.) It is important to understand that each individual is unique and the program below is an example of the complex multilayered approach that is needed to put enough pressure on cancer cells to drastically reduce their aggressive nature. Each individual is evaluated to determine the protocol that is appropriate for them.

IV Protocol, Week 1:

Monday: Photodynamic therapy (PDT) using platelet derived nano particles mixed with thymosin alpha-1, mistletoe, methylene blue, and ICG; high dose vitamin C with DMSO, artesunate, IV endolaser (red 20 minutes, infrared 20 minutes, 10 minutes ultraviolet, blue, green, yellow).

Tuesday: PDT with nano ICG, Poly-MVA, DCA, curcumin, IV, endolaser (red 20 minutes, infrared 20 minutes, 10 minutes ultraviolet, blue, green, yellow).

Wednesday: PDT with nano ICG 5, high dose vitamin C with DMSO, artesunate, hydrogen peroxide, IV endolaser (red 20 minutes, infrared 20 minutes, 10 minutes ultraviolet, blue, green, yellow).

Thursday: Poly-MVA, DCA, curcumin, IV, endolaser (red 20 minutes, infrared 20 minutes, 10 minutes ultraviolet, blue, green, yellow).

Friday: RHP ozone therapy, IV endolaser (red 20 minutes, infrared 20 minutes, 10 minutes ultraviolet, blue, green, yellow).

Week 2:

Monday: PDT with platelet derived nano particles mixed with thymosin alpha-1, mistletoe, methylene blue, and ICG; high dose vitamin C with DMSO, artesunate, IV endolaser(red 20 minutes, infrared 20 minutes, 10 minutes ultraviolet, blue, green, yellow)

Tuesday: Poly-MVA, DCA, curcumin, IV endolaser (red 20 minutes, infrared 20 minutes, 10 minutes ultraviolet, blue, green, yellow).

Wednesday: High dose vitamin C with DMSO, artesunate, hydrogen peroxide, IV endolaser(red 20 minutes, infrared 20 minutes, 10 minutes ultraviolet, blue, green, yellow)

Thursday: Poly-MVA, DCA, curcumin, IV endolaser (red 20 minutes, infrared 20 minutes, 10 minutes ultraviolet, blue, green, yellow).

Friday: RHP ozone therapy, IV endolaser (red 20 minutes, infrared 20 minutes, 10 minutes ultraviolet, blue, green, yellow).

Additional Services, Week 1:

Monday: HOCATT, laser bed, ionic foot bath with LED, shock wave right after infusion of methylene blue/ ICG, sonodynamic therapy (10 minutes ultrasound 2-3 MHz over tumor site(s), laser shower head IR 500-1000 mW over tumor (s) 20-30 minutes, 10 minutes fiber coupled laser system laser treatment over tumor site(s) at comfortable intensity, nutritional testing, evaluation, and consultation.

Tuesday: Interstitial injection around tumor site with nano ICG, HOCATT, laser bed, ionic foot bath with LED, colonic, shock wave right after infusion of ICG, sonodynamic therapy (10 minutes ultrasound 2-3 MHz over tumor site(s)), laser shower head IR 500-1000 mW over tumor (s) 20-30 minutes, 10 minutes fiber coupled laser system laser treatment over tumor site(s) at comfortable intensity, and applied psychoneurobiology (APN).

Wednesday: HOCATT, laser bed, ionic foot bath with LED, colonic, shock wave right after infusion of ICG, sonodynamic therapy (10 minutes ultrasound 2-3 MHz over tumor site(s)), laser shower head IR 500-1000 mW over tumor (s) 20-30 minutes, 10 minutes fiber coupled laser system laser treatment over tumor site(s) at comfortable intensity.

Thursday: HOCATT, laser bed, ionic foot bath with LED, sonodynamic therapy (10 minutes ultrasound 2-3 MHz over tumor site(s)), laser shower head IR 500-1000 mW over tumor (s) 20-30 minutes, 10 minutes fiber coupled laser system laser treatment over tumor site(s) at comfortable intensity. APN.

Friday: HOCATT, laser bed, ionic foot bath with LED, colonic, sonodynamic therapy (10 minutes ultrasound 2-3 MHz over tumor site(s)), laser shower head IR 500-1000 mW over tumor (s) 20-30 minutes, 10 minutes fiber coupled laser system laser treatment over tumor site(s) at comfortable intensity.

Week 2:
Monday: HOCATT, laser bed, ionic foot bath with LED, shock wave right after infusion of methylene blue/ ICG, sonodynamic therapy (10 minutes ultrasound 2-3 MHz over tumor site(s)), laser shower head IR 500-1000 mW over tumor (s) 20-30 minutes, 10 minutes fiber coupled laser system laser treatment over tumor site(s) at comfortable intensity, nutritional testing and evaluation.

Tuesday: Interstitial injection around tumor site with methylene blue, Hocatt, laser bed, ionic foot bath with LED, colonic, sonodynamic therapy (10 minutes ultrasound 2-3 MHz over tumor site(s)), laser shower head IR 500-1000 mW over tumor (s) 20-30 minutes, 10 minutes fiber coupled laser system laser treatment over tumor site(s) at comfortable intensity, APN.

Wednesday: HOCATT, laser bed, ionic foot bath with LED, colonic, sonodynamic therapy (10 minutes ultrasound 2-3 MHz over tumor site(s)), laser shower head IR 500-1000 mW over tumor (s) 20-30 minutes, 10 minutes fiber coupled laser system laser treatment over tumor site(s) at comfortable intensity.

Thursday: HOCATT, laser bed, ionic foot bath with LED, sonodynamic therapy (10 minutes ultrasound 2-3 MHz over tumor site(s)), laser shower head IR 500-1000 mW over tumor (s) 20-30 minutes, 10 minutes fiber coupled laser system laser treatment over tumor site(s) at comfortable intensity, APN.

Friday: HOCATT, laser bed, ionic foot bath with LED, colonic, sonodynamic therapy (10 minutes ultrasound 2-3 MHz over tumor site(s)), laser shower head IR 500-1000 mW over tumor (s) 20-30 minutes, 10 minutes fiber coupled laser system laser treatment over tumor site(s) at comfortable intensity.

In addition, during this two-week protocol, I will often use various peptides along with repurposed drugs, both of which are discussed below. I also monitor my patients' progress with the following lab tests: CBC, CMP, hsCRP, LDH, ESR, fibrinogen, ferritin, CEA, A1C, ultra-sensitive insulin, the specific cancer maker tests for the type of cancer they have (see Chapter 1), vitamin D, DHEA-S.

Other specialty lab tests that I recommend include the chemical immune reactivity screen (Cyrex 11) and the pathogen-associated immune reactivity screen (Cyrex 12) from Cyrex Laboratories, the micronutrient test from SpectraCell Laboratories, the Chronic Inflammation Test, as well as the other diagnostic and screening tests discussed in Chapter 5.

Obviously, two weeks is not enough time to reverse cancer, but by undergoing the two-week protocol patients will often make significant progress in halting the progression of cancer and shrinking tumors while simultaneously improving their overall immune and mitochondrial function. Once this protocol is completed, using the same therapies above, my staff and I continue to see and treat cancer patients on an ongoing, follow-up basis, the frequency of which is determined by how well they continue to progress towards a full recovery, particularly if they are local.

For patients who are not local, I conduct follow up telehealth visits, while continuing to monitor their progress with lab tests, imaging, and their symptom presentation. All patients will remain on their tailor-made diet and supplement protocol unless we need to pivot. I encourage all nonlocal patients to find local resources in their area that are able to administer high dose IV vitamin C treatments and, if possible, hyperbaric oxygen therapy (HBOT) treatments to saturate their bodies with oxygen, two to three times each week for two months. In some cases, I may suggest that patients return to The Karlfeldt Center for more photodynamic therapy six to eight weeks after the initial two-week protocol. Patients also frequently continue with mistletoe injections, and in some cases I will shift them towards doing a protocol using high dosing of pancreatic enzymes per the Kelley protocol. (When following the Kelley protocol, they cannot do high dose vitamin C.)

What follows are overviews of each of the above anticancer therapies, as well as an explanation of how and why they can be so helpful in aiding patient recovery.

Dietary and Nutritional Interventions

A healthy diet combined with the appropriate use of nutritional and herbal supplements needs to be a cornerstone of any cancer treatment. My staff and I spend time educating patients on the importance of healthy eating and, if necessary, we test them for any food allergies or sensitivities they may have. Genetic DNA testing to determine the best foods for patients to eat based on their genotype, as well as what foods they should avoid, may also be done.

For many of the cancer patients that I see, I recommend either the ketogenic (keto) or GAPS diets. For other patients, a plant-based, Mediterranean style diet may be more appropriate. In some cases, I may choose a diet based on the Kelley Protocol. As you learned in Chapter 8, the Kelly protocol was developed by William Kelley, DDS, who used it to cure himself of pancreatic cancer and then went on to treat approximately 30,000 other cancer patients, achieving a success rate of over 50 percent. My staff and I have been trained by and continue to collaborate with Pamela McDougle, who worked directly with Dr. Kelley during the last seven years of his life. Using the Kelley protocol, she achieved a similar success rate with the over 6,000 cancer patients she treated, most of whom had previously failed conventional cancer therapies.

For more information about these diets, as well as my overall healthy eating recommendations, please refer back to Chapter 8.

The use of nutritional and herbal supplements to address nutritional deficiencies or imbalances, and to boost the body's ability to fight cancer is also an important element of my approach to treating cancer. The nutrients and herbs I most regularly use for this are discussed in Chapter 9.

In addition, I may also employ hyper-oxidative therapy (HOP), which involves combining high doses of vitamin C with various other nutrients and herbs, along with ozone (discussed later in this chapter). This HOP protocol creates a highly pro-oxidative effect in the body that is designed to create oxidative stress in cancer cells, pushing them to die. Cancer cells are full of their own supply of antioxidants. The dosage levels of the nutrients used in HOP cause the antioxidants in cancer cells to shift into pro-oxidants, causing the cells to weaken and die. (Remember, cancer cannot thrive in an oxygen-rich environment. Pro-oxidants increase oxygen levels.)

In addition to vitamin C and ozone, the HOP protocol may include vitamin K3, artemisia, borage seed oil, magnesium, butyrate, and vanadium, along with Tylenol.

Photodynamic Therapy (PDT)

In addition to dietary and nutritional interventions, at the core of The Karlfeldt Center's integrative oncology program is PDT, a relatively new approach for treating cancer, as well as infections and other diseases.

Photodynamic therapy uses specific non-toxic dyes and natural agents called photosensitizers that are administered locally or systemically and introduced intravenously, interstitially, and orally. These photosensitizers have the ability to accumulate in cancer cells and tumors. After the introduction of a photosensitizer, the cancer cells are exposed to powerful laser light that triggers oxidation of the cancer cells, killing them. Intravenous and interstitial PDT illumination with ultraviolet, visible, or infra-red laser light excites the photosensitizers as they interact with the body's oxygen supply. This interaction produces reactive oxygen species (ROS), causing cytotoxic effects that weaken and destroy cancer cells. The photosensitizers in the cancer cells intensify the impact of laser light on cancer cells.

A significant benefit of PDT is that the same laser light that triggers oxidation of cancer cells supports the health of non-cancerous cells. Cancer cells, as well as malignant infectious cells, can be selectively killed by this approach.

To maximize the saturation of photosensitizers in cancer cells, the Karlfeldt Center uses a platelet-derived nanoparticle delivery system. The microenvironment of a tumor is highly inflammatory, and platelets are drawn to areas of inflammation. The small size of the nanoparticles allows them to penetrate cancer tissues to offload the photosensitizer in the tumor microenvironment.

To enhance the efficacy of photodynamic thereby, we combine it with oxidative therapies, such as IV infusions of ozone, hyperbaric oxygen therapy (HBOT), and/or HOCATT, to elevate the level of oxygen in the cancer cells and tumors, along with the intravenous use of the photosensitizers such as methylene blue, riboflavin, curcumin and the powerful nano ICG, which accumulate in cancer cells and, in the case of nano ICG, remains in them for approximately two weeks, while patients also receive intravenous and interstitial laser light, along with high dose vitamin C, hydrogen peroxide, and artesunate to support further oxidation of cancer cells. I also employ Poly-MVA and dicholoracetate (DCA) to inhibit cancer metabolism and support mitochondrial activation of the death switch of cancer cells. Mistletoe is used to promote enhanced immune system activity, and curcumin, Boswellia, and DMSO are used to reduce the activity of tumor-promoting cancer drivers. All of these substances are discussed later in this chapter.

PDT can be administered in the following ways.

Intravenous PDT: Intravenous PDT brings light directly to the bloodstream through optic fibers that are inserted through a catheter in a vein. The blood is then exposed to different colors and wavelengths of laser light. This process is also known as blood irradiation. Since the catheter is in the vein, the treatment is in a sterile environment compared to other versions of light therapy where blood is extracted and treated outside of the body. Additionally, the blood will pass by the optic fibers in the vein about once every minute. This means that in a 60 minute therapy session the whole blood volume gets treated about 60 times. Intravenous PDT enhances the body's immune response and is effective for killing cancer cells, including circulating tumor cells and cancer stem cells, including stems cells that have escaped the tumor site(s) to circulate in the bloodstream.

Due to the tumor's inefficient use of energy sources, and it's very high metabolic activity, it requires a large influx of nutrients to feed its existence and growth. To satisfy this energy expenditure, it requires the creation of a extensive network of blood vessels. Without this network, the cancer would starve to death. PDT supports the destruction of this network of blood vessels. This is an added method where PDT supports cancer cell death. One of the challenges with cancer is its ability to hide from the immune system and even recruit the immune system to promote its activities. When PDT triggers cancer cell death, the dead fragments of the cancer cells enter the circulation allowing the immune system to analyze the specific aspects of the cancer and trigger the production of targeted antibodies. Cancer continually evolves to adjust to changes in its environment. A major benefit of PDT is that enables the immune system to manufacture the antibodies specific to how cancer expresses itself at that moment, producing a vaccine-like effect that is not manufactured from how the cancer was expressing a week ago, but at this exact moment. In addition, intravenous PDT helps to eliminate infections that are co-factors in cancer.

Ultrasound Guided Interstitial Laser Therapy: This method of PDT was first introduced as a method of interventional oncology in 2004 in a published study by researchers from the Faculty of Interventional Oncology at the University of Frankfurt, Germany. In their study, the researchers sought to overcome the problem of limited penetration depth by using fiber optic laser catheters inserted directly into tumor tissue or in metastases. Using this approach, they were able to document an effective and controlled necrosis and apoptosis (both forms of cancer cell death), and convincingly demonstrated that this method of PDT was effective as a treatment for metastases in the liver. Furthermore, they also proved that one of the key advantages of this treatment modality is that it causes little to no pain and is almost entirely free of other harmful side effects.

External (Shower Head) Laser Therapy: In this PDT method, so-called laser needles are painlessly placed on the skin without puncturing, or combined with special applicators for the treatment of larger body surfaces. The combination of red, infrared, green, and blue laser light provides various depths of laser light penetration while simultaneously providing a multitude of beneficial effects in and on body tissue without any side effects.

Photosensitizer Nano-ICG: ICG stands for indocyanine green, a water-soluble dye often used in medical diagnostics. The use of nano-ICG as a photosensitizer creates an "over-heating" effect on tumor tissue. ICG absorbs infrared light at a depth of 810 nanometers (approximately two inches), enabling the light to penetrate more deeply beneath the skin. Besides activation of ICG with production of singlet oxygen, tumor tissue will be warmed up, or overheated as the photodynamic reaction occurs, helping to destroy the tumor (a process sometimes referred to as "tumor melting") without damaging the surrounding healthy tissue. This combination of PDT and overheating is also called photo-thermodynamic therapy (PTDT) or photo-thermo ablation due to its ability to generate a hyperthermia effect (the overheating) in tumor tissue.

As an illustration of the potential PDT therapy has, consider the case of a patient who came to me presenting with cancerous tumors in her lungs. After only one month of treatment with PDT, scans showed that her lungs were completely free of cancer. While this remarkable recovery is not the norm, it is still a powerful example of what is possible when PDT is used as a cancer treatment.

Intravenous (IV) Therapy

Intravenous, or IV, therapy is a method feeding vitamins, minerals, amino acids, and other substances directly into the bloodstream. It is used to help correct intracellular nutrient deficiencies and enables the body to more readily and completely absorb critical nutrients.

IV therapy typically supplies high doses of these substances. Oral intake of such high doses is not possible due to the absorption limitations of the gastrointestinal tract. A single IV therapy treatment can supply up to ten times the amount of nutrients that oral intake allows. For example, while it is well known that vitamin C can be useful to treat health conditions caused by viruses, its antiviral effects are not effective until at least

10 to 15 mg/dL blood levels of vitamin C are reached. This can only be achieved via IV vitamin C therapy, since taking vitamin C orally only results in blood levels between 1.2 to 4 mg/dL. In comparison, blood levels of 50 to 90 mg/dL can be achieved in a single IV vitamin C treatment.

In addition to the benefits IV therapy has been shown by research to provide cancer patients, studies also demonstrate that this therapy can help a wide variety of other conditions. In addition to vitamin C, other substances that I use in IV therapy for my cancer patients include artesunate, curcumin, DMSO, mistletoe, and Poly-MVA.

Vitamin C: High dose vitamin C has been studied as a treatment for patients with cancer since the 1970s. All healthy cells require vitamin C to fuel their metabolic activity. Simply put, vitamin C is the fuel on which healthy cells run. Inside cells, where the antioxidant glutathione plays a prominent role, vitamin C is needed to maintain glutathione in its active state. When the body's supply of vitamin C is severely depleted, disease inevitably follows. Because vitamin C is water soluble, the body cannot store it, so it must be replenished on a daily basis via diet and supplementation.

While vitamin C is essential for maintaining the health of normal cells, in a high dose, it has the opposite effect on cancer cells and tumors because of the oxidative stress it causes them. Unlike normal cells, cancer cells and tumors accumulate iron and hydrogen peroxide. When vitamin C in sufficient dosages comes in contact with cancer cells, it causes oxidative stress by generating highly reactive hydroxyl free radicals capable of killing cancer cells. In contrast, the only effect of vitamin C on normal cells is decreased oxidative stress. When enough vitamin C is present and maintained in the body, normal cells cannot accumulate iron and hydrogen peroxide and are therefore unable to turn cancerous.

In addition to its anticancer effects, IV vitamin C also helps prevent the side effects chemotherapy can cause because of how it protects healthy cells from the damaging effects of chemo drugs. To be most effective in this regard, I recommend that IV vitamin C be given the day before and a couple of days after chemotherapy treatments. If given on the same day after the chemo, it is powerful enough to neutralize the chemo and potentially negate some of the desired effect of the chemo.

Artesunate: Artesunate is a medication that is most commonly used to treat malaria. It is derived from the wormwood herb (artemesinin - see Chapter 9). Like artemesinin itself, artesunate has been found to possess potent anticancer properties.

Artesunate administered intravenously causes little to no side effects, even at high doses. For cancer patients, it can be used alone or in combination with IV vitamin C. Research shows that IV artesunate improves tumor sensitivity to chemotherapy drugs, thereby enhancing their effectiveness. It has also been shown to reduce chemo's side effects. Other benefits include improved energy and appetite, an overall improved quality of life, and, most importantly, increased survival times.

Among the studies demonstrating artesunate's anticancer benefits, research conducted at the Bastyr Integrative Oncology Research Center found that the combination of IV artesunate and IV vitamin C is a viable treatment for advanced cancer. In that research, women diagnosed with stage 4 breast cancer who were given this combination IV therapy had a 90 percent survival rate.

Curcumin: Curcumin is discussed in more detail in Chapter 9. It can safely be taken orally, but because of its many potent anticancer properties, I often administer it intravenously, as well. It is also a highly effective and selective natural photosensitizer that can be used in combination with photodynamic therapy.

DMSO: DMSO (dimethyl sulfoxide) is a sulfur compound that is used worldwide as a treatment for many serious illnesses, including cancer. Among its uses, it acts as a carrier that can bring other substances into cancer cells. It is especially useful in this regard due to its ability to quickly and easily infiltrate tumors in otherwise hard to reach places in the body. Because of this property, DMSO is very effective as part of a combination therapy that also incorporates other anticancer agents, better enabling them to reach and penetrate cancerous tumors. On its own, it works as a cancer therapy by promoting cellular differentiation (the process by which primitive, rapidly growing cancer cells are transformed back into slow-growing normal cells). It has also been shown to reduce tumor cell invasion and metastases by stimulating a tumor-suppressing protein called HLJ1.

Mistletoe: Mistletoe, also known as Iscador, has been used as a cancer treatment for many years, especially in Europe, where in many countries it is considered mainstream because of its anticancer benefits, low risk of serious side effects (common minor side effects when it is administered via IV are temporary inflammation, soreness, and pain around the injection site, as well as fever and chills), and its low cost. It can also be given subcutaneously via injection under the skin (usually on the abdomen) or delivered via IV. It can also be taken orally, though the effect will be decreased due to it having to travel through the digestive tract.

The first injectable mistletoe treatment occurred in 1917 by Dutch physician Ita Wegman. Since then, studies primarily conducted in Europe have shown that mistletoe used as a cancer treatment can improve patient quality of life, improve remission and long-term survival rates, and reduce the side effects caused by conventional cancer treatments, thereby enhancing their effectiveness.

Mistletoe is noted for its benefit to the immune system and its ability to improve the overall quality of life of cancer patients. It is suitable as a treatment for nearly all types of tumors. Following injection into the tumor site, a rash is created, signaling the mounting of an immune system attack.

Mistletoe increases the production of several white blood cell types. These white blood cells release immune-enhancing cytokines such as tumor necrosis factor-alpha, interleukin-1, and interleukin-6. Mistletoe also allows for the synthesis of proteins in specified cells to facilitate the natural destruction of cancer cells (apoptosis).

One of the more remarkable outcomes of mistletoe as a cancer treatment was reported in *Johns Hopkins Magazine*, a publication of Johns Hopkins University. An excerpt from that report follows:

"In September 2008, Ivelisse Page, a 37-year-old mother of four, was diagnosed with colon cancer. Several weeks later, she had 15 inches of her colon and 28 lymph nodes removed. But in December of that same year, Page's doctor, Luis Diaz, an associate professor of oncology in the Johns Hopkins School of Medicine, had to deliver the devastating news that the cancer had spread to her liver. He told her that she had just an 8 percent chance of surviving for more than two years.

"Page had more surgery to remove 20 percent of her liver, but instead of undergoing conventional chemotherapy, she pondered the suggestion of another of her doctors, Peter Hinderberger of Baltimore's Ruscombe Mansion Community Health Center. A specialist in using complementary therapies, Hinderberger had seen positive effects from injections of mistletoe extract.

"Page and Diaz had never heard of the treatment. Diaz...reviewed several European studies on the extract and somewhat reluctantly gave Page the green light. 'I'm an oncologist who treats with chemotherapy—and I'm really good at it—and here's somebody who says not only do I not want chemotherapy, but I still want you to be my oncologist while I'm getting mistletoe,' Diaz says. 'I reviewed the literature on mistletoe in other parts of the world and there is some acceptance of it. I was willing to work with her.'

"The next time the doctor saw his patient, he was amazed. 'The one thing I noticed was that as soon as she went on it, she started feeling better,' he recalls. 'That's a universal feature I've seen in all patients who get mistletoe. Their [color] improves; they have more energy.'

"Page has been cancer-free since the operation on her liver and attributes her turnaround to a combination of surgery, diet and exercise, and the mistletoe." You can hear her powerful story on my podcast Integrative Cancer Solutions with Dr. Karlfeldt. It is available at https://

integrative-cancer-solutions-with-dr-karlfeldt.simplecast.com/episodes/ivelisse-page-publishes-6-29.

Between 1993 and 2000, a retrospective cohort study was performed with 800 patients to examine mistletoe extract for its benefits as an adjuvant treatment for chemotherapy and/or radiation therapy for colorectal cancer. The study found that those patients treated with mistletoe experienced a reduction in adverse events, improved symptom relief, and increased disease-free survival rates versus those patients who did not receive mistletoe therapy.

Another study, conducted in 2013, examined mistletoe's usefulness for advanced or metastatic pancreatic cancer patients. Best supportive care practices were used and patients received random assignments for mistletoe or another anti-cancer approach. The study found that the 200 patients who received mistletoe therapy experienced improved survival rates and reduced rates of symptoms such as weight loss, fatigue, anxiety, diarrhea, nausea, and pain compared to those patients who did not receive mistletoe therapy.

Poly-MVA: Poly-MVA's anticancer benefits are recounted in Chapter 9. Poly-MVA can be taken as an oral supplement, and higher doses that are more absorbable can be administered intravenously. Poly-MVA can also be used in conjunction with photodynamic therapy. When taken orally, I recommend a daily dose that is determined by the severity of a patient's cancer. For IV and PDT treatments, it typically is administered a few times per week.

Ozone/Oxygen Therapy

Ozone is one of the most versatile forms of healing oxygen on the planet. In healthcare, ozone therapy has been used since the 1950s. It's a versatile treatment that can be used for many diseases, both acute and chronic, including cancer. Its main benefit as an anticancer treatment is its ability to create an oxygen-rich cellular environment in which cancer cells and tumors can no longer survive.

Ozone also has the potential to fight infection, and can also help the body to produce its own antioxidant system. It can also re-oxygenate blood, tissues, and organs. Additionally, ozone relaxes the nervous system by essentially resetting the nerves. This creates a sense of well-being in patients from the oxygenation of the body, helping to bring it into balance.

Another reason why ozone therapy helps fight cancer is because ozone reacts instantaneously with proteins and cell membranes to create organic compounds called ozonides. As they are created, these ozonides carry out oxidative processes as they circulate in the body. Though healthy cells have protection against oxidative damage, cancer cells, as well as bacteria, fungi, and viruses—all of which can be contributing factors for cancer—do not. In addition, the ozonides help stimulate the immune system to more effectively target and eliminate cancer cells and these infectious agents.

Ozone therapy also enhances the body's biochemical pathways that support basic cellular functions, such as cellular repairs, detoxification, and energy metabolism. All of these benefits are why ozone therapy is used in many medical clinics around the world as one of the main treatments for cancer patients. Moreover, ozone therapy has been scientifically proven to diminish tumor size while helping to restore homeostasis (balance) in the body, as well as diminishing pain and improving appetite. It also has been shown to reduce or eliminate the toxic side effects caused by chemotherapy and radiation therapy.

Ozone therapy can be delivered in various ways. The primary methods my staff and I employ at my clinic are ozone IV, also known as ultraviolet blood irradiation (UBI), recirculatory hemoperfusion (RHP) ozone therapy, and HOCATT. In addition, I also use hyperbaric oxygen therapy (HBOT) to further help saturate the body with oxygen.

Ozone IV (UBI): The UBI ozone procedure involves inserting a small catheter into a vein in the forearm, similar to donating blood. A small amount of blood (approximately two to four ounces) is then removed using a sterile syringe. The blood is inserted into a saline bag along with an equal amount of ozone. The ozone will oxidize pathogens, cancer cells and toxins in the blood. The ozonated fluid in the bag is returned to the body intravenously. As it is returned it passes through a flat quartz cuvette (a small tube-like container) and is irradiated with ultraviolet light in a closed, airtight, sterile circuit. The ultraviolet light further kills pathogens and cancer cells and excites red blood cells with a massive amount of energy. As the destroyed pathogens, cancer cells, and oxidized toxins enter the bloodstream the immune system is able to evaluate the harmless fractions of these previously harmful agents and signal for a specific and targeted immune response. Additional benefits include an increased delivery of oxygen and blood that operates from an elevated energetic state. The entire procedure typically takes less than an hour.

Recirculatory Hemoperfusion (RHP) Ozone Therapy: RHP Ozone therapy essentially acts as whole blood and body/cell purification system that ozonates and oxygenates almost the entire blood volume of a patient. Blood passes from the veins of one arm of the patient through a machine that ozonates/oxygenates the blood into the patient's opposite arm. Through RHP, enhanced oxygen reaches all of the body's organs and tissues, including the bones, and crosses the blood/brain barrier very effectively.

RHP itself is a dialysis-like method in which the patient's blood is treated in an extracorporeal loop before being re-infused back into the patient over repeated cycles during the same treatment session. The RHP device synthesizes the combining ratios of stabilized concentrations of oxygen, ozone, and other oxygen molecules. This is achieved by passing pure medical grade oxygen through a corona discharge, which creates the stabilized forms of recombinant oxygen atoms at specific frequencies and Hertz settings. Then the device injects the enhanced oxygen into the bloodstream in a precise computer chip-controlled measured dosage and flow rate, timed to body weight and other medical therapy treatment parameters, for circulation through the patient's blood throughout all the veins, arteries, and capillaries.

RHP uses a highly negatively charged molecule that naturally attaches to the patient's hemoglobin in red blood cells and transports the enhanced oxygen throughout the bloodstream. Being highly attracted to positively charged cancer and other diseased cells, the hemoglobin and enhanced oxygen molecules react immediately upon encountering these diseased cellular structures. Enhanced oxygen molecules move into these infected areas and, upon contact with diseased cells, react by ionization and oxidation to eradicate them. In some cases, concentrated enhanced oxygen may be injected directly into cancer tumors and the surrounding affected area of the body.

RHP treatment sessions typically run from 60 minutes to 120 minutes, after which patients can immediately carry on with their everyday lives.

HOCATT: The HOCATT is a multi-modality health device that synergistically combines medical ozone therapy, carbonic acid therapy, whole body hyperthermia, far infrared therapy, steam sauna therapy, electrotherapy, ultrasonic therapy, oxygen breathing, photon light, color therapy, and aromatherapy into one system. This combination of therapies are sequenced to provide a gentle, yet powerful treatment experience.

The overall health benefits HOCATT treatments provide include:

- Increased sexual vitality and stamina
- Increased metabolism and improved ability to maintain healthy weight
- Smoother and more youthful skin
- Improved mental clarity and memory
- Elimination of cellulite.

HOCATT also helps the body to inactivate viruses, bacteria, yeast, fungi, parasites, and protozoa, stimulate the immune system and speed healing, clean arteries and veins to improve circulation, oxidize toxins and facilitate their excretion, normalize hormone and enzyme production, reduce inflammation, reduce pain and calm nerves, and help the body dissolve fat.

For people battling cancer, HOCATT supports the immune system, helping it target cancer cells and tumors as HOCATT floods the body with oxygen and ozone. This causes tumors to shrink and helps inhibit further tumor growth (metastasis), while also improving white blood cell counts. In addition, HOCATT therapy helps detoxify the body down to the cellular level, further strengthening the immune system.

HOCATT treatments have also been found to reduce the side effects caused by conventional cancer therapies, thus enhancing their effectiveness. Patients who receive HOCATT treatments while also undergoing chemo and/or radiation therapy typically experience less nausea and hair loss, have more energy, and recover more quickly than patients who undergo conventional treatments alone. HOCATT can also be effective as a stand-alone treatment when conventional treatments are contraindicated.

Hyperbaric Oxygen Therapy (HBOT): HBOT refers to the medical use of oxygen in a pressurized environment. When breathing under pressure, much higher levels of oxygen are able to reach and saturate the bloodstream, well beyond the levels of oxygen intake from breathing in a normal environment. The majority of air in a normal environment is only about 21 percent oxygen. The delivery of 100 percent oxygen under pressure during hyperbaric oxygen treatments provides up to 20 times normal oxygen levels to all tissues within the body, and increases stem cell circulation by eight times. This can stimulate healing on all levels by promoting the production of therapeutic chemicals in the body, creating an environment where tissue regeneration and overall healing is greatly increased.

One way that HBOT helps to fight and eliminate cancer cells and tumors is by reducing the low-oxygen (hypoxia) environment that is common in cancer and in which cancer cells and tumors thrive. HBOT also significantly decreases inflammation by stimulating the body's own anti-inflammatory defenses. This is shown by reductions in C-reactive protein (CRP) levels. CRP measures the body's overall level of inflammation and is also a marker for cancer.

In addition, HBOT promotes the growth of new, healthy blood cells. This increase in blood cell growth does not benefit the growth of cancer cells and tumors, however, because cancer growth happens through anaerobic (low-oxygen) activity.

HBOT, until recently, was only available at certain hospitals and medical clinics. In recent years, however, portable HBOT units have come to market, some of which are available on a rental basis, potentially making them suitable for in-home care for cancer and other patients, providing patients and their caregivers are properly trained in their use. You can find more information about such units online.

Detoxification Therapies

Supporting the body's detoxification system is also crucial for properly treating cancer. When our bodies are able to efficiently detoxify, they turn on and enhance their innate anticancer defenses and other mechanisms of action. As detoxification occurs, the body becomes better able to destroy cancer cells, shrink tumors, and finally heal.

Detoxification therapies help the body to clear away all of the toxic build-up that occurs due to all of the environmental toxics we are all exposed to on a daily basis, including in our food and water. The human body was perfectly designed to handle and eliminate normal amounts of natural toxins, but the massive amount of man-made environmental toxins is far too much for the body to manage without therapeutic support. This is especially true for people with cancer and other chronic, degenerative diseases.

According to the Environmental Working Group (EWG), of the nearly 85,000 man-made chemicals in the United States that are currently approved for use, more than 1,400 chemicals or chemical groups "are known or likely carcinogens. Through industrial applications, consumer products and food, water and air, Americans are exposed daily to these cancer-causing compounds, which invade the body and build up in blood and urine." The abundance of heavy metals and other toxins further burdens the body to increase the risk of cancer. This is why detoxification therapy is so important.

In my clinic, the primary detoxification therapies I use are coffee enemas and colon hydrotherapy, laser energetic detoxification, ionic foot baths, diet, and specific detoxification promoting supplements.

Coffee Enemas and Colon Hydrotherapy: Both coffee enemas and colon hydrotherapy can improve gut motility and the frequency of bowel movements, while also helping to remove toxic mucoid plaque stuck to the colon walls. They can also stimulate the removal of parasites in the gut.

The use of an enema for health was first recorded in 1500 BC in an Egyptian document called the *Eber Papyrus*. In earlier times, people implemented enema treatments in a river by using a hollow reed to induce water to flow into the rectum. It is recorded that before the departure of Lewis and Clarke expedition, a physician instructed them in the appropriateness of using enemas in cases of fever and illness.

Coffee enemas have been used to improve health since the 1800s. They are performed by adding two to three cups of room temperature organic coffee to an enema bag or bucket. The coffee enema solution is delivered through the enema tubing into the rectum, where it is retained for ten to 15 minutes before being expelled into the toilet.

Coffee enemas can improve energy levels, prevent and relief bloating, and reduce the toxicity of the whole body by prompting liver cleansing and tissue repair. Another benefit of coffee enemas is that they promote the production of glutathione in the liver. This powerful antioxidant protects cellular damage to DNA and stimulates the removal of toxic waste out of the cells. Cancer patients and individuals with digestive issues, autoimmune conditions, liver conditions, gallstones, and low energy can all benefit from coffee enemas because of how they can clean and purify the gastrointestinal tract in a short period of time. Specific enema kits can be purchased using stainless steel bucket and specific tubing to prevent leaching of plastic into the enema fluid before entering into the colon.

Colon hydrotherapy, also known as colonics or colon irrigation, is a safe, effective, and controlled method of cleansing the colon using a mechanical flow of warm, pure-filtered and temperature-regulated water that is infused gently into the colon by a sterile rectal nozzle. This process softens and loosens waste in the large intestine, resulting in its elimination through natural peristalsis. Colon hydrotherapy has an antiseptic and solvent action on the impacted fecal matter, other toxins, and parasites that it helps remove from the colon. Accumulated waste along the lining of the colon is readily absorbed into the blood supply causing autointoxication.

Other benefits of colon hydrotherapy include increasing the water level and diuretic action of the body, which increases blood volume and circulation; improving liver detoxification and overall liver function; restoring the natural shape of the colon (impacted fecal matter typically causes the colon to become distorted over time, causing various colon problems); improving muscle tone; and improving functioning of the body's lymphatic system.

As cancer tissue is destroyed through oxidative therapies, it is important to eliminate the debris of the destroyed cancer cells. The risk is that current and potentially new tumor sites can use the old debris of destroyed cancer tissue as building materials to rapidly support the growth of tumors. This is an additional reason why detoxification strategies are so important.

While coffee enemas can be performed at home, colon therapy requires the services of a skilled colonic therapist.

Laser Energetic Detoxification: Laser energetic detoxification, also known as LED therapy, was developed by Lee Cowden, MD, MD(H). It is a gentle, rapid, and non-invasive method of addressing chemical toxicities, heavy metal burdens, sulfur intolerances, nutritional deficiencies, chemical and hormonal imbalances, genetic dysfunctions, chronic infections, and much more.

Among his achievements, Dr. Cowden is an expert in homeopathy. In conventional homeopathy, remedies are taken as pellets or liquid drops under the tongue. In LED, a clear glass treatment vial of water and alcohol is imprinted with homeopathic-like frequencies. A low-powered laser light is then shone through the treatment vial onto the patient's body with a sweeping motion. This creates a physiological impact, the effects of which include the release of toxins, activation of the immune system, and the balancing of hormones. It can also be used to balance enzymes, neurotransmitters, and other biochemicals in the body.

As the laser shines through the homeopathic vial, the information in the vial piggy backs onto the light beam into the body. If it is a homeopathic mercury vial, the body will immediately start releasing mercury; if the vial is imprinted with the spirochete borrelia, the immune system will gain the information needed about this infectious agent to more effectively fight it off. LED therapy is an extremely powerful healing technique, and I find it to be an excellent tool for helping the body release toxins. At our center we will use a vial imprinted with the frequency of the cancer the patient is dealing with and through a process called autonomic response testing be able to identify if the cancer is associated with a specific pathogen, toxin, nutritional deficiency, or other factor. We will then pair the two vials and then use LED to educate the body about what the cancer is connected with to call on the body's innate intelligence to correct the cancer-causing factor.

Ionic Foot Baths: Ionic foot baths are becoming more popular in the integrative medical space, as well as in health and beauty spas. These detoxifying cleanses are easy to do, non-invasive, and effective.

Chemicals and pathogens, heavy metals, and other toxins all have specific electrical charges. These charges interfere with the body's ability to operate normally, and as toxicity builds up in the system, illness frequently occurs. The ionic foot bath provides opposite charges that cause the toxic materials within the body to break loose and leave the body through the feet. The benefits of ionic foot baths can be increased by pairing it with laser energetic detoxification treatments. LED works to open up the detoxification pathways and to loosen toxic elements within the body, while the ionized water of the footbath helps to pull the toxins out.

Ionic foot baths also work well in conjunction with the IV therapies discussed earlier in this chapter, all of which also help facilitate detoxification. The bath provides an outlet for the toxic waste that the body is working to remove. I recommend implementing an ionic footbath protocol along with other detoxification therapies to increase the effectiveness of those therapies.

Yet another benefit of the ionic foot bath is the alkalizing effect it produces in the body. The ionization in the water reduces the body's acidity and shifts it to a more alkaline state. It is well known that many diseases cannot exist in an alkaline environment. This therapy provides a simple, effective way for the body to reach a healing, balanced alkaline condition.

Critics of ionic foot baths point out that the water used in an ionic foot bath will change colors even if feet have not been placed in the water. This is because all water contains some impurities that will be affected by the charge produced during the bath. The toxins that come out of the feet are indicated by particles of varying colors that the procedure draws out, depending on the body's impacted energy pathways or meridians. In addition to the toxins eliminated during the therapy session, ion channels are opened up to promote detoxification for many days. This has been shown in studies where toxins in the urine have been measured several days post an ionic foot bath.

Peptides and Repurposed Drugs

Certain peptides and repurposed drugs can also be important supportive aids for fighting cancer.

Peptides are compounds composed of two or more amino acids that are linked together in a chain. If the chain is longer than 40 amino acids, it is called a protein. If it has fewer than 40 amino acids, it is called a peptide.

Peptides control and modulate most systems in the body in a tissue- and cell-specific manner. Among their many functions, peptides regulate hormone production, immune function, the body's sleep cycle, the production of inflammatory mediators, DNA replication, cell division and renewal, cancer cell destruction and apoptosis, libido and sexual arousal, weight loss, lean muscle gain, mitochondrial function, cognitive function, mood, energy and other metabolic activities, tissue healing, and specific biological functioning of the brain, skin, eyes, urinary and reproductive systems, aging and longevity, and many more.

Compared to medications and hormones, peptides tend to be more selective in terms of their mechanisms of action in the body, and much less likely to cause serious adverse side effects.

The peptides I find most useful as anticancer agents are thymosin Alpha-1, met-enkaphalin, and GHK-Cu.

Thymosin Alpha-1 (TA1): Among its many benefits, TA1 stimulates the immune system, including markedly improving the functional maturation of dendritic cells (DCs). One of the main functions of DCs is to process antigen material and present it on the cell surface to the T cells of the immune system. In this capacity, DCs act as the immune system's "sentinels". They also serve as messengers between the body's innate and adaptive immune systems.

In addition to its effects on DCs, TA1 significantly improve the killing rate of T lymphocytes by increasing their cytotoxicity in response to cancer cells and infectious microorganisms. TA1 also enhances effector T-cell responses, increases CD4 and CD8 count and natural killer (NK) cell function, enhances cell mediated immunity, and increases the efficiency of antigen presenting cells.

Like the other peptides in this section, TA1 is administered by subcutaneous injection. A typical dose for cancer patients is 35 units twice a week.

Met-Enkaphalin: This peptide, also known as metenkefelin, is produced by the adrenal medulla in the adrenal glands. It regulates normal cell growth while inhibiting abnormal cell growth. It also modulates cell functionality and mounts an antitumor effect by regulating dendritic cells. Like TA1, it too increases and activates cytotoxicity against tumor cells. In addition, it stimulates the P16 and P21 inhibitory pathways of cancer cell division, thereby help to suppress and halt the spread of cancer cells.

In vitro studies have found that met-enkaphalin kills cancer cells in the colon, pancreas, brain (neuroblastoma), kidneys, ovaries, and the breast (triple negative breast). A phase 1 human trial of 16 pancreatic cancer patients showed that met-enkaphalin improved survival time compared to standard 5-FU or gemcitabine chemotherapy drugs, with good pain control.

GHK-Cu: GHK-Cu has been shown to alter oncogene expression and lower inflamasome activity (inflamsomes are involved in the inflammatory response, which can be a contributing factor in cancer). Research also found that GHK-Cu suppresses RNA production in 70 percent of 54 genes that are over-expressed in cancer patients, and that it has health-promoting effects on gene regulation of multiple cancer promoting pathways, resetting gene activity, and reactivating the body's apoptosis system that is lost in cancer.

Like TA1, a typical dose of GHK-Cu for cancer patients is 35 units twice weekly by subcutanous injection.

The repurposed drugs I most recommend for cancer patients are ivermectin, mebendazole, metformin, doxycycline, low dose naltrexone, dichloroacetate sodium, and the statin drugs atorvastatin, simvastatin or lovastatin.

Ivermectin (IVM): IVM has been shown to trigger apoptosis in cancer cells. It does this primarily through the cells' mitochondrial pathway, where it changes the balance between pro- and anti-apoptosis-related proteins. IVM also induces autophagy, the process by which the body eliminates old and diseased cells, thus preventing such cells from turning cancerous. Research also suggests that IVM could inhibit cancer stem cells (CSCs).

A typical dosage of ivermectin for cancer patients is 12 mg twice a day, cycling four days on, three days off, and then repeating this cycle. Side effects can include tiredness, loss of energy, stomach pain, loss of appetite, nausea, vomiting, diarrhea, dizziness, sleepiness or drowsiness, and itchiness.

Mebendazole (MBZ): Several in vitro studies suggest that MBZ inhibits a wide range of factors involved in tumor progression, including angiogenesis, cancer cells' pro-survival pathways, and their multi-drug resistance protein transporters. Mebendazole on its own not only exhibits direct cytotoxic activity on cancer cells and tumors, but also acts synergistically with radiation therapy and different chemotherapeutic agents to stimulate an enhanced anti-tumor immune response when used in conjunction with these therapies.

A typical dose is 100 mg daily. Possible side effects include diarrhea, stomach pain, abdominal discomfort or swelling, nausea, vomiting, and loss of appetite.

Metformin: Metformin is widely used to treat type II diabetes, a condition known to be a causative factor for numerous types of cancer, including cancers of the colon, rectum, pancreas, and liver. Research also shows that metformin has various anticancer benefits. According to a comprehensive review of data regarding metformin and cancer, published in the peer-reviewed medical journal *Cancer Management and Research*, "Generally, metformin can: 1) reduce the incidence of cancers, 2) reduce the mortality from cancers, 3) increase the response to treatment in cancer cells when using radiotherapy and chemotherapy, 4) optimize tumor movement and reduce the malignancy, 5) reduce the likelihood of relapse, and 6) reduce the damaging effects of ADT." (ADT stands for androgen deprivation therapy, which is primarily used to treat prostate cancer.)

When taking metformin, cancer patients should begin with a dose of 500 mg with dinner for the first two weeks. From the third week on, they can increase the dose to 500 mg taken with breakfast and again with dinner. Taken metformin with a meal will reduce the risk of stomach upset. Common side effects include diarrhea, nausea, flatulence, indigestion, headache, lack of energy, and taste disturbances. While using metformin, patients' blood sugar and vitamin B12 levels, as well as kidney function, should all be monitored.

Doxycycline: Doxycycline is a broad-spectrum antibiotic most commonly used to treat bacterial infections ranging from bacterial acne,

Chlamydia and cholera to Lyme disease, syphilis, and typhus, as well as parasites. It can help treat cancer because of its ability to inhibit mitochondrial ribosomes and protein translation, which blocks the formation of new mitochondria in cancer cells. It also inhibits the activity of matrix metalloproteinases (MMPs), a class of enzymes involved in tissue invasion by cancer cells and tumors. In addition, doxycycline blocks transcription factor Myc, a family of oncogenes involved in cancer cell progression, and suppresses key developmental cancer stem cell factors.

Research has found that doxycycline's anticancer benefits can be significantly increased when it is taken along with vitamin C. Studies show that this combination therapy is up to ten times as effective compared to the use of doxycycline alone, particularly with regard to targeting and killing cancer stem cells.

The recommended dose for cancer patients is 100 mg a day. Common side effects include headache, nausea, dyspepsia, joint or back pain, nasal and sinus congestion, or a rash.

Dichloroacetate sodium (DCA): DCA is an inexpensive drug compound that shares similarities with vinegar and salt when they are combined together. It has been used widely and safely for decades in human beings to treat a variety of conditions, including cancer.

Non-toxic to healthy cells, DCA is targets cancer cells by disrupting their fermentation cycles. This, in turn, protects the body from lactate, a metabolic by-product of energy production in cancer cells. Lactate produced during the cancer cells' fermentation process converts surrounding tissue to cancer and promotes metastasis. DCA turns that mechanism off.

Unlike chemotherapy, which targets cells that grow and divide quickly, DCA restores natural cell apoptosis. It does this by blocking the function of the enzyme pyruvate dehydrogenase kinase (PDK), which is critical for cancer cell proliferation. Cells are then returned to a state of normal cellular metabolic activity.

DCA also interferes with cancer cells' use of glucose by removing glucose from cancer cells. DCA does not, however, deprive glucose to healthy cells in the body. In addition, DCA restores "bad" metabolism in cancer cells by activating their damaged mitochondria. By doing so, DCA increases the production of reactive oxygen species (ROS) in cancer cells, which causes them to cease spreading and die, while simultaneously shrinking tumors and alleviating various cancer symptoms, such as pain, loss of appetite, and unhealthy weight loss, and improving survival outcomes.

DCA is also an excellent enhancer of various other cancer therapies, both conventional and integrative, including chemotherapy and radiation, as well as IV vitamin C, IV artesunate, hyperbaric oxygen therapy (HBOT), and various other oxygen/ozone therapies. It also enhances the effects of a ketogenic diet.

DCA is typically safe to use long-term, presenting little risk for serious side effects. In some cases, however, it can cause peripheral neuropathy. In such cases, stopping DCA reverses this condition. This risk can also be reduced by taking vitamin B1 and alpha-lipoic acid along with DCA. When using DCA, liver function should also be monitored because in a small percentage of patients its use can cause an asymptomatic but reversible elevation of liver enzymes.

A typical dose of DCA is between 300 to 500 mg per day at a recurring cycle of two weeks on and one week off. During the weeks that DCA is used, taking 300 mg of vitamin B1 and 900 mg of alpha-lipoic acid is also advisable.

A more recent discovery has been to couple the use of DCA with Poly-MVA to reduce the potential for peripheral neuropathy. Since I began using this combination, all of my patients have safely been able to use DCA without the concern for peripheral neuropathy. As it turns out, the combination of the two is much more powerful in addressing the metabolic pathways of cancer than either one of them alone.

Because of its safety profile, it may be advisable to continue using DCA for at least five years in lower doses after cancer has gone into remission, along with follow-up checkups every three to five months, to help ensure that cancer does not come back.

Low Dose Naltrexone (LDN): Naltrexone is a pharmaceutical drug that the FDA approved in the 1980s. It was originally used to treat opioid and heroin addiction. However, research conducted by Dr. Bernard Bihari, MD, in the 1980s and 1990s revealed that its use created an improved immune response in his HIV patients and led to improved outcomes for those diagnosed with pancreatic cancer and lymphoma, and also lupus patients. Bihari also found that many who received conventional cancer therapies and failed to respond could benefit from the administration of low dose naltrexone.

Since 1985 when the first immunotherapy findings were produced, researchers led by Ian Zagon, MS, PhD, at Pennsylvania State Medical School published 300 papers showing that LDN use causes an increase in endorphin production and stimulates an immune response, in particular, in the creation of natural killer cells (NK). Generally speaking, over 60 percent of those who have been diagnosed with cancer may experience marked benefits from administration of LDN for their disease.

LDN works to increase endorphins that the body produces during exercise and other physical activities. These compounds not only provide the "high" experienced during physical exertion, but also support and improve immune function and overall well-being. Low dose naltrexone has the ability to affect the opioid growth factor (OGF), which stimulates the growth of cancer cells. In one study, 31 types of cancer revealed high levels of OGF. LDN's effectiveness in impacting the opioid receptors in tumors and possibly even contributing to death in cancerous cells has been well-noted by cancer researchers.

Some cancer types that show high levels of OGF include lung, breast, endometrial, pancreatic, prostate, uterine, throat, ovarian, bladder, liver, colon and rectal cancers, lymphocytic leukemia, glioblastoma, neuroblastoma, malignant melanoma, myeloid leukemia, multiple myeloma, renal cell carcinoma, carcinoid tumors (tumors of the neuroendocrine system), head and neck squamous cell carcinoma, and blood and lymphatic system cancers such as Hodgkin's and non-Hodgkin's lymphoma.

In a 2011 study using animal subjects published in an issue of Experimental Biology and Medicine, researchers found that over a six hour period, administration of naltrexone every second day lowered the development of DNA and replicating malignant cells in the ovaries. In another case, ovarian cancer cell growth was shown to be restricted and mice were observed to have tumors that decreased in size by 45 percent.

Researchers have also found that LDN is useful as a supportive therapy along with traditional chemotherapy drugs such as Cisplatin. In some case studies, those experiencing late stage pancreatic cancer were successfully administered intravenous alpha-lipoic acid which has typically been used as a secondary support to primary cancer therapy, in conjunction with LDN, with no adverse effects as well as increased survival times reported.

LDN is believed to fight cancer and reduce tumor growth by:

Creating an increase in the density and number of opiate receptors on cell membranes of the tumor. This produces an increased response to growth-inhibiting effects of endorphin levels, which then triggers apoptosis in cancer cells.

Creating an increase of natural killer (NK) cell numbers and corresponding activity in those cells, as well as lymphocyte activated CD8. These are observed to be highly responsive to a rise in endorphin levels

LDN has also been shown to not only provide pain relief for cancer patients, but also fortification of the body's defense mechanisms while fighting cancer. In addition, it modifies certain genes related to cancer and promotes the death of cancer cells. It also inhibits cancer cell division and directly blocks toll-like receptors which are known to produce inflammatory compounds that stimulate the growth of cancer cells and encourage spreading (metastases). It can also be helpful as a treatment for cancers that have failed to respond to conventional therapies.

Naltrexone has minimal side-effects when administered at low-doses and is extremely cost-effective. A typical dose schedule is 1.5 mg taken at night in week 1, then increasing to 3 mg at night during weeks 2 and 3, and to 4.5 mg at night during week 4 and beyond.

Note: LDN is contraindicated for cancer and other patients who have been prescribed opioid drugs such as morphine because LDN can behave as an antagonist to these types of medications.

Statins: Statin drugs have been used for decades to reduce cholesterol levels to help prevent heart disease. Although the side effects that statins can cause can be more serious than the side effects typically caused by the drugs mentioned above, statins can still be beneficial.

In recent years, research indicates that stain drugs may provide anticancer benefits. As one study noted, "Statins appear to enhance the efficacy and address the shortcomings associated with conventional cancer treatments, suggesting that statins should be considered in the context of combined therapies for cancer."

One of the most studied aspects of statins with regard to cancer is their effects on what is known as the mevalonate pathway. The fluctuation of this pathway is an essential requirement for all cells, including cancer cells. Statins block the mevalonate pathway and inhibit YAP and TAZ, both of which are master transcriptional regulators (regulatory proteins that are predominantly responsible for regulating the expression of multiple genes) of both normal organ and tumor growth. By inhibiting YAP/TAZ-dependent transcriptional responses by blocking the mevalonate pathway, statins also inhibit the development of cancer cells. Among their other anticancer benefits, statins also reduce cytokines, and thus cancer-promoting inflammation and metastasis.

The statin drugs I most commonly use for cancer are atorvastatin, simvastatin, or lovastatin at a dose of 40 mg once a day for two weeks, then twice daily. Their use must be monitored carefully, however, because of the side effects they can cause. Common side effects include diarrhea, muscle spasm and weakness, urinary tract infection, insomnia, limb and musculoskeletal pain, myalgia, and nausea. But they also carry a risk of hemorrhagic stroke, a life-threatening condition caused when a blood vessel in the brain ruptures and bleeds.

Additional Support Therapies

The following therapies are also offered at The Karlfeldt Center to further support cancer patients.

Applied Psycho-Neurobiology (APN): I introduced you to APN and explained how it works and is effective for healing unresolved emotional issues and traumas in Chapter 7. Any emotionally-charged event and the unhealthy or limited beliefs surrounding it can have a strong, negative impact on your health, behavior, relationships, and life choices. When dealing with difficult life events, a common coping mechanism is to suppress the emotions associated with them. But if they are not resolved, suppressed emotions can trigger and perpetuate physiological changes that can cause chronic disease, including cancer. In fact, suppressed emotions are quite common among cancer patients.

APN enables practitioners trained in its use to communicate with their patients' subconscious mind to identify unresolved emotions and the life events that caused them, as well as identifying where in the body they are causing dysfunction. APN can then be used to help resolve the emotions and balance the affected organs so that they can begin to heal. Combining APN with the other therapies I use to treat cancer can often speed patient recovery.

Sonodynamic Therapy: Sonodynamic therapy involves the use of drugs that only become toxic to cells upon exposure to ultrasound. Since ultrasound can be focused into small tissue volumes within the body, it provides a means of localizing treatment and reducing the risk of side effects elsewhere in the body. In this respect, sonodynamic therapy is similar to photodynamic therapy (PDT), which uses light for drug activation. A number of drugs are known to be sensitive to and activated by both light and sound. The main advantage of sonodynamic therapy over PDT is the much greater tissue depth that can be reached noninvasively by ultrasound compared to light.

Upon activation, sonodynamic therapy drugs, known as sonosensitizers, produce reactive oxygen species (ROS) that generate a cytotoxic effect on cancer cells and tumors. Ultrasonic irradiation in combination with the presence of a photosensitizer in the cancer cells can trigger a cavitation effect, producing shock waves and micro jets, which can destroy tumor microvascular structures, damage endothelial cells, and even cause the breakdown of cancer cell membranes (a process known as lysis). Cytotoxicity has been shown to be significantly increased in the presence of ultrasound contrast agents, particularly when these are loaded with oxygen. As the sonosensitizers accumulate in tumor cells, focused ultrasound eliminates the tumor by forcing the tumor cells to undergo apoptosis. Sonodynamic therapy has been shown to be effective in the treatment of tumors in both in vitro (lab testing of specimens) and human studies. It is also being explored for other applications, including its potential as a treatment bacterial and other microbial infections.

Pulsed Electromagnetic Field (PEMF) Therapy: Science has established that the Earth has a pulsing electromagnetic field of 7.8 hertz, and that this field is what is required for our planet to support life. Science has also proven that the human body produces its own electromagnetic field, and that all of the body's systems work because of exchanges that occur within this field, including the electromagnetic signals that the brain uses to communicate with the body's other systems.

The underlying principle of PEMF therapy is that providing the body's cells with the proper and sufficient electromagnetic charge enables the body to more effectively maintain and repair itself and remain healthy. By contrast, disruption of the cells' electromagnetic energy impairs cell function and metabolism, setting the stage for cancer and other diseases to occur. PEMF therapy uses pulsed electromagnetic fields to stimulate and energize the body on a cellular level by delivering beneficial, health-enhancing frequencies to the body that penetrate every cell, tissue, organ, and even bones, to enhance the body's numerous electrical and chemical processes.

Research shows that PEMF helps support the body's repair and restorative mechanisms, while also helping to improve circulation, reduce pain and inflammation, boost immunity, and assist detoxification by enabling cells to release metabolic waste products. PEMF therapy devices provide these health benefits by directing electromagnetic pulses and signals to the body, either to local targeted areas or as a whole body treatment delivered by laying on a PEMF mat.

A growing body of in vitro, animal, and human studies demonstrate the potential EMF therapy has as an adjunctive treatment for cancer, and also as a means to help prevent cancer. Many health clinics around the world, including mine, offer PEMF therapy using various PEMF devices. Various units are also available for home use, as well. However, before choosing a PEMF device, should you decide to purchase one, it is important to first educate yourself about how they work and which ones are most appropriate for your needs. One of the world's leading educators and researchers about PEMF therapy and PEMF devices is William Pawluk, MD, MSc, who provides a wealth of information about PEMF therapy at his website, www.DrPawluk.com and in his book, *Supercharge Your Health With PEMF Therapy*.

Hyperthermia with Far Infrared Sauna: Certain types of tumor cells are more sensitive to heat damage than healthy cells, and are unable to adapt to higher temperatures. When exposed to higher temperatures, cancer cells are unable to grow and they also weaken, making them more susceptible to other cancer therapies. In many cases, however, high heat alone can be enough to destroy cancer cells. When core body temperature rises to between 107 to 111 degrees Fahrenheit, cancer cells and tumors begin to destruct. In some cases, tumors can be destroyed when core body temperature of 111 degrees Fahrenheit is sustained for half an hour. Because of this fact, hyperthermia, which is a method for temporarily increasing the body's core temperature, has been used as cancer treatment for many years in various clinics and hospitals around the world.

Even mild fevers are known to result in natural immune system defenses against cancer cells, in much the same way that the body generates fever in response to invading pathogens and other microorganisms. Far infrared sauna therapy is a hyperthermia method that elevates the heat within the body's tissues to create a fever-like condition. This causes cancer cells to produce heat shock proteins. As they do so, the immune system stimulates a tumor-specific immune response to attack the weakened cancer cells. With repeated far-infrared treatments, cancer cells and tumors have a better chance of being destroyed. Far-infrared treatments are also effective in enhancing the anticancer properties of chemotherapy when both treatments are used concurrently. Another advantage of this combination approach is that it often allows for lower doses of chemotherapy to be used that are still effective, yet less likely to cause severe side effects.

In my clinic, I use HOCATT to administer far-infrared sauna therapy to my patients because of the other therapies HOCATT also provides at the same time.

A Further Word About Prayer, Spirituality and Family Support

As effective as all of the therapies that you've learned about in this chapter can be for treating cancer—both as part of an overall integrative cancer treatment plan and, in many cases, on their own—I cannot over-emphasize the importance of prayer and other spiritual practices, as well as the support of family and other loved ones, and the positive effects they can have on patient outcomes.

During my many years of clinical practice as a naturopathic doctor with a focus on oncology, I have repeatedly witnessed seeming miracle recoveries among patients with a prayerful attitude who committed to enlisting God as their primary ally as they journeyed through cancer. Doing so enabled them to not only meet their challenges head on, with less fear and more faith, but often to even cheerfully face those challenges as they kept their focus on God and being grateful for the blessings in their lives. For many of them, their prayers and faith transformed even cancer into one of those blessings because of all they learned and discovered about themselves as they underwent their treatments, and how the love their families and friends gave them and which they returned grew even deeper during their shared journey.

As a physician with decades of clinical practice under my belt, I have come to realize that prayer and spirituality and the abiding love that God bestows on everyone of us is truly the most powerful and "best medicine" above all of the wonderful therapies that are available to us today. Please keep that in mind when facing any challenges you may be presented with. No matter what, God is always there for you, and calling on God for help can make all the difference.

Recovery and Remission

Patients in remission often return to good health after receiving cancer treatments, especially if they underwent an integrative treatment approach. However, in order to maintain their long-term health so that they can enjoy the years ahead as cancer survivors, it is essential that they continue to follow an anticancer lifestyle, as well as regularly being tested and evaluated by their physicians and receiving further recommended treatments on a preventive basis to best ensure that they remain cancer-free. Along the way, they should also continue to make general improvements and fine-tune their diets, nutrition, and overall lifestyle choices to adapt to the inevitable challenges and stresses that all of us face as part and parcel of our human existence.

My hope for everyone with cancer is that they are able to avail themselves of the treatments and therapies covered in this chapter. I realize that this is not yet possible for many patients due to issues of availability of these therapies in their local areas, as well as for financial reasons, given that many of these therapies are yet to be covered by their health insurance. Yet I also remain hopeful that as more physicians and patients alike learn about these treatments and come to understand how and why they work and can significantly improve cancer outcomes and survival rates, that the demand for them will one day soon make them more widely available and that insurance companies will choose to provide coverage for them.

My ultimate hope is that all cancer patients triumph over cancer and can attest to their success in much the same way that that so many of my patients are able to. I end this chapter with one such testament from one of my patients to illustrate what is possible when cancer patients are able to receive comprehensive, integrative cancer treatments.

A Cancer Patient's Story: "Looking back today, I can see that I'd been having symptoms of esophageal cancer for a while. I'd just been ignoring or downplaying them as typical issues that most people develop as they get older. However, after an unexpected scare of passing out on the bathroom floor and my wife finding me, I was rushed to the hospital, where I underwent a day and a half of tests that concluded I had cancer and that it had spread to one of my lymph nodes. While the prognosis was terrifying, to say the least, I knew that I needed to create a game plan to beat this. That's why I decided to contact the Karlfeldt Center. Working around my chemotherapy, I cannot say enough about the Center's entire staff of professionals. The Karlfeldt team was brilliant at developing a customized treatment plan to address the underlying issues contributing to my cancer. I really counted on their guidance in outsmarting my cancer and building a course of action. I am still on my healing journey, but I've been in remission now for almost five years. I am grateful for every day and grateful for the team that has supported me." ~ J.M.

Chapter 13

Creating A Cancer Prevention Lifestyle

It's been said that the best way to treat cancer is to prevent it from happening. In this chapter, you will learn the essential steps you need to take to help ensure that you are never faced with a cancer diagnosis.

What We Can Learn From Patients Who Survived Cancer

It may seem counterintuitive, but learning from patients who successfully recovered from cancer, especially from patients who triumphed over advanced cases of cancer for which there was seemingly no hope, can provide important clues about what can be done to prevent cancer. The steps they took to recover are among the same important steps we can take to keep cancer at bay.

These steps, or key factors, that are common among patients who defied their prognosis and achieved long-term survival were identified by Kelly A. Turner, PhD, author of the book *Radical Remission: Surviving Cancer Against All Odds*. Dr. Turner spent more than ten years studying and analyzing over 1,500 cases of cancer patients who defied the odds of their dire prognoses to achieve complete and lasting remission. As she did so, she discovered that what all of the patients had in common, besides their recoveries, were nine factors that they all employed during their journey back to health. I have found that these same factors are common among my own patients who beat cancer, as well.

The nine factors are:

1. Improving your diet, often to a radical degree, if necessary.
2. Becoming proactive and taking control of your health.
3. Connecting with and heeding your intuition, or inner guidance.
4. Discovering and using nutritional supplements, herbs, and other anticancer products that are most appropriate for your unique nutritional needs.
5. Uncovering and releasing suppressed emotions.
6. Focusing on experiencing and increasing positive emotions.
7. Embracing social support.
8. Deepening your spiritual connection.
9. Discovering and connecting with your life's purpose in order to have strong reasons for living.

As you can see, these traits or factors align closely with the information I've provided you in this book's previous chapters, particularly Chapters 6 through 11. To them, I would add managing stress, evaluating your exposure to toxins in your environment and personal care products, making sure that you get enough regular exercise, practicing self-care detoxification measures, ensuring healthy hormone balance, monitoring your health using the various tests discussed in Chapters 1 and 5, and working with an integrative physician who can provide you with some of the therapies I discussed in Chapter 12 on a preventative medicine basis.

Creating Your Very Own Cancer Prevention Lifestyle

As you consider the above traits of long-term cancer survivors, let's recap and review the action steps you learned in this book that you can apply them to create an ongoing action plan to protect you and your loved ones from cancer.

In Chapter 1, you learned what cancer is and the three dominant theories that currently shape cancer research and cancer treatments: that cancer is a genetic disorder, a metabolic disorder involving damaged or dysfunctional mitochondria, or a survival mechanism initiated by the body in response to an ongoing onslaught of toxins, chronic stress, nutritional deficiencies, and other factors.

You also learned that, more than these theories, what is most important is to recognize the numerous factors that have been identified as causes of cancer, as well as cancer's early warning signs. Doing your best to minimize these cancer drivers, and being alert to any changes in your body and health that could be indications of cancer is vital for preventing cancer and for catching it in its earliest stages, should it occur, so that it can more easily and effectively be treated. You also learned about the many conventional diagnostic tests doctors use to confirm a diagnosis of cancer.

In Chapter 2, you learned how and why chronic inflammation is a primary cause of cancer. You also learned the causes of chronic inflammation, including iron overload and insulin resistance. In addition, you learned about the best tests that screen for and monitor inflammation levels, as well as important steps you can take on your own to prevent and reverse chronic inflammation. As part of your overall cancer prevention lifestyle plan, I recommend that you be tested for chronic inflammation on an annual or semi-annual basis while also implementing the action steps I shared in Chapter 2.

Eliminating, or at least minimizing, the additional cancer risk factors that you learned about in Chapter 3 is also something you must work towards in order to reduce your risk of ever developing cancer. You can start by implementing the action steps I shared in Chapter 3, which I repeat here:

1. Learn how to better manage and alleviate stress, exploring and improving your mindset, and getting help to heal your emotions are vitally important.

2. Commit to eating healthy and improving your body's nutritional status.

3. Avoid second- and third-hand smoke. If you smoke, seek help so you can quit.

4. Commit to regularly exercising or engaging in other physical activities.

5. Maintain a healthy weight. If you are overweight, work with your health practitioner to help your lose excess weight.

6. Beware of infections and do all you can to avoid them and boost your immunity.

7. Become aware of environmental toxins in your home and workplace and do your best to minimize your exposures to them, creating healthier home and workplace environments.

8. Minimize your exposures to EMFs, especially during bedtime.

9. Avoid exposures to ionizing radiation and test your home for radon.

10. Get at least seven hours of restorative sleep each night, and work with your doctor or a sleep specialist if you suffer from sleep problems.

11. Maintain healthy hormone balance by working with your doctor or another hormone specialist to test your hormone levels and keep them optimal.

12. Practice safe sex and avoid being promiscuous.

In Chapter 4, you learned about cancer stem cells (CSCs) and circulating tumor cells (CTCs), both of which are primary drivers of cancer and cancer recurrence. In Chapter 5, you learned about various tests that are effective for detecting CSCs and CTCs, as well as some of them that can detect cancer and when the body is starting to shift into a precancerous condition. Given how prevalent cancer is today, as part of your annual physical exam, I recommend that you ask your doctor to include some of these early detection tests, such as thermography, the Chronic Inflammation Test, and the Cancer Profile©, the Galleri(R), and, for men, the free PSA test, IsoPSA, the 4K score, and/or the prostate health index (PHI) tests to screen for prostate cancer.

In addition to the above tests, I also recommend an annual or semi-annual comprehensive health assessment to determine and monitor your current health status. This can be done using a variety of other lab tests that your physician can advise you about and order for you. These tests provide important insights into various factors related to your health and can alert you and your doctor to early signs of health issues before they become serious. Checking for underlying infections, toxicity levels, inflammation markers, immune system function, genetic predisposition, and hormone levels can help identify any potential areas that need attention. If lab tests reveal imbalances in thyroid, adrenal, or sex hormones, targeted nutritional support and, if necessary, bioidentical hormone therapy may be beneficial.

Regular lab tests can also reveal any nutritional deficiencies, allowing for tailored dietary adjustments or supplementation as needed. Undergoing an annual or semi-annual comprehensive health evaluation is an essential element of preventive health care. See Chapter 9 for more about these lab tests.

In addition, also periodically review check lists and answer the cancer risk assessment questionnaire I shared in Chapter 5 to better ensure that you are doing all you can to reduce your cancer risk.

Other important action steps that you need to incorporate into your life on a preventive basis include the following.

Improving Your Diet

As you learned in Chapter 8, an unhealthy diet is one of the most significant causes of cancer, as well as disease in general. Improving your diet is therefore one of the most important action steps you can take to safeguard your health and help prevent cancer. In order to do so, I recommend that you start by taking an inventory of the foods you habitually eat and eliminating from your diet all foods that fall into the following categories:

- Genetically modified foods (GMOs) aka bioengineered (BE) foods.
- Sugar and simple/refined carbohydrate foods.
- Conventionally raised meats, poultry, and fish laced with antibiotics and growth hormones.
- Foods laced with pesticides and herbicides. (Visit www.EWG.org, the website of the Environmental Working Group to see which commercially grown foods contain the lowest amounts of pesticides and herbicides.)
- Fast foods and processed foods that contain artificial food additives and preservatives, trans- and hydrogenated oils and fats, and excessive amounts of omega 6 essential fatty acids.
- Nonorganic dairy products.
- Iron-enriched foods.
- Sodas and other unhealthy beverages, such as nonorganic fruit and vegetable juices, sports drinks, nonherbal teas, and alcohol.
- Also avoid foods sold in plastic wraps or in plastic food containers.

In place of such foods, focus on eating a variety of different colored, ideally organic, vegetables in each of your meals, along with wild caught fish and free-range meats and poultry food free of hormones and antibiotics. For snacks, eat non-starchy fruits away from meals.

In general, an organic, Mediterranean-style, anti-inflammatory diet, also known as a "rainbow diet", that emphasizes fruits, vegetables, lean proteins, healthy fats, and whole grains is an appropriate dietary solution for most people. It's rich in antioxidants and can reduce inflammation, two key factors in preventing cancer and promoting overall health.

Also include foods rich in healthy fats, as well as fermented foods, and vary your meals to ensure that you supply your body with a wide variety of nutrients, and to minimize the risk of developing food allergies and sensitivities.

In place of unhealthy beverages, drink pure filtered water throughout the day, but avoid doing so when eating so that you don't dilute stomach acid and digestive enzymes, thus impairing digestion. In place of coffee, drinking organic herbal teas, especially organic green tea is also advisable. Finally, get in the habit of adding more spice to your diet by including spices such as cayenne pepper, cinnamon, garlic powder, ginger, and turmeric, all of which have anticancer properties.

The Ketogenic diet, Kelley protocol, and a stricter plant-based diet can be incorporated as needed to achieve specific therapeutic goals. Refer back to Chapter 8 for further tips on how you can most effectively optimize your diet and eating habits in order to prevent cancer.

Evaluating Your Exposure to Toxins in Your Environment and Personal Care Products

Understanding your personal and family toxic exposure is another crucial step to take. This includes evaluating your personal and family history to determine previous exposures you may have incurred. Were you or your parents before you were born exposed to mold, chemicals or heavy metals in work environment, hobby or living location? Also, assess your current living and work environment for any potential carcinogens, such as tobacco smoke, radiation, certain chemicals, and specific viruses, all of which were discussed in Chapter 3.

And take a closer look at the products you use regularly, such as detergents, cleaning products, and personal hygiene items. Many commercial products contain potentially harmful chemicals. Opt for items marked as non-toxic and organic when possible, to reduce your overall toxin exposure.

Detoxification practices can help rid the body of toxins. Techniques such as coffee enemas, sauna sessions, Epsom salt baths, and colonic therapy can assist in detoxification. Dry skin brushing and deep breathing exercises are also useful, as they enhance circulation and oxygenation, respectively. Regular fasting, juicing, and consumption of clean water can further support the body's natural detoxification processes.

Becoming Proactive and Taking Control Of Your Health

Your health is your responsibility. Doctors and other health practitioners can guide you in making your health choices, but it is up to you to learn all you can about how to improve and maintain your health and, most importantly, to implement what you learn on a consistent basis.

Neither health nor disease "just happens". By and large, they are both outcomes that are determined by your life choices and habits. Acknowledging that fact and then act accordingly is vitally important if you want to minimize your risk of cancer.

Becoming proactive about your health begins with making an honest assessment of your current health status and lifestyle choices. Take a moment to answer these questions:

- How healthy is your diet?
- Are you getting enough exercise or other physical activities on a regular basis?
- Do you get regular exposure to healthy sunlight outdoors?
- Are you overweight? If so, by how much?

- Are you achieving at least 7 hours of deep, restorative sleep each night?

- How content are you in your daily life?

- Do you habitually feel stressed out and/or subject to unhealthy emotions?

- When was the last time you had a comprehensive health checkup? (Ideally, you should have one at least once a year.)

- Do you feel that you are living your life purpose?

Your answers to these and similar health assessment questions provide important clues about various factors in your life that may require your attention so that you can improve them. Once you have identified what needs improvement, commitment to working on each area to the best of your ability, ideally with the assistance of a naturopathic or other type of integrative physician.

As you move forward towards a healthier lifestyle, don't try to accomplish everything at once. Instead, focus on one or two areas at first and do your best to improve upon them one step at a time. Then, as you progress, begin to work on additional areas that may require improvement. By taking this consistent approach, you may be pleasantly surprised how much better you look and feel within a few months, which will further incentivize you to keep at it.

Connecting With and Heeding Your Intuition

Intuition is something all of us can tap into and be guided by at any time. All that is required is to become aware of how intuition "speaks" to you so that you can become better able to perceive its guidance. For most people, one of the most common forms of intuitive communication occurs as a "gut feeling". Such feelings can be messages of caution or warnings, or they can be signals that show us how to most effectively move in the direction of our desires and dreams in order to achieve them.

What all gut feelings have in common are palpable feelings that literally seem to be located in the gut, or solar plexus area of our bodies. Learning how to recognize your gut feelings when they occur can aid you make better decisions about all areas of your life, including your health.

To gain a better sense of your gut feelings try this simple experiment that next time you go grocery shopping. Go to the aisles that sell healthy fruits, vegetables, and other foods. Pick up a piece of food, get still, and take moment to notice how you feel as you hold it. Mostly likely, you will feel positive emotions. Now go to an aisle where unhealthy foods are sold, such as pastries or packaged foods full of preservatives and other additives. Pick up one of these foods and again notice how you feel as you hold it. Then notice the difference between those feelings and the feelings you experienced when you held the healthy food.

Another simple way to improve your ability to "listen to your gut" is to get still and then state out loud something that you know to be true, such as stating "My name is [state your name]. Notice how you feel as you do so. Then repeat the same statement, but insert a name that isn't yours. Again, notice how you feel.

With practice, both of these exercises can make it easier for you to perceive your gut feelings and recognize and be guided by their messages.

Gut feelings are hardly the only way that intuition can "speak" to us. Often they can occur as an "inner voice," a flash of vision, guidance in dreams, or a sudden sense of clarity and knowingness that you feel in the depths of your being. You can also cultivate your intuition through prayer and meditation, asking for guidance as you engage in such practices.

The more that you practices such methods, the more proficient you will become at making intuition a regular part of your daily life experience and gain the guidance and other benefits that come from it.

Discovering the Nutritional Supplements, Herbs, and Other Anticancer Products That Are Most Appropriate For You

As I explained in Chapter 9, a healthy diet, while of paramount importance to good health and for keeping cancer at bay, is no longer enough to ensure that our bodies obtain all the nutrients they require to stay healthy due to pollution, stress, commercial farming methods, and other factors. For most people, supplementing with nutritional, herbal, and other products is also necessary.

However, rather than adopting a willy-nilly approach of supplementation without knowing what supplements your body actually needs—and, just as critically, in what dosages—is unwise. Before using any type of supplement, you need to first know your body's current nutritional status. This knowledge can be easily obtained by using the tests and testing methods I shared with you in Chapter 9. If possible, working with a nutritionally-oriented physician or other health practitioner, especially one skilled in the use of Autonomic Response Testing (ART), which I also explained in Chapter 9, can also be very helpful.

Once you obtain your test results, you will have a much better idea of which supplements your body needs. You can then track how well your nutritional status is improving by periodically repeating your tests.

Commit To Daily Exercise and Physical Activity

Cardiovascular exercises like walking, jogging, cycling, or swimming can improve heart health and overall stamina. Strength training, on the other hand, can build muscle mass, improve balance, and enhance metabolic health. Both contribute to overall wellbeing and lower the risk of numerous diseases, including certain types of cancer. Aim for a minimum of 30 minutes of moderate intensity activity most days of the week. Consider activities that also promote relaxation, like yoga or tai chi. See Chapter 10 for further exercise recommendations.

Uncovering and Releasing Suppressed Emotions/Focusing On Experiencing and Increasing Positive Emotions

Because of traumatic experiences and other difficult challenges that can affect us during the course of our lives, it is all too easy for people to fall prey to unhealthy emotions and then to suppress them as they struggle to move past such incidences. All too often, they many also lose hope that they will ever recover their sense of well-being that existed before trauma struck. This sense of hopelessness can lead to feelings of depression, sorrow, and even anger.

It is now well-established that suppressed emotions can significantly impair immune function and negatively impact your body's ability to stay healthy and heal should cancer or any other disease strike. Uncovering and releasing such emotions is essential for good health, whereas not doing so can lead to disease and other unhealthy life issues.

I encourage you to refer back to Chapter 7 and the checklist of questions that can help you to determine if suppressed or unresolved are affecting you, and to answer each question truthfully. Also assess how stress may be affecting you by examining the stress checklist in Chapter 7. Then make use of the various self-care options for optimizing your mindset and emotions that I shared in that chapter.

At the same time, as you work on releasing and healing the emotions that no longer serve you, begin to focus on cultivating positive emotions so that they become an increasing part of your daily life. Positive emotions such as happiness, joy, gratitude, and peace have been shown to directly and powerfully enhance immune function, as well as the functioning of many other body systems, thereby contributing to our well-being, both physically and psychologically.

In my experience, one of the most powerful ways to cultivate positive emotions is by taking time each day to practice gratitude. You can do this in the morning when you wake up, before you go to bed, or at any other time during the day. By committing yourself to make time to appreciate the blessings that come your way each day, you will likely be surprised by how much there is for you to be grateful for.

In addition to practicing gratitude, there are many other ways you can cultivate positive emotions in your life. These include engaging in hobbies you like, exercising, gardening, getting together with loved ones for fun times, and anything else that brings you happiness and joy. Find the activities and pursuits that you most enjoy and incorporate them into your life on a regular basis.

Mindfulness practices, such as meditation or prayer, are also important measures for reducing stress and enhancing your mental and emotional wellbeing. Embracing the act of forgiveness also contributes to psychological wellness. Additionally, spending time in nature and the sunshine can provide therapeutic benefits by further reducing stress and increasing vitamin D levels, respectively.

Embracing Social Support

As the famous saying goes, "No man is an island." The importance of healthy relationships to good health is also well documented by medical researchers. Additionally, good relationships with others can make a significant positive difference in how well we are able to respond to life challenges with resiliency.

I encourage my patients to turn to their families and friends when they feel they need support, and I recommend that you do the same. I also recommend that you reciprocate and do your best to be there for your loved ones when they need you. Doing so helps to take your attention off of your own problems. Many patients report that their pain, fatigue, and various other health symptoms tend to be forgotten or diminished when they are enjoying themselves with those they love.

Another important, yet often under-appreciated relationship that I encourage you to cultivate is the one you have with your physician and other health care providers. The ideal relationship between patient and doctor should be a partnership. Be an active participant in your professional health care treatment, and be willing to share what you are going through in your health journey so that your doctor can best meet your needs.

The more that you can surround yourself with understanding loved ones the happier you will be and the more supported you will feel as go about your life.

Deepening Your Spiritual Connection

In Chapter 6, I highlighted how important developing spiritual awareness and a connection with God. I encourage you to assess your current state of spiritual health scoring your answers to the questionnaire I provided in that chapter.

I believe that nearly everyone, at some point in their lives, will experience a connection with the God or the Divine. Even so, people often forget to call on God to guide them as they go about their lives. Yet, when they remember to do so, they very often find that their lives improve. This fact is borne out by a variety of scientific studies that have examined the relationship between spirituality and health and disease.

As I shared in Chapter 6, research confirms that people who believe in God, or a Higher Power, and regularly engage in religious or spiritual practices derive significant health benefits. This is particularly evident should they become sick compared to patients who are not religiously or spiritually oriented. This is why I encourage all of my patients to engage in religious or spiritual practices that they are comfortable with, and to actively call upon God to aid them in their healing journey. By turning your life over to God, I am confident that you will derive similar benefits.

For me, prayer is the most powerful spiritual tool for cultivating a relationship with God. There are many ways to pray. I find that the most effective ways are those that combine prayer with gratitude for the blessings we already have, and a positive expectation that what we pray for is already becoming reality. By praying in this manner, you will start to receive answers to your problems and become better aware of the role God is playing in your life.

Maintaining a positive vision as you pray is also very important. It is helpful to see yourself as you want to be—whole, healthy, and happy. Your body has an amazing capacity to try to recreate whatever images your mind projects to it. Therefore, it is vital that you keep positive healing images in your mind as you pray, especially when you are tempted to feel discouraged. Dwelling on positive images of yourself and your future helps positive things come to you by the law of attraction. Positive thinking also helps you to avoid victim thinking, which is characterized by helplessness, negativity, complaining, anger, self-pity, and depression. By choosing not to be a victim and actively putting your trust in God, you make it possible for what you ask for to be "given unto you."

Meditation, spending time in nature, practicing forgiveness, and attending spiritual services are also effective ways for deepening your spiritual connection. Find the way or ways that you are most comfortable with and make them a regular part of your life. And remember, God is always ready to answer and guide you.

Discovering and Connecting With Your Life's Purpose

To me, discovering and living out your life's purpose, is a natural outgrowth of having a connection with God. After all, it is from God that all of the talents we have come. Putting those talents to use in ways that both enables you to forge a life that fulfills you and makes a positive contribution and difference to your loved ones and your community is one of the best ways you can honor God. It is also one of the very best ways for keeping yourself healthy. Because when you find and live your life purpose, the fulfillment you will derive from doing so will keep stress at bay while providing you feelings of happiness and joy, and the knowingness that you are doing what you are meant to be doing.

If you are unsure of your life purpose, please revisit Chapter 7 for tips on how you can go about discovering it. Then, once you realize what it is, pray to God to guide you in how best to make it your reality.

Keep Learning

In concluding this chapter, I want to emphasize how important it is for all of us to do our best to keep abreast with the latest findings related to health and disease care, including the latest developments in cancer care. As Albert Einstein said, "Once you stop learning, you start dying."

I have learned much about how to treat cancer in the decades since I began my naturopathic practice, yet I realize every day that there remains still much more for me to learn. That recognition excites me and fuels my passion to continue learning about new discoveries related to health and new treatment options that may enable to me to be of even greater help and service to my patients. When it comes to your health and keeping yourself healthy, I encourage you to do the same.

One way that you can do so is to subscribe to my free online newsletter, which you can do on the home page of my website, www.thekarlfeldtcenter.com. There, you will also find articles and videos on my blog.

You can also stay informed and continue your learning by listening to my podcast. There, I have the good fortune to interview many leading physicians and other health experts, as well as people who have survived cancer. I learn a lot of valuable and practical information from these guests, and I am confident you will do. You can listen to my podcast and find archives of my past interviews at https://integrative-cancer-solutions-with-dr-karlfeldt.simplecast.com.

You will find other sources of information that can help keep you informed in this book's References and Recommended Reading sections.

Conclusion

This book serves as a comprehensive guide designed to empower and equip you with knowledge and practical steps to enhance your body's inherent ability to ward off and combat cancer. We have explored a wide array of topics that collectively serve as a blueprint for optimal health and cancer prevention. From understanding your past and present environmental exposures to managing emotional wellness, we have established the interconnected aspects of overall health and their significance in relation to cancer. We have journeyed through different practices that range from the familiar, such as exercise, diet, immune system support and nutritional supplementation to the possibly lesser-known, like targeting cancer drivers, importance of the mitochondria and addressing cancer stem cells. By exploring and addressing each of these facets, we can form a holistic strategy to maintain health and prevent disease. My wish is that you implement that strategy as an integral part of your daily life so that you and your loved ones remain cancer-free.

Chapter 14

Frequently Asked Questions

This chapter covers the questions I am often asked about cancer and my approach to treating it as a naturopathic oncologist, and provides my answers to those questions.

Although you treat patients with a wide range of health conditions, you are increasingly treating many patients with cancer. How did you move into this area of medicine?

I've been in clinical practice since 1987. In the beginning of my naturopathic career, I didn't set out to treat cancer; I planned on practicing a traditional type of naturopathy in which you deal with pretty much any type of condition under the sun. Then I learned that my father passed away from colon cancer. It was a shock because we hadn't been in communication for a number of years. He did standard conventional cancer care therapies and just wilted away to nothing before he passed. I wish I could have been there and maybe in some way changed the outcome. In addition, when I began my practice I was witnessing the frustration of cancer patients who came to see me at a time when there were really no solutions, just the same type of standard conventional care that to this day continues to have a poor overall record of success, especially for advanced cases of cancer. So that gave me an extra desire to learn more about cancer and how to best treat it, to spare others from what my father went through. Not all that much has changed in the conventional cancer field since that time, so I continue to be motivated to find a better way. Today, being a naturopathic integrative oncologist is what I love to do because I regularly witness what a significant difference it can make in my patients' lives.

What are the latest areas that you are looking into with regard to preventing and treating cancer?

One of my biggest passions is sharing ideas and learning from other leading integrative cancer doctors from all over the world. I've had the benefit to collaborate with and interview many of them on my radio show, podcasts, and at cancer summits so I can communicate with them as to what is out there that is working. You know, we can have a lot of theoretical ideas and hypotheses, but at the end of the day all that really matters is if the patient gets rid of cancer or not. Getting the chance to pick each other's brains about what we are finding to be the most effective approaches for treating our patients advances our overall knowledge base and hopefully makes what we are doing more well known and acceptable to other oncologists so that they can provide their own patients with similar benefits and more positive outcomes.

Obviously, nobody can say, "I can cure cancer," because we're not there yet. But there are amazing tools now that are available that we didn't have 30 years ago. There's been an explosion in regard to integrative oncology and the choices and options that are now available. I wrote my book to inform more patients and doctors alike about them.

One of your specialties is treating cancer using photodynamic therapy along with various photosensitizing agents. What is the rationale behind that approach?

Photodynamic therapy, or PDT, is proving to be a very important noninvasive, nontoxic tool within the overall cancer treatment protocols that I employ, based on my patients' specific needs. The goal of PDT is to attract a strong amount of laser light into tumors to trigger oxidation of cancer cells. As oxidation occurs, cancer cells die. The photosensitizing agents that I use increase the ability of PDT to kill off cancer cells by further concentrating the laser light into the tumor and using the type of photosensitizer, such as nano-ICG, that concentrates in the tumor for an extended period of time to increase treatment time.

Injecting a photosensitizer to a tumor site enables an accumulation of light in the tumor over a longer period of time and creates a stronger pull of whatever laser that we're using to trigger really strong oxidative stress within the tumor. The issue with many of the traditional photosensitizers is that they clear out of the system in about 40 minutes or so. We want them to be able to concentrate in tumor tissue for a longer period of time, so that when laser light is applied, there is enough of the photosensitizer present to intensify the light to the point of cancer cell death. If it clears out in 40 minutes, then it doesn't have the time to accumulate in the tumor tissue and less of the desired effect is achieved.

The issue with PDT when it's used alone is that the light clears out of the system in about 40 minutes or so. We want it to be able to concentrate in tumor tissue longer than that. If it clears out in 40 minutes, then it doesn't have the time to accumulate in the tumor tissue. Injecting a photosensitizer to a tumor site enables an accumulation of light in the tumor over a longer period of time and creates a stronger pull of whatever laser that we're using to trigger really strong oxidative stress within the tumor.

Both chemotherapy and radiation therapy are also therapies that oxidate tumors and cancer cells, but they also harm healthy cells, which accounts for the toxic side effects they are known to cause. The beauty of PDT is that it is beneficial for healthy cells and supports their mitochondria while it is creating oxidative stress on the cancer cells to kill them, especially when we intensify PDT with these photosensitizers.

Another significant benefit is how versatile PDT is. You can combine it with intravenous therapies to treat the body, or you can use it with optic needles that break the skin barrier to get closer to, and even inside, the tumor, depending on the tumor location. In addition, you can also combine PDT with ultrasound, or sonotherapy, with the photosensitizers to pull both light and sound frequencies into the tumor to really stress cancer cells. The ultrasound creates cavitation bubbles within the cancer cells, which causes them to rupture. I always wonder why more physicians aren't incorporating PDT and sonotherapy into their cancer treatments because they can both be effective and neither of them have any negative downsides or anything like that.

How many patients each day are you able to see, given all these different therapies and protocols that you use?

I usually see about 20 to 30 patients a day. Along with my personal patient interaction, I am very blessed to have an excellent staff around me to ensure that each patients get the best possible care.

Can the diagnostic tests that you use in your practice be used to replace x-rays and CT and MRI scans to detect cancer cells or cancer recurrences after all conventional treatments have been concluded?

The different diagnostic tools each have their place. I like using tests that screen for circulating tumor cells and allow me to assess my patients' health status before, during, and after treatment. But as of yet, there is nothing out there that is able to look at everything. Even CT and MRI scans are not capable of looking at and assessing everything, and they also carry the risk of causing cancer—CT scans because of the radiation they emit, and MRIs because the dyes they use can also be cancer-causing. The toxic impact on genes and cancer causing effect of MRIs by themselves are still under discussion.

I use a wide range of blood and inflammation marker tests, as well, in order to get a more complete picture of my patients' health status. CT and MRI scans and other conventional imaging tests certainly have their place, but they are not 100 percent accurate in detecting cancer, especially in its early stages. Just because you don't see cancer on an image doesn't mean that it doesn't exist. It takes many millions of cancer cells in the body before you're even able to see cancer on any kind of image. So you can't rely on imaging alone.

Conventional oncologists tend to focus on tumors, whereas you take a somewhat different approach. Why is that?

When you deal with cancer, it is not always the tumor that is the most important thing that you want to be concerned about. It's often the inner terrain in the body that the tumor exists within that needs the most attention. It's just as important to shift the terrain into an environment that is not conducive to cancer as it is to attack tumors. When you do both, you usually get better results and longer lasting outcomes, which is why I make sure to educate my patients on all that they can do to keep their inner terrain and microbiome healthy during and after treatment.

You use methylene blue in your clinic, both as a photosensitizer for PDT therapy, and also as an IV. What are your thoughts about taking it orally for cancer patients?

I am a proponent of methylene blue. It does so many things just by itself. In addition to being a photosensitizer, it turns on mitochondria, is a potent antiviral agent, and does so many other things, including shifting the body away from being in a chronic inflammatory state. Inflammation always shows up before cancer, so when you address inflammation, you address cancer at the same time. That's why when my cancer patients come my center and do my two week intensive, I use methylene blue as a photosensitizer both orally and intravenously. We inject methylene blue locally around the tumor sites, as well. And if we have access to the tumor, there is benefit to inject it there along with using other therapies such as IV vitamin C.

Taking methylene blue orally is something that I think pretty much everyone should also consider. I recommend five milligrams twice a day, depending on the individual. And if you can combine that at the same time with light therapy, such as an infrared sauna or a BioMat or other kind of infrared device at home, you will benefit from the photodynamic effect. First you take methylene blue, and then 30 minutes later you can do a session of infrared therapy. Combining methylene blue with some kind of light therapy on a fairly regular basis is a good idea for anybody.

Why do you use ionic foot baths as part of your cancer treatment programs?

Ionic foot baths are an easy tool to use. Some people are skeptical of them because of videos online showing that they change the color of water whether feet are placed in them or not. That's due to the ionization of the water as it's reacting with the minerals that are already in water. That's where the debunking videos come from. But what those videos don't show you is that the water turns a lot darker when feet are placed in them.

What ionic foot baths do is open up the ion channels in the body. These channels play a role in transporting nutrients throughout the body, and are also where a lot of detoxification takes place. When these channels are blocked then the transportation of nutrients is not functioning the way that it should and the body's ability to detoxify is impaired.

Proper transport of nutrients, as well as efficient detoxification, are both important for preventing and treating cancer. So one of the biggest benefits of ionic foot baths is that they support your ability to detoxify and support your ability to move nutrients from one location to the other. This makes them a valuable tool to use in combination with other therapies. For example, as an aid to IV vitamin C therapy. The use of IVs gets vitamins directly into the bloodstream, but we also want to ensure that the vitamins pass through the ion channels to get into the cells and tissues, where they are most needed. Ionic foot baths aid in that process.

Another important benefit of the foot baths is their ability to reduce the body's load of toxic heavy metals and other harmful chemicals. Tests of urine samples collected several days after an ionic foot bath session show that you pee out more heavy metals and chemicals that are being collected in the urine than you do without a foot bath session. This means that the benefits of ionic foot baths don't just happen during a session. They continue for days afterward. That is important.

Ionic foot baths are contraindicated for some people, however. They are not advised for pregnant and nursing woman, organ transplant recipients, people wearing pacemakers or other battery operated implants. People taking heart or blood pressure medications, and people using various antidepressant and antipsychotic drugs should be monitored by their doctor. I also recommend only using a high quality ionic foot bath to ensure you are getting the most benefit, and that you work with a skilled practitioner trained in their use.

With so many nutritional supplements and herbs and other products known to have anticancer properties, how do you know which ones to use for your patients?

That's a very good question. Although there are indeed many nutrients, herbs, and other supplement products that can be beneficial for cancer patients, knowing which ones are most useful for each individual patient is the key. That's why I use the various blood tests, hormone panels, gene testing, and automatic response testing (ART) to determine the most appropriate supplement plan for each of the patients I treat.

In addition, patients have different needs that must be addressed and prioritized. This means evaluating each patient from a logistic perspective to determine which are the most important supplements to give them first, and then monitoring their effects and making adjustments and perhaps adding other supplements as needed along the way. With some cancer patients, there is only so much that their bodies can take. For example, some patients who receive chemotherapy can barely handle food, so care must be taken to determine the best supplement approach. If they are having trouble eating, then capsules and pills aren't always advisable. So maybe nutrients delivered in fluids is the best way to go, or perhaps nutritional IV treatments. The approach I take varies depending on each patient's situation. Proper testing and evaluation is essential for determining the best solution.

What advice do you have for using dichloroacetate sodium (DCA)?

DCA is a fascinating substance and it can be very helpful for cancer patients, as a growing body of published research confirms. To understand why it works we need to look at fermentation. The way that the cancer cells produce energy is by fermenting glucose. For healthy cells, this is a very inefficient way of producing energy, but it is very good for the cancer cells. DCA helps to block that process, impairing the ability of cancer cells to get energy through the fermentation cycle. Essentially, DCA causes cancer cells to starve, making them much more susceptible to any kind of stress, including the oxidative stress that many of the other cancer therapies I use subject cancer cells and tumors to.

But one of the issues that can occur with DCA is a risk for neuropathy. If you are using DCA and starting to notice neuropathy, then you should immediately stop using it. When you do, the neuropathy should stop. But if you continue using DCA after you start to experience neuropathy it could lead to chronic neuropathy, which may not be reversible.

So the question with DCA is how do you reduce the risk of neuropathy? Utilizing things that support mitochondria, like taking vitamin B1, CoQ10, alpha lipoic acid, and L-carnitine with DCA can help. But thanks to what I learned from Dr. Paul Anderson, I combine DCA with Poly-MVA. They work together like a marriage made in heaven. By doing that, I have not seen any neuropathy or any other complications. And I've administered thousands of doses now. My protocol is to administer Poly-MVA via IV before administration of IV DCA, doing two weeks on, then one week off, twice a week with both Poly-MVA and DCA. You do that for four cycles. DCA via IV tends to be safer and more effective than taking DCA orally.

What are your thoughts about ketosis and a ketogenic diet for cancer?

Ketosis is one of those things that we have really been learning more and more about in regards to cancer. It is important. Each healthy cell should have what's called metabolic flexibility, where it's able then to shift in response to what kind of fuel source that it needs. With the standard American diet, which is loaded with sugar and refined carbohydrates, cells lose this flexibility and become stuck. Both healthy and cancer cells have a lot of insulin receptors along their walls that pull sugar into them, because that's the primary way that energy in both of these cell types are produced. Through the metabolism of glucose. Because cancer cells are so inefficient in producing energy and is so reliant on producing energy through glucose fermentation, a cancer cell have a much larger quantity of insulin receptors than a normal cell.

Shifting how cells produce energy by using ketones instead of glucose does not impair energy production in healthy cells, whereas cancer cells are not as able to use ketones for energy. They are still able to produce some degree of energy, but not very efficiently, so they become much more vulnerable to any type of cancer therapy when the body shifts into a state of ketosis. Combining a ketogenic diet with anticancer therapies can be very powerful.

However, it's very important to recognize that the body still requires a wide range of nutrients, some of which ketogenic diets do not provide. So a ketogenic diet needs to be undertaken prudently, and you can pulse it so you don't have to be on it all the time. You follow it for a few weeks and then you can go off it, eating a healthy, ideally organic, other type of diet for a bit, and then returning to a ketogenic diet. This keeps the cancer cells guessing and prevents them from being able to effectively produce energy.

One thing I want to point out about ketogenic diets is the importance of what I call clean eating. Because a ketogenic diet can be comprised of just unhealthy food, with a lot of dairy, unhealthy fats, and too much meat, and still be ketogenic by definition. In the short term, eating an unhealthy ketogenic diet may leave you feeling like you have more energy but after a while you won't feel as good as you did initially, because you won't be getting all the nutrients you need, and likely further compromising your health by consuming unhealthy fats and so forth. So, as with any dietary approach, you need to ensure that you are eating healthy foods when you go keto. And even then, for most people, it is important to pulse it by alternating it with another healthy diet, such as the Mediterranean diet, rather than staying on it all the time. Because our bodies also need the fiber and phytonutrients that fruits and vegetables and other healthy foods provide.

The ketogenic diet can be an important tool for fighting cancer, but how effective it will be depends on the individual and where they're at in their journey through cancer.

Do you have any recommendations on how to deal with the side effects of radiation therapy during treatments and afterwards, if the side effects linger?

Yes, there are certain things that you can do to support your body while maximizing the beneficial effects of radiation. One of them is as simple as taking a niacinamide, a form of vitamin B3. Unlike niacin, niacinamide does not produce a flushing effect, which can be discomforting. One of the aspects of radiation therapy, as well as of chemotherapy, and also many of the therapies I use, is that it is an oxidative type of therapy. Remember, to treat cancer effectively, you need to get oxygen within the tumor in order to weaken and hopefully destroy it. In order to be able to do that, you want to support circulation in the body. Niacinamide is a really powerful tool for doing that.

At the same time, to help bind the various components given off by radiation therapy that can cause side effects, and help rid them from the body, you can use Pecta-Sol, the form of modified citrus pectin developed by Dr. Isaac Eliaz. Other agents such as magnesium, selenium, and zinc are also helpful because they enhance the effects of radiation therapy and support the body through that process.

Berberine is also useful during radiation, as well as any other therapy that produces an oxidative effect, because it helps reduce the amount of glucose that enters cancer cells, helping to stress and starve them. There are different repurposed drugs, such as metformin, that you can use to also starve the cancer at the same time.

Taking high doses of essential fatty acids (EFAs) can also help. EFAs help to support the lipid membranes, or walls, of cells. You want to keep the lipid membranes as healthy and pliable as possible so that when you are receiving radiation the healthy cells can withstand that better, versus what takes place with the cancer cells.

Fasting prior to receiving radiation therapy or chemo can also help, since it further reduces cancer cells' ability to obtain sustenance. Fasting also triggers autophagy, the mechanism by which the body rids itself of old and diseased cells.

If you have also the access to oxygen therapies, such as hyperbaric oxygen therapy, receiving oxygen therapy prior to radiation will push oxygen into cancer cells and tumors, so that the radiation will have an even greater beneficial impact. The same is true for receiving oxygen therapy before chemo.

Before and after radiation therapy, IV therapies using substances like vitamin C, glutathione, and/or curcumin can also be very helpful to support tissues and repair tissue damage caused by radiation therapy. With radiation, you're burning tissues, so you, you want to support the healthy cells and tissues as much as possible to minimize radiation's side effects.

You also want to keep your blood sugar levels in a healthy range, which is another way that metformin can help. I want my cancer patients to have blood sugar levels in the mid-80s, and their A1C level between 4.8 and 5.2. Your doctor should also monitor your insulin levels because if you need a lot of insulin, that means that your insulin receptors are not functioning very well. I want to keep my patients fasting insulin levels at 10 or below. In addition to metformin, berberine, chromium, vanadium, and other nutrients help to support healthy blood sugar and insulin levels.

After radiation treatments are completed, you can continue to use these integrative approaches to enhance your body's ability recover and reduce the risk of lingering side effects.

Lymph nodes are often involved in cancer, since cancer can often spread there. Any advice about keeping the lymphatic system healthy?

Proper lymphatic system function is very important, both as a way of helping to prevent cancer, and also to help reverse cancer. Anytime that you deal with lymph, just as anytime that you deal with blood, you need to look at it systemically. Unlike other systems in the body, the lymphatic system needs our assistance to ensure the proper flow of lymph.

The lymphatic system is the body's filtration system. And just like filtration systems in swimming pools and so forth, you want to keep it clear and unclogged. If it does become clogged and lymph flow becomes sluggish, you want to see what is getting trapped in that filtering system. Is it infections, heavy metals or other toxins? Has cancer taken hold in one or more lymph nodes?

Whatever the answer is, you need to eliminate that component. There are many ways to do this, such as IV vitamin C, ozone therapies, and laser therapies, all of which I use. Juice fasts, coffee enemas, colonics, and other detoxification therapies can also make a significant difference, as can sweating, especially when it is induced by far infrared and other sauna therapies. Anything that promotes detoxification is really important. Chlorella can also help, especially if heavy metals are involved, as can bentonite clay and activated charcoal tablets. Great herbs to support the purification of the lymphatic system are burdock, sarsaparilla, Echinacea, red clover, Oregon grape, poke root, and chaparral.

Self-care tools to maintain healthy lymph flow and prevent it from becoming sluggish include deep diaphragmatic breathing done periodically throughout the day, regular exercise and physical activity, and dry brushing of the arms, legs, and upper torso. Drinking high quality water and staying hydrated is also very important.

One of the most effective exercise methods for supporting healthy lymph flow is bouncing or jogging in place on a mini-trampoline, also called a rebounder, for five to ten minutes a few times each day.

Find the self-care methods that you most enjoy and be consistent in performing them on a daily basis, including after you complete your cancer treatments.

What advice would you give to people who have just been told that they have cancer?

Obviously, being given a diagnosis of cancer is a major life-changing event, and it's quite understandable that when patients are first told they have cancer they may feel fear and even become overwhelmed by it. Despite all of the advances that have been made in how we treat cancer, and the longer survival rates that are being achieved, many people still regard cancer as a death sentence. I want to assure people that it is not.

My first piece of advice is, if you feel fear and are afraid, acknowledge that. Don't try to deny your fears or whatever other emotions may come up for you, because that will only cause more stress. But don't succumb to fear.

I also want to emphasize two very important points: Today, more than at any other time in history, there are very good reasons to set aside your fears and have hope, because of the advances that continue to be made when cancer is addressed using a truly integrative approach. My fellow integrative oncologists and I witness the successes such an approach can achieve all the time. Cancer is NOT a death sentence. That's point number one.

Point number two is even more important, and that is that you are not alone in this journey through cancer. Whether or not you are religious or spiritually oriented, God is always with you, and when you invite Him into your life and ask for His help, He will provide it. I cannot over-emphasize how important this is. Find a way to connect with God in whatever way suits you best. Doing so doesn't necessarily mean attending religious services. Cultivate your relationship with God in your own way.

Another essential step newly diagnosed cancer patients need to take is to do all they can to educate themselves about their specific type of cancer and the treatments that are available to them. This doesn't necessarily mean spending long hours conducting research on the Internet, although that can help. It also means asking questions of your doctor and getting more than one professional opinion. Don't settle for a one-size-fits-all, cookie cutter approach for your treatment. If at all possible, seek the help of an integrative oncologist who can provide you with many viable therapies that conventional oncologists do not utilize.

The conventional approach is to focus on and target cancer cells. In my experience, it is far more effective to focus on your body's healthy cells and your body's inner terrain, doing all that you can to strengthen them so that your body becomes better able to fight and recover from cancer. Surgery, chemo, and/or radiation may be necessary, but there is much that you can also do to improve their effectiveness if they are required, as well as when they are not. In addition, if possible, seek out and speak to cancer survivors, especially those who were diagnosed with and triumphed over your type of cancer.

Also, remember that you are in charge of your life, not anyone else. Take responsibility for that and trust your own inner guidance and "gut feelings" as you consider your treatment options. Research proves that the patients who take the most proactive approach when facing cancer are the ones who typically achieve the best outcomes and longest survival rates. This is especially true of proactive patients who also call on God to help them.

Are you available for consultations?

Yes. My staff and I offer a free 15-minute consultation by phone that you can schedule on my website. Visit www.thekarlfeldtcenter.com/contact-us and under the Select box, choose the "Schedule a consultation" or "Speak with an expert" option. I also provide telemedicine consultations via Zoom or phone.

You can also listen to the many interviews I've conducted with cancer doctors and other health experts, as well as with patients who conquered cancer to learn more about the full range of treatment options available to you. Visit https://integrative-cancer-solutions-with-dr-karlfeldt.simplecast.com.

Resources

The Karlfeldt Center
www.thekarlfeldtcenter.com
3451 E. Copper Point Drive
Meridian, ID 83642
(208) 338-8902

Visit my website to learn more about the full range of services my team and I provide. You can also sign up for my free newsletter on the homepage. My library of free articles is also available at this site (www.thekarlfeldtcenter.com/blog)

To schedule a free 20-minute consultation to see how my medical team and I may help you, visit www.thekarlfeldtcenter.com/contact-us

Dr. Karlfeldt's Podcast
Integrative Cancer Solutions with Dr. Karlfeldt
https://integrative-cancer-solutions-with-dr-karlfeldt.simplecast.com
Dr. Karlfeldt's YouTube Channel
https://www.youtube.com/c/healthmade

Naturopathic Physicians and Naturopathic Oncologists
American Board of Naturopathic Oncology (ABNO)
www.fabno.org
American Association of Naturopathic Physicians
www.naturopathic.org
Oncology Association of Naturopathic Physicians (OncANP)
https://oncanp.org
Ontario Association of Naturopathic Doctors (OAND)
https://oand.org

Cancer Organizations
American Cancer Society
www.cancer.org
National Cancer Institute
www.cancer.gov
National Breast Cancer Foundation, Inc
www.nationalbreastcancer.org

Environmental Health Organizations
American Academy of Environmental Medicine (AAEM)
www.aaemonline.org
EM-Radiation Research Trust
www.radiationresearch.org
Environmental Health Trust
www.ehtrust.org
Environmental Protection Agency
www/epa.gov
Environmental Working Group
www.ewg.org
Natural Resources Defense Council
www.nrdc.org

Cancer Tests
American Metabolic Laboratories Cancer Profile© Test
AmericanMetabolicLaboratories.com
Chronic Inflammation Test
https://chronicinflammationtest.com
Galleri® Test
www.galleri.com

Thermography (aka Thermology) Organizations
American Academy of Thermology
https://aathermography.org
Institute for the Advancement of Medical Thermography
https://iamtonline.org
Professional Academy of Clinical Thermology
https://medicalthermology.org

Genetic Testing
The DNA Company
www.TheDNACompany.com
Nutrition Genome
NutritionGenome.com
Self Decode
SelfDecode.com

Additional Lab Testing Resources
The following companies offer the lab tests that you can order on your own (restrictions may apply for residents of certain states).

Everly Well
www.everlywell.com
Life Extension Foundation for Longer Life (LEF)
www.lef.org/Vitamins-Supplements/Blood-Tests/Blood-Tests
Quest Diagnostics
https://questdirect.questdiagnostics.com
Request A Test
https://requestatest.com
SpectraCell Laboratories
www.spectracell.com
(The innovative and unique micronutrient test, or MNT, SpectraCell offers can only be ordered from a provider in SpectraCell's nationwide network of physicians.)

Verisana
www.verisana.com

Other Helpful Websites
The Annie Appleseed Project
www.annieappleseedproject.org
Believe Big
www.believebig.org
The Beljanski Foundation
www.beljanksi.org
Nasha Winter's Metabolic Terrain Institute of Health
www.mtih.org

Other Resources
Autonomic Response Testing (ART)
https://klinghardtinstitute.com
GAPS Diet
www.gapsdiet.com
Kaufmann Diet
www.knowthecause.com
Kelley Diet
https://drkelley.info/dr-kelleys-metabolic-typing.
Exercise Guidelines for Cancer Patients
www.movingthroughcancer.com
Pulsed Electromagnetic Field (PEMF) Therapy
www.DrPawluk.com
Tension and Trauma Releasing Exercises (TRE(R))
www.TraumaPrevention.com
Body Mass Index Calculator
www.calculator.net/bmi-calculator.html

Anticancer Products
Fermented Wheat Germ Extract (FWGE)
www.americanbiosciences.com

fwgeresearch.org

Modified Citrus Pectin (Pecta-Sol^(R))
www.dreliaz.org

Perfect Amino
www.bodyhealth.com

Poly-MVA
PolyMVA.com

www.polymvasurvivors.com/scientific_research.html

Recommended Reading

A More Excellent Way by Dr. Henry W. Wright. Whitaker House, 2009.

Beating Cancer With Nutrition, 5th Edition by Patrick Quillin, PhD. Nutrition Times Press, Inc. 2021.

Cancer as a Metabolic Disease by Thomas Seyfried. Wiley, 2012.

Cancer: The Journey From Diagnosis To Empowerment by Paul Anderson, NMD. Lioncrest Publishing, 2020.

Cracking Cancer Toolkit by Jeffrey Dach, MD. Medical Muse Press, 2020.

Heal Breast Cancer Naturally 2nd ed. by Veronique Desaulniers, DC. Self Published 2019.

Holistic Cancer Medicine by Henning Saupe, MD. Chelsea Green Publishing, 2022.

Hope For Cancer by Antonio Jimenez, MD, ND. Envision Health Press, 2022.

How to Starve Cancer…and Then Kill It With Ferroptosis by Jane McLelland. Agenor Publishing 2021.

I Used to Have Cancer by James Templeton. Square One Publishers, 2019.

Medical Low-Level-Laser Therapy-Foundations and Clinical Applications 2nd ed by Michael Weber, MD, Robert Weber and Martin Junggebauer. Self Published 2015.

Mistletoe and the Emerging Future of Integrative Oncology by Steven Johnson, DO, and Nasha Winters, ND. Portal Books, 2021.

Moving Through Cancer by Kathryn Schmitz, PhD. Chronicle Prism, 2021.

Naturopathic Oncology, 4th Edition by Neil McKinney, ND. Liaison Press, 2020.

Outside The Box Cancer Therapies by Mark Stengler, NMD, and Paul Anderson, NMD. Hay House, Inc, 2020.

Radical Remission by Kelly A. Turner, PhD. HarperOne, 2015.

Stop Fighting Cancer by Kevin Conners, DC. Self Published 2012.

Textbook of Naturopathic Oncology by Gurdev Parmar, ND and Tina Kaczor, DN. Medicatrix Holdings Ltd, 2020.

The Breakthrough Code by Tom McCarthy. Self Published, 2022.

The Cancer Revolution by Leigh Erin Connealy, MD. De Capo, 2016.

The Germ That Causes Cancer by Doug Kaufmann. Media Trition, 2002.

The Metabolic Approach to Cancer by Nasha Winters, ND, and Jess Higgins Kelly. Chelsea Green Publishing, 2017.

The Revolutionary Trauma Release Process by David Bercelli, PhD. Namaste Publishing, 2008.

The Survival Paradox by Isaac Eliaz, MD. Lioncrest Publishing, 2021

The Undying Soul by Stephen Iacoboni. SJI Publishing, 2010

Winning the War on Cancer by Sylvie Beljanski. Morgan James Publishing, 2018

GAPS Introduction Diet Cookbook by Andre Parker. Stretford Publishing, 2017.

Gut and Physiology Syndrome by Natasha Campbell-McBride, MD. Medinform Publishing, 2020.

Supercharge Your Health With PEMF Therapy by William Pawluk, MD. Gatekeeper Press, 2021.

The Acid-Alkaline Food Guide by Susan Brown, PhD and Larry Trivieri Jr. Square One Publishers, 2013.

References

Introduction

Chow, RD. Bradley EH, Gross, CP. Comparison of Cancer-Related Spending and Mortality Rates in the US vs 21 High-Income Countries. JAMA Health Forum. 27 May 2022;3(5):e221229.

Chapter 1

Abboud C. William Stewart Halstead (1852-1922). The Embryo Project Encyclopedia. (2017-07-23) ISSN: 1940-5030. https://hpsrepository.asu.edu/handle/10776/12963

Brand RA. Biographical Sketch: Otto Heinrich Warburg, PhD, MD. *Clin Orthop and Relat Res.* Nov 2010; 48(11): 2831-2832.

Cameron JL. William Stewart Halsted. Our surgical heritage. *Ann Surg.* May 1997;225(5):445-58.

Coller HA. Is cancer a metabolic disease? *Am J Pathol.* Jan 2014;184(1):4-17.

GBD 2019 Cancer Risk Factors Collaborators. The global burden of cancer attributable to risk factors, 2010-19: a systematic analysis for the Global Burden of Disease Study 2019. *The Lancet.* Aug 20, 2022; 400 (10352):563-591.

History Of Cancer. *The Cancer Atlas.* canceratlas.cancer.org/history-cancer

Israel L. Tumour progression: Random mutations or an integrated survival response to cellular stress conserved from unicellular organisms? *J Theor Biol.* 1996;178:375-80.

Ji S. Is Cancer An Ancient Survival Program Unmaked? Feb13, 2012. *GreenMedInfo.* https://greenmedinfo.com/blog/cancer-ancient-survival-program-unmasked2017

Johnson G. Cancer Has Afflicted People Since Prehistoric Times. *Discover.* Jul 20, 2013. www.discovermagazine.com/health-/cancer-has-afflicted-people-since-prehistoric-times

Ledford, H. End of cancer-genome project prompts rethink. *Nature* 517, 128–129 (2015).

Lineweaver C, Davies PCW, Vincent M. Targeting cancer's weaknesses (not its strengths): Therapeutic strategies suggested by the atavistic model. *Bioessays.* Sept 2014; 36(9):827-835.

Majumdar B. An Ancient Approach of Understanding Cancer: Atavism Hypothesis. *Enviro Dental Journal.* Jan 9, *2021*;02(1):01-03.

McKinney, Neil. ND. *Naturopathic Oncology*, 4th ed. Vancouver, Canada: Liason Press, 2020.

Nobel Prize In Physiology or Medicine, 1931. nobelprize.org/prizes/medicine/1931/summary

Otto Warburg Biographical. nobelprize.org/prizes/medicine/1931/warburg/biographical

Report by the Surveillance Branch of the Department of Epidemiology and Surveillance, American Cancer Society, Atlanta, GA. *CA—A Cancer Journal for Clinicians* 45:1 (1995), 8-28.

Sandhir R., Halder A., Sunkaria A. Mitochondria as a centrally positioned hub in the innate immune response. *Biochim. Biophys. Acta Mol. Basis Dis.* 2017;1863:1090–1097.

Seyfried TN. Cancer as a mitochondrial metabolic disease. *Front Cell Dev Biol.* Jul 7 2015;3:43. doi: 10.3389/fcell.2015.00043.

Trigos AS, Pearson RB, Papenfuss AT, Goode DL. How the evolution of multicellularity set the stage for cancer. *Brit J Cancer*. 2018; 118:145-152.

Tumor Markers In Common Use. National Cancer Institute. www.cancer.gov/about-cancer/diagnosis-staging/diagnosis/tumor-markers-list

Tumor Marker Tests. American Society of Clinical Oncology (ASCO). www.cancer.net/navigating-cancer-care/diagnosing-cancer/tests-and-procedures/tumor-marker-tests

Twelve Major Cancers. *Scientific American*. September 1996; 126-132.

Understanding What Cancer Is: Ancient Times To Present. American Cancer Society. www.cancer.org/treatment/understanding-your-diagnosis/history-of-cancer/what-is-cancer.html

Vincent M. Cancer: A de-repression of a default survival program common to all cells?: A life-history perspective on the nature of cancer. *Bioessays*. Jan 2012;34(1):72-82.

What Is Cancer? National Cancer Institute. www.cancer.gov/about-cancer/understanding/what-is-cancer

Weinberg SE, Sena LA, Chandel NS. Mitochondria in the regulation of innate and adaptive immunity. *Immunity*. 2015;42:406–417.

Zajicek, G. A New Cancer Hypothesis. *Medical Hypotheses*. 1996; 47: 111-115.

Chapter 2

Ahmed H, Guha P, Kaptan E, Bandyopadhyaya G. Galectin-3: a potential target for cancer prevention. *Trends Carbohydr Res*. 2011;3(2):13-22.

Aggarwal BB. Nuclear factor-kappaB: the enemy within. *Cancer Cell*. Sep 2004;6(3):203-8.

Arcidiacono B, Iiritano S, Nocera A, et al. Insulin resistance and cancer risk: an overview of the pathogenetic mechanisms. *Exp Diabetes Res*. Jun 4, 2012;2012:789174.

Balkwill F, Mantovani A. Inflammation and cancer: back to Virchow? *Lancet* 2001;357:539-45.

Blanc JF, Bioulac-Sage P, Balabaud C. Surcharge en fer et cancer [Iron overload and cancer]. *Bull Acad Natl Med*. 2000;184(2):355-63. French. PMID: 10989544.

Brieger K, Schiavone S, Miller FJ Jr, Krause KH. Reactive oxygen species: from health to disease. *Swiss Med Wkly*. 2012 Aug 17;142:w13659.

Buonacera A, Stancanelli B, Colaci M, Malatino L. Neutrophil to Lymphocyte Ratio: An Emerging Marker of the Relationships between the Immune System and Diseases. *Int J Mol Sci*. Mar 26, 2022;23(7):3636.

Byun JS, Gardner K. Wounds that will not heal: pervasive cellular reprogramming in cancer. Am J Pathol. 2013 Apr;182(4):1055-64.

Chan JC, Chan DL, Diakos CI, Engel A, Pavlakis N, Gill A, Clarke SJ. The Lymphocyte-to-Monocyte Ratio is a Superior Predictor of Overall Survival in Comparison to Established Biomarkers of Resectable Colorectal Cancer. *Ann Surg*. Mar 2017;265(3):539-546.

Chandel NS, Maltepe E, Goldwasser E, Mathieu CE, Simon MC, Schumacker PT. Mitochondrial reactive oxygen species trigger hypoxia-induced transcription. *Proc Natl Acad Sci USA*. Sep 29, 1998;95(20):11715-20.

Chang HY, Sneddon JB, Alizadeh AA, et al. Gene expression signature of fibroblast serum response predicts human cancer progression: similarities between tumors and wounds. *PLoS Biol*. 2004 Feb;2(2):E7.

Chiefari E, Mirabelli M, La Vignera S, et al. Insulin Resistance and Cancer: In Search for a Causal Link. *Int J Mol Sci*. Oct 15, 2021;22(20):11137.

Cupp MA, Cariolou M, Tzoulaki I, et al. Neutrophil to lymphocyte ratio and cancer prognosis: an umbrella review of systematic reviews and meta-analyses of observational studies. *BMC Med.* Nov 20, 2020;18(1):360.

Dubeau MF, Iacucci M, Beck PL, Moran GW, Kaplan GG, Ghosh S, Panaccione R. Drug-induced inflammatory bowel disease and IBD-like conditions. *Inflamm Bowel Dis.* 2013 Feb;19(2):445-56.

Dvorak HF (1986) Tumors: Wounds that do not heal: Similarities between tumor stroma generation and wound healing. *N Engl J Med* 1986;315:1650–59.

Guo YH, Sun HF, Zhang YB, Liao ZJ, Zhao L, Cui J, Wu T, Lu JR, Nan KJ, Wang SH. The clinical use of the platelet/lymphocyte ratio and lymphocyte/monocyte ratio as prognostic predictors in colorectal cancer: a meta-analysis. *Oncotarget.* Mar 21, 2017;8(12):20011-20024.

Helicobactor pylori and Cancer. National Cancer Institute. www.cancer.gov/about-cancer/causes-prevention/risk/infectious-agents/h-pylori-fact-sheet

Huang X. Iron overload and its association with cancer risk in humans: evidence for iron as a carcinogenic metal. *Mutat Res.* Dec 10,2003;533(1-2):153-71.

Kamp DW, Shacter E, Weitzman SA. Chronic Inflammation and Cancer: The Role of Mitochondria. *Oncology* (Williston Park) Apr 30, 2011;25(5):400-10,413.

Karin M. Nuclear factor-kappaB in cancer development and progression. *Nature.* May 25 2006;441(7092):431.

Kumar A, Takada Y, Boriek AM, et al. Nuclear factor-κB: its role in health and disease. *J Mol Med* 82, 434–448 (2004).

Kunnumakkara AB, Shabnam B, Girisa S, et al. Inflammation, NF-κB, and Chronic Diseases: How are They Linked? *Crit Rev Immunol.* 2020;40(1):1-39.

Li M, Deng Q, Zhang L, He S, Rong J, Zheng F. The pretreatment lymphocyte to monocyte ratio predicts clinical outcome for patients with urological cancers: A meta-analysis. *Pathol Res Pract.* Jan 2019;215(1):5-11.

Lu H, Ouyang W, Huang C. Inflammation, a key event in cancer development. *Mol Cancer Res.* 2006 Apr;4(4):221-33.

Malhab LJB, Saber-Ayad MM, Al-Hakm R, Nair VA, Paliogiannis P, Pintus G, Abdel-Rahman WM. Chronic Inflammation and Cancer: The Role of Endothelial Dysfunction and Vascular Inflammation. *Curr Pharm Des.* 2021;27(18):2156-2169.

Missiroli S, Genovese I, Perrone M, Vezzani B, Vitto VAM, Giorgi C. The Role of Mitochondria in Inflammation: From Cancer to Neurodegenerative Disorders. *J Clin Med.* 2020 Mar 9;9(3):740.

Modica-Napolitano JS, Singh KK. Mitochondrial dysfunction in cancer. *Mitochondrion.* Sep 2004;4:755-762.

Prescott SM, Fitzpatrick FA. Cyclooxygenase-2 and carcinogenesis. *Biochim Biophys Acta.* Mar 27, 2000;1470(2):M69-78.

Radić M, Martinović Kaliterna D, Radić J. Drug-induced vasculitis: a clinical and pathological review. *Neth J Med.* 2012 Jan;70(1):12-7.

Ren H, Liu X, Wang L, Gao Y. Lymphocyte-to-Monocyte Ratio: A Novel Predictor of the Prognosis of Acute Ischemic Stroke. *J Stroke Cerebrovasc Dis.* Nov 2017;26(11):2595-2602.

Sandhir R, Halder A, Sunkaria A. Mitochondria as a centrally positioned hub in the innate immune response. *Biochim Biophys Acta Mol Basis Dis.* 2017 May;1863(5):1090-1097.

Shacter E, Weitzman SA. Chronic inflammation and cancer. *Oncology* (Williston Park). 2002 Feb;16(2):217-26.

Steele VE, Hawk ET, Viner JL, Lubet RA. Mechanisms and applications of non-steroidal anti-inflammatory drugs in the chemoprevention of cancer. *Mutat Res.* Feb-Mar 2003;523-524:137-44.

Stevens RG, Graubard BI, Micozzi MS, Neriishi K, Blumberg BS. Moderate elevation of body iron level and increased risk of cancer occurrence and death. *Int J Cancer.* Feb 1, 1994;56(3):364-9.

The Mount Sinai Hospital/Mount Sinai School of Medicine. "Reducing Consumption of Glycotoxins From Heat-processing Of Foods Reduces Risk Of Chronic Disease." *ScienceDaily.* 4 November 2009. www.sciencedaily.com/releases/2009/11/091104000929.htm

Torti SV, Manz DH, Paul BT, Blanchette-Farra N, Torti FM. Iron and Cancer. *Annu Rev Nutr.* 2018;38:97-125.

Tsujii, M., Kawano, S., & Dubois, R. N. (1997). Cyclooxygenase-2 expression in human colon cancer cells increases metastatic potential. *Proceedings of the National Academy of Sciences of the United States of America, 94*(7), 3336-3340.

Vlassara H, Cai W, Goodman S, et al. Protection against loss of innate defenses in adulthood by low advanced glycation end products (AGE) intake: role of the antiinflammatory AGE receptor-1. *J Clin Endocrinol Metab.* Nov 2009;94(11):4483-91.

Wang D, DuBois RN. Immunosuppression associated with chronic inflammation in the tumor microenvironment. *Carcinogenesis.* 2015 Oct;36(10):1085-93.

Wang L, Li YS, Yu LG, et al. Galectin-3 expression and secretion by tumor-associated macrophages in hypoxia promotes breast cancer progression. *Biochem Pharmacol.* Aug 2020;178:114113.

Weinberg SE, Sena LA, Chandel NS. Mitochondria in the regulation of innate and adaptive immunity. *Immunity.* 2015;42:406–417.

Williams CS, Mann M, DuBois RN. The role of cyclooxygenases in inflammation, cancer, and development. *Oncogene.* Dec 20,1999;18(55): 7908-16.

Wound-healing genes influence cancer progression, researchers say. https://med.stanford.edu/content/sm/news/all-news/2004/01/wound-healing-genes-influence-cancer-progression-researchers-say.html

Wu T, Sempos CT, Freudenheim JL, Muti P, Smit E. Serum iron, copper and zinc concentrations and risk of cancer mortality in US adults. *Ann Epidemiol.* Mar 2004;14(3):195-201.

Chapter 3

232 Toxic Chemicals in 10 Minority Babies(full report available at: www.scribd.com/document/23503846/EWG-2009-Minority-Cord-Blood-Report) and *Toxic Chemicals Found in Minority Cord Blood.* Environmental Working Group. Dec 2, 2009.

2008-2009 Annual Report. President's Cancer Panel. *Reducing Environmental Cancer Risk.* Available at www.cleanwater.org/files/publications/mn/president_cancer_panel_report_08-09_508.pdf

American Cancer Society. *Cancer Prevention & Early Detection Facts & Figures 2019-2020.* Atlanta: American Cancer Society.

American Cancer Society. *Does Body Weight Affect Cancer Risk?* www.cancer.org/healthy/cancer-causes/diet-physical-activity/body-weight-and-cancer-risk/effects.html

American Cancer Society: The Cancer Atlas. Environmental & Occupational Exposures. https://canceratlas.cancer.org/risk-factors/environment

American Cancer Society: The Cancer Atlas. Globally, one half of cancer deaths are caused by potentially modifiable risk factors. https://canceratlas.cancer.org/risk-factors

Anttila T, Saikku P, Koskela P, et al. Serotypes of Chlamydia trachomatis and risk for development of cervical squamous cell carcinoma. *JAMA*. 2001;285:47–51.

Bloom J. *Tumors Have A "Fungal Biome" - Implications For Powerful New Cancer Screens*. American Council On Science and Health. Oct 3, 2022. www.acsh.org/news/2022/10/03/tumors-have-fungal-biome-implications-powerful-new-cancer-screens-16588

Centers for Disease Control and Prevention (CDC). *Overweight and Obesity.* www.cdc.gov/obesity/index.html and www.cdc.gov/nchs/fastats/obesity-overweight.htm

DiNicolantonio JJ, O'Keefe JH. Importance of maintaining a low omega–6/omega–3 ratio for reducing inflammation. *Open Heart* 2018;5:e000946.

García-Bustos V, Salavert M, Blanes R, Cabañero D, Blanes M. Current management of CMV infection in cancer patients (solid tumors). Epidemiology and therapeutic strategies. *Rev Esp Quimioter.* Oct 2022;35 Suppl 3:74-79.

GBD 2019 Cancer Risk Factors Collaborators. The global burden of cancer attributable to risk factors, 2010-19: a systematic analysis for the Global Burden of Disease Study 2019. *The Lancet*. Aug 20,2022;400(10352):563-591.

Grabovac I, Smith L, Yang L, et al. The relationship between chronic diseases and number of sexual partners: an exploratory analysis. *BMJ Sexual & Reproductive Health* 2020;46:100-107.

Holzinger F, Z'graggen K, Büchler MW. Mechanisms of biliary carcinogenesis: a pathogenetic multi-stage cascade towards cholangiocarcinoma. *Ann Oncol.* 1999;10 Suppl 4:122-6.

Islami F, Goding Sauer A, Miller KD, et al. Proportion and number of cancer cases and deaths attributable to potentially modifiable risk factors in the United States. *CA Cancer J Clin.* 2018;68:31-54.

International Agency for Research on Cancer and World Health Organization. *IARC classifies radiofrequency electromagnetic fields as possibly carcinogenic to humans.* Press Release. May 31, 2011. www.iarc.who.int/wp-content/uploads/2018/07/pr208_E.pdf

Jeffay N. Fungus is a telltale cancer sign, possibly screenable by blood test: Israel-US study. *Times Of Israel.* Oct 2, 2022. www.timesofisrael.com/fungus-is-telltale-cancer-sign-possibly-screenable-by-blood-test-israel-us-study/

Joshi SM. The sick building syndrome. *Indian J Occup Environ Med.* 2008 Aug;12(2):61-64.

Lawler SE. Cytomegalovirus and glioblastoma; controversies and opportunities. *J Neurooncol.* Jul 2015;123(3):465-71.

Michaelis M, Doerr HW, Cinatl J. The story of human cytomegalovirus and cancer: increasing evidence and open questions. *Neoplasia.* Jan 2009;11(1):1-9.

National Cancer Institute. Helicobacter pylori and Cancer. www.cancer.gov/cancertopics/factsheet/risk/h-pylori-cancer.

National Cancer Institute. Hormones. www.cancer.gov/about-cancer/causes-prevention/risk/hormones

National Cancer Institute. Infectious Agents. https://www.cancer.gov/about-cancer/causes-prevention/risk/infectious-agents

National Cancer Institute. Obesity and Cancer. www.cancer.gov/about-cancer/causes-prevention/risk/obesity/obesity-fact-sheet

Narunsky-Haziza L, Sepich-Poore G, Livyatan L, et al. Pan-cancer analyses reveal cancer-type-specific fungal ecologies and bacteriome interactions. *Cell.* Sept 29, 2022;185:3789–3806.

Okedele OO, Nelson HH, Oyenuga ML, Thyagarajan B, Prizment A. Cytomegalovirus and cancer-related mortality in the national health and nutritional examination survey. *Cancer Causes Control.* Jun 2020;31(6):541-547.

Palamaner Subash Shantha G, Kumar AA, Cheskin LJ, Pancholy SB. Association between sleep-disordered breathing, obstructive sleep apnea, and cancer incidence: a systematic review and meta-analysis. *Sleep Med.* 2015 Oct;16(10):1289-94.

Pall ML. Microwave frequency electromagnetic fields (EMFs) produce widespread neuropsychiatric effects including depression. *J Chem Neuroanat.* 2016 Sep;75(Pt B):43-51.

Renehan AG, Tyson M, Egger M, Heller RF, Zwahlen M. Body-mass index and incidence of cancer: A systemic review and meta-analysis of prospective observational studies. *Lancet.* 2008;371:569-578.

Rock CL, Thomson C, Gansler T, et al. American Cancer Society guideline for diet and physical activity for cancer prevention. *CA Cancer J Clin.* 2020;70(4):245-271.

Silins I, Ryd W, Strand A, et al. Chlamydia trachomatis infection and persistence of human papillomavirus. *Int J Cancer.* 2005;116:110–115.

US Department of Health and Human Services. 2018 Physical Activity Guidelines Advisory Committee Scientific Report. health.gov/paguidelines/second-edition/report

Weinstein AL, et al. Breast Cancer Risk and Oral Contraceptive Use: Results from a Large Control Study. *Epidemiology.* Sept 1991;2(5):353-58.

Wilson LF, Antonsson A, et al. How many cancer cases and deaths are potentially preventable? Estimates for Australia in 2013. *Int J Cancer.* Feb 15, 2018;142(4):691-701.

World Cancer Research Fund/American Institute for Cancer Research. *Diet, Nutrition, Physical Activity, and Cancer: A Global Perspective.* Continuous Update Project Expert Report 2018. www.wcrf.org/dietandcancer

World Cancer Research Fund International. *Obesity, weight gain and cancer risk.* www.wcrf.org/diet-activity-and-cancer/risk-factors/obesity-weight-gain-and-cancer

Chapter 4

Ajani JA, Song S, Hochster HS, Steinberg IB. Cancer stem cells: the promise and the potential. *Semin Oncol.* Apr 2015;42 Suppl 1:S3-17.

Azvolinsky A. Cancer Stem Cells: Cancer's Roots. *J Natl Cancer Inst.* Oct 1, 2012;104(12):893-95.

Batlle E, Clevers H. Cancer stem cells revisited. *Nat Med.* Oct 2017:6;23(10):1124-1134.

Bork U, Rahbari NN, Schölch S, et al. Circulating tumour cells and outcome in non-metastatic colorectal cancer: a prospective study. *Br J Cancer.* Mar 31,2015;112:1306-1313.

Chang AI, Schwertschkow AH, Nolta JA, Wu J. Involvement of mesenchymal stem cells in cancer progression and metastases. *Curr Cancer Drug Targets.* 2015;15(2):88-98.

Cohen SJ, Punt CJ, Iannotti N, et al. Relationship of circulating tumor cells to tumor response, progression-free survival, and overall survival in patients with metastatic colorectal cancer. *J Clin Oncol.* Jul 1, 2008;26(19):3213-21.

Danila DC, Heller G, Gignac GA, et al. Circulating tumor cell number and prognosis in progressive castration-resistant prostate cancer. *Clin Cancer Res.* Dec 1, 2007;13(23):7053-8.

Diehn M, Cho RW, Lobo NA, et al. Association of reactive oxygen species levels and radioresistance in cancer stem cells. *Nature.* Apr 9, 2009;458(7239):780-3.

Fillmore CM, Kuperwasser C. Human breast cancer cell lines contain stem-like cells that self-renew, give rise to phenotypically diverse progeny and survive chemotherapy. *Breast Cancer Res.* 2008;10(2):R25.

Furth J, Kahn MC, Breedis C. 1937. The transmission of leukemia of mice with a single cell. *The Amer J Cancer.* 1937;31(2):276-282.

Grillet F, Bayet E, Villeronce O, Zappia L, et al. Circulating tumour cells from patients with colorectal cancer have cancer stem cell hallmarks in *ex vivo* culture. *Gut.* Oct 2017;66(10):1802-1810.

Halabi S, Small EJ, Hayes DF, Vogelzang NJ, Kantoff PW. Prognostic significance of reverse transcriptase polymerase chain reaction for prostate-specific antigen in metastatic prostate cancer: a nested study within CALGB 9583. *J Clin Oncol.* Feb1, 2003;21(3):490-95.

Hayes DF, Cristofanilli M, Budd GT, et al. Circulating tumor cells at each follow-up time point during therapy of metastatic breast cancer patients predict progression-free and overall survival. *Clin Cancer Res.* Jul 15, 2006;12(14 Pt 1):4218-24.

Houghton J. Bone-marrow-derived cells and cancer--an opportunity for improved therapy. *Nat Clin Pract Oncol.* Jan 2007;4(1):2-3.

Krishnamurthy S. Circulating tumour cells in non-metastatic breast cancer: a prospective study. *Lancet Oncol.* Jul 2012;13(7):688-95.

Kuukasjärvi T, Karhu R, Tanner M, et al. Genetic heterogeneity and clonal evolution underlying development of asynchronous metastasis in human breast cancer. *Cancer Res.* Apr 15,1997;57(8):1597-604.

Lagadec C, Vlashi E, Della Donna L, Dekmezian C, Pajonk F. Radiation-induced reprogramming of breast cancer cells. *Stem Cells.* May 2012;30(5):833-44.

Lagadec C, Vlashi E, et al. Survival and self-renewing capacity of breast cancer initiating cells during fractionated radiation treatment. *Breast Cancer Res.* 2010;12(1):R13.

Lagerqvist EL, Lunke S, Charafe-Jauffret E, et al. Circulating tumour cells from patients with colorectal cancer have cancer stem cell hallmarks in *ex vivo* culture. *Gut.* Oct 2017;66(10):1802-1810.

Liu T, Xu H, Huang M, et al. Circulating Glioma Cells Exhibit Stem Cell-like Properties. *Cancer Res.* Dec 12018;78(23):6632-6642.

Lobo NA, Shimono Y, Qian D, Clarke MF. The biology of cancer stem cells. *Annu Rev Cell Dev Biol.* 2007;23:675-99.

Lucci A, Hall CS, Lodhi AK, Bhattacharyya A, et al. Circulating tumor cells predict survival in patients with metastatic prostate cancer. *Urology.* Apr 2005;65(4):713-8.

Massagué J, Obenauf AC. Metastatic colonization by circulating tumour cells. *Nature.* Jan 21, 2016;529(7586):298-306.

Mukherjee, Siddhartha. *The Cancer Sleeper Cell.* Oct 29, 2010. Adapted from his book *Emperor of All Maladies: A Biography of Cancer.* New York: Scribner. 2010.

Nagrath S, Sequist LV, Maheswaran S, et al. Isolation of rare circulating tumour cells in cancer patients by microchip technology. *Nature.* Dec 2007;20;450(7173):1235-39.

Nassar D, Blanpain C. Cancer Stem Cells: Basic Concepts and Therapeutic Implications. *Annu Rev Pathol.* May 23, 2016;11:47-76.

Pachmann K, Dengler R, Lobodasch K, Fröhlich F, et al. An increase in cell number at completion of therapy may develop as an indicator of early relapse: Quantification of circulating epithelial tumor cells (CETC) for monitoring of adjuvant therapy in breast cancer. *J Cancer Res Clin Oncol.* Jan 2008;134(1):59-65.

Phillips TM, McBride WH, Pajonk F. The response of CD24(-/low)/CD44+ breast cancer-initiating cells to radiation. *J Natl Cancer Inst.* Dec 20, 2006;98(24):1777-85.

Pound CR, Partin AW, Eisenberger MA, Chan DW, Pearson JD, Walsh PC. Natural history of progression after PSA elevation following radical prostatectomy. *JAMA.* 1999;281:1591-97.

Quintela-Fandino M, López JM, Hitt R, et al. Breast cancer-specific mRNA transcripts presence in peripheral blood after adjuvant chemotherapy predicts poor survival among high-risk breast cancer patients treated with high-dose chemotherapy with peripheral blood stem cell support. *J Clin Oncol.* Aug 1, 2006;24(22):3611-18.

Skoda J, Neradil J, Veselská R. Funkční testy pro detekci nádorových kmenových buněk [Functional assays for detection of cancer stem cells]. *Klin Onkol.* 2014;27 Suppl 1:S42-7. Czech.

Tombal B, Van Cangh PJ, Loric S, Gala JL. Prognostic value of circulating prostate cells in patients with a rising PSA after radical prostatectomy. *Prostate.* Aug 1, 2003;56(3):163-70.

University of Massachusetts Amherst. Several FDA-approved anti-cancer drugs induce stem cell tumors, perhaps thwarting therapy. *Medical Express*. Mar 10, 2014. https://medicalxpress.com/news/2014-03-fda-approved-anti-cancer-drugs-stem-cell.html

Vlashi E, Pajonk F. Cancer stem cells, cancer cell plasticity and radiation therapy. *Semin Cancer Biol*. Apr 2015;31:28-35.

Xiao Y, Ye Y, Yearsley K, Jones S, Barsky SH. The lymphovascular embolus of inflammatory breast cancer expresses a stem cell-like phenotype. *Am J Pathol*. Aug 2008;173(2):561-74.

Yin W, Wang J, Jiang L, James Kang Y. Cancer and stem cells. *Exp Biol Med (Maywood)*. Aug 2021;246(16):1791-1801.

Yu Z, Pestell TG, Lisanti MP, Pestell RG. Cancer stem cells. *Int J Biochem Cell Biol*. Dec 2012;44(12):2144-51.

Chapter 5

Albin, Richard with Ronald Piana. *The Great Prostate Hoax: How Big Medicine Hijacked the PSA Test and Caused A Public Health Disaster.* New York: St. Martin's Press. 2014.

Bielawska B, Hookey LC, et al. Anesthesia assistance in outpatient colonoscopy and risk of aspiration pneumonia, bowel perforation, and splenic injury. *Gastroenterology*. 2018;154:77-85.e3.

Bretthauer M, Loberg M, et al. Effect of Colonoscopy Screening on Risks of Colorectal Cancer and Related Death. *N Engl J Med* Oct 27, 2022;387:1547-1556.

Clebak K, Nickolich S, Mendez-Miller M. Multitarget Stool DNA Testing (Cologuard) for Colorectal Cancer Screening. *Am Fam Physician*. 2022;105(2):198-200.

Dobielewski M, Hauser J, Beck O, Stemme G, Roxhed N. Blood cell quantification on dry blood samples: toward patient-centric complete blood counts. *Bioanalysis.* 2022 May;14(10):693-701.

Ekici S, Jawzal H. Breast cancer diagnosis using thermography and convolutional neural networks. *Med Hypotheses.* 2020 Apr;137:109542.

Fraiman, J., Brownlee, S., Stoto, M.A. et al. An Estimate of the US Rate of Overuse of Screening Colonoscopy: a Systematic Review. *J Gen Intern Med. 2022;* 37, 1754–1762.

Garber, Judith. As many as 25% of screening colonoscopies are unnecessary, study finds. Lown Institute. Feb 28, 2002. https://lowninstitute.org/as-many-as-25-of-screening-colonoscopies-are-unnecessary-study-finds

Imperiale TF, et al. Multitarget stool DNA testing for colorectal-cancer screening. N Eng J Med. 2014;370:1287.

Kalager M, et al. Effect of Screening Mammography on Breast-Cancer Mortality in Norway. *New Eng J Med* Sept 23, 2010; 363:1203-1210.

Klein EA, Richards D, Cohn A, et al. Clinical validation of a targeted methylation-based multi-cancer early detection test using an independent validation set. *Ann Oncol.* 2021 Sep;32(9):1167-1177.

Ko CW. Colonoscopy Risks: What Is Known and What Are the Next Steps. *Gastroenterology.* Feb 1, 2018;154(3):473-75.

Kulis M, Esteller M. DNA methylation and cancer. Adv Genet. 2010; 70:27–56.

Levin TR, Zhao W, Conell C, et al.Complications of colonoscopy in an integrated health care delivery system. *Ann Intern Med.* 2006;145: 880-886.

Liu MC, Oxnard GR, Klein EA, et al. CCGA Consortium. Sensitive and specific multi-cancer detection and localization using methylation signatures in cell-free DNA. *Ann Oncol.* 2020;31(6):745–59.

Miglioretti DL, Lange J, van den Broek JJ, et al. Radiation-Induced Breast Cancer Incidence and Mortality From Digital Mammography Screening: A Modeling Study. *Ann Intern Med.* 2016 Feb 16;164(4):205-14.

Miller AB, Wall C, et al. Twenty-five tear follow-up for breast cancer incidence and mortality of the Canadian National Breast Screening Study: randomised screening trial. *BMJ.* 2014;348:g366.

Robertson DJ, Selby K. Fecal Immunochemical Test: The World's Colorectal Cancer Screening Test. *Gastrointest Endosc Clin N Am.* Jul 2020;30(3):511-526.

Royce TJ, Hendrix LH, Stokes WA, Allen IM, Chen RC. Cancer Screening Rates in Individuals With Different Life Expectancies. *JAMA Intern Med.* 2014;174(10):1558–1565.

Singh D, Singh AK. Role of image thermography in early breast cancer detection- Past, present and future. *Comput Methods Programs Biomed.* 2020 Jan;183:105074.

Chapter 6

Akbari M, Hossaini SM. The Relationship of Spiritual Health with Quality of Life, Mental Health, and Burnout: The Mediating Role of Emotional Regulation. *Iran J Psychiatry.* 2018 Jan;13(1):22-31.

Alimujiang A, Wiensch A, Boss J, et al. Association Between Life Purpose and Mortality Among US Adults Older Than 50 Years. *JAMA Netw Open.* 2019;2(5):e194270.

Balboni TA, VanderWeele TJ, Doan-Soares SD, et al. Spirituality in Serious Illness and Health. *JAMA.* 2022;328(2):184–197.

Basso JC, McHale A, Ende V, Oberlin DJ, Suzuki WA. Brief, daily meditation enhances attention, memory, mood, and emotional regulation in non-experienced meditators. *Behav Brain Res*. 2019 Jan 1;356:208-220.

Bengtson VL, Whittington FL. From Ageism to the Longevity Revolution: Robert Butler, Pioneer, *The Gerontologist*, 2014 Dec;54(6):1064–1069.

Biegler KA, Chaoul MA, Cohen L. Cancer, cognitive impairment, and meditation. *Acta Oncol*. 2009;48(1):18-26.

Bredle JM, Salsman JM, Debb SM, Arnold BJ, Cella D. Spiritual well-being as a component of health-related quality of life: the functional assessment of chronic illness therapy-spiritual well-being scale (FACIT-Sp). *Religions* 2011;2:77–94.

Bruce M et al. Church attendance, allostatic load and mortality in middle aged adults. *PLOS One,* 2017 May 16;12(5):e0177618.

Dahl CJ, Lutz A, Davidson RJ. Reconstructing and deconstructing the self: cognitive mechanisms in meditation practice. *Trends Cogn Sci*. 2015 Sep;19(9):515-23.

Fehring RJ, Miller JF, Shaw C. Spiritual well-being, religiosity, hope, depression, and other mood states in elderly people coping with cancer. *Oncol Nurs Forum* 1997;24:663–71.

Galante J, Galante I, Bekkers MJ, Gallacher J. Effect of kindness-based meditation on health and well-being: a systematic review and meta-analysis. *J Consult Clin Psychol*. 2014 Dec;82(6):1101-14.

Gard T, Hölzel BK, Lazar SW. The potential effects of meditation on age-related cognitive decline: a systematic review. *Ann N Y Acad Sci*. 2014 Jan;1307:89-103.

Goncalbes J, Lucchetti G, et al. Religious and spiritual interventions in mental health care: A systematic review and meta-analysis of randomized controlled clinical trials. *Psych Med.* 2015 Jul 3;45(14):2937-49.

Goyal M, Singh S, Sibinga EM, Gould NF, et al. Meditation programs for psychological stress and well-being: a systematic review and meta-analysis. *JAMA Intern Med.* 2014 Mar;174(3):357-68.

He X, Shi W, Han X, Wang N, Zhang N, Wang X. The interventional effects of loving-kindness meditation on positive emotions and interpersonal interactions. *Neuropsychiatr Dis Treat.* 2015 May 25;11:1273-7.

Hekmati Pour N, Hojjati H. The relationship between praying and life expectancy in cancerous patients. *J Med Life.* 2015;8(Spec Iss 4):60-64.

Holland JC, Passik S, Kash KM, et al. The role of religious and spiritual beliefs in coping with malignant melanoma. *Psychooncology* 1999; 8:14–26.

Hurley RV, Patterson TG, Cooley SJ. Meditation-based interventions for family caregivers of people with dementia: a review of the empirical literature. *Aging Ment Health.* 2014;18(3):281-8.

Jantos M, Kiat H. Prayer as medicine: how much have we learned? *Med J Aust.* 2007 May 21;186(S10):S51-3.

Johnson, K.A. Prayer: A Helpful Aid in Recovery from Depression. *J Relig Health* 2008 Jan 30;57:2290–2300.

Khalsa DS. Stress, Meditation, and Alzheimer's Disease Prevention: Where The Evidence Stands. *J Alzheimers Dis.* 2015;48(1):1-12.

Koenig HG. An 83-year-old woman with chronic illness and strong religious beliefs. *JAMA.* 2002 Jul 24-31;288(4):487-93.

Lindsay EK, Young S, Brown KW, Smyth JM, Creswell JD. Mindfulness training reduces loneliness and increases social contact in a randomized controlled trial. Proc Natl Acad Sci U S A. 2019 Feb 26;116(9):3488-3493.

Manning LK. Spirituality as a Lived Experience: Exploring the Essence of Spirituality for Women in Late Life. *The International Journal of Aging and Human Development*. 2012;75(2):95-113.

Mehta R, Sharma K, Potters L, Wernicke AG, Parashar B. Evidence for the Role of Mindfulness in Cancer: Benefits and Techniques. *Cureus*. 2019 May 9;11(5):e4629.

Meraviglia MG. Prayer in people with cancer. *Cancer Nurs*. 2002 Aug;25(4): 326-31.

Meisenhelder JB, Schaeffer NJ, Younger J, Lauria M. Faith and mental health in an oncology population. *J Relig Health*. 2013 Jun;52(2):505-13.

Mickley JR, Soeken K, Belcher A. Spiritual well-being, religiousness and hope among women with breast cancer. *Image J Nurs Sch* 1992;24: 267–72.

Meditation and Mindfulness: What You Need To Know. National Center for Complementary and Integrative Health. https://www.nccih.nih.gov/health/meditation-and-mindfulness-what-you-need-to-know

Movafagh A, Heidari MH, Abdoljabbari M, et al. Spiritual Therapy in Coping with Cancer as a Complementary Medical Preventive Practice. *J Cancer Prev*. 2017 Jun;22(2):82-88.

Norris CJ, Creem D, Hendler R, Kober H. Brief Mindfulness Meditation Improves Attention in Novices: Evidence From ERPs and Moderation by Neuroticism. *Front Hum Neurosci*. 2018 Aug 6;12:315.

Ong JC, PhD, Manber R, et al. A Randomized Controlled Trial of Mindfulness Meditation for Chronic Insomnia, *Sleep*, 2014 Sept 1;37(9): 1553–1563.

Paul Victor CG, Treschuk JV. Critical Literature Review on the Definition Clarity of the Concept of Faith, Religion, and Spirituality. *Jf Holistic Nursing*. 2020 Dec 20;38(1):107-113.

Rura N. Spirituality linked with better health outcomes, patient care. *The Harvard Gazette*. Jul 12, 2022. news.harvard.edu/gazette/story/2022/07/spirituality-linked-with-better-health-outcomes-patient-care

Shanshan Li, Meir J. Stampfer, David R. Williams, Tyler J. VanderWeele. Association of Religious Service Attendance With Mortality Among Women. *JAMA Internal Medicine*, 2016 June; 176(6):777-785.

Singh Y, Goel A, Kathrotia R, Patil PM. Role of yoga and meditation in the context of dysfunctional self: a hypothetico-integrative approach. *Adv Mind Body Med*. 2014 Summer;28(3):22-5.

Sood A, Jones DT. On mind wandering, attention, brain networks, and meditation. *Explore (NY)*. 2013 May-Jun;9(3):136-41.

Spirituality in Cancer Care (PDQ®)–Patient Version. National Cancer Institute. cancer.gov/about-cancer/coping/day-to-day/faith-and-spirituality/spirituality-pdq

Tsai SY, Jaiswal S, Chang CF, Liang WK, Muggleton NG, Juan CH. Meditation Effects on the Control of Involuntary Contingent Reorienting Revealed With Electroencephalographic and Behavioral Evidence. *Front Integr Neurosci*. 2018 May 15;12:17.

Wachholtz AB, Sambamthoori U. National Trends in Prayer Use as a Coping Mechanism for Depression: Changes from 2002 to 2007. *J Relig Health* 2012 O0ct 6;52:1356–1368.

Whitehead BR, Bergeman CS, Coping with Daily Stress: Differential Role of Spiritual Experience on Daily Positive and Negative Affect, *The Journals of Gerontology: Series B*. 2012 Jul;67(4):456–9.

Weil A. *Health and Healing*. Boston: Houghton Mifflin, 1998.

Zimmer J. Another possible benefit of going to church: A 33 percent chance of living longer. *Washington Post*. May 16, 2016.

Chapter 7

Avvenuti G, Baiardini I, Giardini A. Optimism's Explicative Role for Chronic Diseases. *Front Psychol*. 2016 Mar 2;7:295.

Berceli, David. *The Revolutionary Trauma Release Process*. Vancouver, CA: Namaste Publishing. 2008.

Bonaz B, Sinniger V, Hoffmann D, Clarençon D et al. Chronic vagus nerve stimulation in Crohn's disease: a 6-month follow-up pilot study. *Neurogastroenterol Motil*. 2016 Jun;28(6):948-53.

Bremner JD, Gurel NZ, Wittbrodt MT et al. Application of Noninvasive Vagal Nerve Stimulation to Stress-Related Psychiatric Disorders. *J Pers Med*. 2020 Sep 9;10(3):119.

Dixit UB, Jasani RR. Comparison of the effectiveness of Bach flower therapy and music therapy on dental anxiety in pediatric patients: A randomized controlled study. *J Indian Soc Pedod Prev Dent*. 2020 Jan-Mar;38(1):71-78.

George MS, Ward HE Jr, Ninan PT et al. A pilot study of vagus nerve stimulation (VNS) for treatment-resistant anxiety disorders. *Brain Stimul*. 2008 Apr;1(2):112-21.

Gerritsen RJS, Band GPH. Breath of Life: The Respiratory Vagal Stimulation Model of Contemplative Activity. *Front Hum Neurosci*. 2018 Oct 9;12:397

Giltay EJ, Zitman FG, Kromhout D. Dispositional optimism and the risk of depressive symptoms during 15 years of follow-up: the Zutphen Elderly Study. *J Affect Disord*. 2006 Mar;91(1):45-52.

Guo YP, McLeod JG, Baverstock J. Pathological changes in the vagus nerve in diabetes and chronic alcoholism. *J Neurol Neurosurg Psychiatry*. 1987 Nov;50(11):1449-53.

Hill PL, Turiano NA. Purpose in life as a predictor of mortality across adulthood. *Psychol Sci*. 2014 Jul;25(7):1482-6.

Howard J. Do Bach flower remedies have a role to play in pain control? A critical analysis investigating therapeutic value beyond the placebo effect, and the potential of Bach flower remedies as a psychological method of pain relief. *Complement Ther Clin Pract*. 2007 Aug;13(3):174-83.

Huikuri HV, Mäkikallio TH, Airaksinen KE et al. Power-law relationship of heart rate variability as a predictor of mortality in the elderly. *Circulation*. 1998 May 26;97(20):2031-36.

Johnson RL, Wilson CG. A review of vagus nerve stimulation as a therapeutic intervention. *J Inflamm Res*. 2018 May 16;11:203-213.

Jungmann M, Vencatachellum S, Van Ryckeghem D, Vögele C. Effects of Cold Stimulation on Cardiac-Vagal Activation in Healthy Participants: Randomized Controlled Trial. *JMIR Form Res*. 2018 Oct 9;2(2):e10257.

Kim ES, Park N, Peterson C. Dispositional optimism protects older adults from stroke: the Health and Retirement Study. *Stroke*. 2011 Oct;42(10):2855-9.

Kim ES, Smith J, Kubzansky LD. Prospective study of the association between dispositional optimism and incident heart failure. *Circ Heart Fail.* 2014 May;7(3):394-400.

Kok BE, Fredrickson BL. Upward spirals of the heart: autonomic flexibility, as indexed by vagal tone, reciprocally and prospectively predicts positive emotions and social connectedness. *Biol Psychol.* 2010 Dec;85(3):432-6.

Krpan KM, Kross E, Berman MG, Deldin PJ, Askren MK, Jonides J. An everyday activity as a treatment for depression: the benefits of expressive writing for people diagnosed with major depressive disorder. *J Affect Disord.* 2013 Sep 25;150(3):1148-51.

Kwon D. Your brain could be controlling how sick you get — and how you recover *Nature.* 2023 Feb 13;614:613-615. nature.com/articles/d41586-023-00509-z

Lange G, Janal MN, Maniker A, Fitzgibbons J, Fobler M, Cook D, Natelson BH. Safety and efficacy of vagus nerve stimulation in fibromyalgia: a phase I/II proof of concept trial. *Pain Med.* 2011 Sep;12(9):1406-13.

Nivethitha L, Manjunath NK, Mooventhan A. Heart Rate Variability Changes During and after the Practice of Bhramari Pranayama. *Int J Yoga.* 2017 May-Aug;10(2):99-102.

Norris P and Porter G. *Why Me? Harnessing the Healing Power of the Human Spirit.* Walpole NH: Stillpoint Publishing. 1985.

Siegler M, Frange C, Andersen ML, Tufik S, Hachul H. Effects of Bach Flower Remedies on Menopausal Symptoms and Sleep Pattern: A Case Report. *Altern Ther Health Med.* 2017 Mar;23(2):44-48.

Simonton OC and Matthews S. *Getting Well Again.* Los Angeles, CA: Jeremy P. Tarcher. 1978.

Sloan DM, Sawyer AT, Lowmaster SE, Wernick J, Marx BP. Efficacy of Narrative Writing as an Intervention for PTSD: Does the Evidence Support Its Use? *J Contemp Psychother.* 2015 Dec;45(4):215-225.

Smyth JM, Johnson JA, Auer BJ, Lehman E, Talamo G, Sciamanna CN. Online Positive Affect Journaling in the Improvement of Mental Distress and Well-Being in General Medical Patients With Elevated Anxiety Symptoms: A Preliminary Randomized Controlled Trial. *JMIR Ment Health.* 2018 Dec 10;5(4):e11290.

Tarn J, Legg S, Mitchell S, Simon B, Ng WF. The Effects of Noninvasive Vagus Nerve Stimulation on Fatigue and Immune Responses in Patients With Primary Sjögren's Syndrome. Neuromodulation. 2019 Jul;22(5):580-585.

Trivieri, Larry Jr. *The American Holistic Medical Association Guide To Holistic Health.* John Wiley & Son: New York, 2001.

Zhang Y, Popovic ZB, Bibevski S, Fakhry I, Sica DA, Van Wagoner DR, Mazgalev TN. Chronic vagus nerve stimulation improves autonomic control and attenuates systemic inflammation and heart failure progression in a canine high-rate pacing model. *Circ Heart Fail.* 2009 Nov;2(6):692-9.

Chapter 8

America's Phytonutrient Report. Nutrilite Health Institute. 2010. Available at www.yumpu.com/en/document/read/44024585/americas-phytonutrient-report-quantifying-the-gap-nutrilite

Amirian ES, Petrosino JF, Ajami NJ, Liu Y, Mims MP, Scheurer ME. Potential role of gastrointestinal microbiota composition in prostate cancer risk. *Infect Agent Cancer.* 2013 Nov 4;8(1):42.

Arumugam M, et al. Enterotypes of the human gut microbiome. *Nature.* 2011 May 12;473(7346):174-80.

Banerjee S, Tian T, Wei Z, Shih N, et al. Distinct Microbial Signatures Associated With Different Breast Cancer Types. *Front Microbiol.* 2018 May 15;9:951.

Benetou V, Trichopoulou A, Orfanos P, Naska A, Lagiou P, Boffetta P, Trichopoulos D; Greek EPIC cohort. Conformity to traditional Mediterranean diet and cancer incidence: the Greek EPIC cohort. *Br J Cancer.* 2008 Jul 8;99(1):191-5.

Canny GO, McCormick BA. Bacteria in the Intestine, Helpful Residents or Enemies from Within. *Infect and Immun.* 2008 Aug;76(8): 3360-3373.

Chattopadhyay I, Dhar R, Pethusamy K, et al. Exploring the Role of Gut Microbiome in Colon Cancer. *Appl Biochem Biotechnol.* 2021 Jun;193(6):1780-1799.

Cohen CW, Fontaine KR, Arend RC, Soleymani T, Gower BA. Favorable Effects of a Ketogenic Diet on Physical Function, Perceived Energy, and Food Cravings in Women with Ovarian or Endometrial Cancer: A Randomized, Controlled Trial. *Nutrients.* 2018; 10(9):1187.

Correa P. Commentary: Is prostate cancer an infectious disease? *Int J Epidemiol.* 2005 Feb;34(1):197-8.

Diop L, Guillou S, Durand H. Probiotic food supplement reduces stress-induced gastrointestinal symptoms in volunteers: A double-blind, placebo-controlled, randomized trial. *Nutrition Research.* 2008; 28(1):1-5.

Fujiki H, Watanabe T, Sueoka E, Rawangkan A, Suganuma M. Cancer Prevention with Green Tea and Its Principal Constituent, EGCG:

from Early Investigations to Current Focus on Human Cancer Stem Cells. *Mol Cells*. 2018 Feb 28;41(2):73-82.

Fujita K, Matsushita M, Banno E, et al. Gut microbiome and prostate cancer. *Int J Urol*. 2022 Aug;29(8):793-798.

Galeone C, Pelucchi C, Levi F, et al. Onion and garlic use and human cancer. *Am J Clin Nutr*. 2006 Nov;84(5):1027-32.

Gianluca I, Silvia P, Valentina G, Antonio G, Giovanni C. Digestive enzyme supplementation in gastrointestinal diseases. *Curr Drug Metab*. 2016;17(2):187-193.

Gopalakrishnan V, Helmink BA, Spencer CN, Reuben A, Wargo JA. The Influence of the Gut Microbiome on Cancer, Immunity, and Cancer Immunotherapy. *Cancer Cell*. 2018 Apr 9;33(4):570-580.

Grosso G, Buscemi S, Galvano F, et al. Mediterranean diet and cancer: epidemiological evidence and mechanism of selected aspects. *BMC Surg*. 2013;13 Suppl 2(Suppl 2):S14.

Heber, D. *What Color is Your Diet?* New York: HarperCollins, 2001.

Herber D, Li Z. Nutrition Intervention in Cancer. *Med. Clinics N. Amer*. 2016 Nov;100(6):1329-40.

Hullar MA, Burnett-Hartman AN, Lampe JW. Gut microbes, diet, and cancer. *Cancer Treat Res*. 2014;159:377-99.

Infectious Agents. National Cancer Institute. www.cancer.gov/about-cancer/causes-prevention/risk/infectious-agents

Jandhyala SM, Talukdar R, Subramanyam C, et al. Role of the normal gut microbiota. *World J Gastroenterol*. 2015 Aug 7;21(29):8787-803.

Jackson DV Jr, Pope EK, McMahan RA, et al. Clinical trial of pyridoxine to reduce vincristine neurotoxicity. *J Neurooncol*. 1986;4:37-41.

Jeon SM, Shin EA. Exploring vitamin D metabolism and function in cancer. *Exp Mol Med.* 2018 Apr 16;50(4):1-14.

Kim J, Lee HK. Potential Role of the Gut Microbiome In Colorectal Cancer Progression. *Front Immunol.* 2022 Jan 7;12:807648.

Klement, R.J. Beneficial effects of ketogenic diets for cancer patients: a realist review with focus on evidence and confirmation. *Med Oncol.* 2017 Jun 26;34:132.

Lee J, Im YH, Jung HH, et al. Curcumin inhibits interferon-alpha-induced NF-kappaB and COX-2 in human A549 non-small cell lung cancer cells. *Biochem Biophys Res Commun.* 2005;334:313-318.

Li Z, Heber D. Ketogenic Diets. *JAMA.* 2020;323(4):386.

Lieu EL, Nguyen T, Rhyne S, Kim J. Amino acids in cancer. *Exp Mol Med.* 2020 Jan;52(1):15-30.

Lin JK, Shih CA. Inhibitory effect of curcumin on xanthine dehydrogenase/oxidase induced by phorbol-12-myristate-13-acetate in NIH3T3 cells. *Carcinogenesis.* 1994;15:1717-2171.

Liontas A, Yeger H. Curcumin and resveratrol induce apoptosis and nuclear translocation and activation of p53 in human neuroblastoma. *Anticancer Res.* 2004;24:987-988.

Liu L, Shah K. The Potential of the Gut Microbiome to Reshape the Cancer Therapy Paradigm: A Review. *JAMA Oncol.* 2022 Jul 1;8(7):1059-1067.

Marx W, Ried K, McCarthy AL, Vitetta L, Sali A, McKavanagh D, Isenring L. Ginger-Mechanism of action in chemotherapy-induced nausea and vomiting: A review. *Crit Rev Food Sci Nutr.* 2017 Jan 2;57(1):141-146.

McDonald TJW, Cervenka MC. The Expanding Role of Ketogenic Diets in Adult Neurological Disorders. *Brain Sciences*. 2018; 8(8):148.

Mentella MC, Scaldaferri F, Ricci C, et al. Cancer and Mediterranean Diet: A Review. *Nutrients*. 2019 Sep 2;11(9):2059.

Milacic V, Banerjee S, Landis-Piwowar KR, et al. Curcumin inhibits the proteasome activity in human colon cancer cells in vitro and in vivo. *Cancer Res*. 2008;68(18):7283-7292.

Morowitz MJ, Carlisle EM, Alverdy JC. Contributions of intestinal bacteria to nutrition and metabolism in the critically ill. *Surg Clin North Am*. 2011 Aug;91(4):771-85, viii.

Mótyán JA, Tóth F, Tőzsér J. Research applications of proteolytic enzymes in molecular biology. *Biomolecules*. 2013;3(4):923-42.

Nagai S, Kurimoto M, Washiyama K, et al., Inhibition of cellular proliferation and induction of apoptosis by curcumin in human malignant astrocytoma cell lines. *J Neurooncol*. 2005;74(2):105-11.

Nakamura Y, Ohto Y, Murakami A, et al. Inhibitory effects of curcumin and tetrahydrocurcuminoids on the tumor promoter-induced reactive oxygen species in leukocytes in vitro and invivo. *Jpn J Cancer Res*. 1998;89:-361-370.

Nicastro HL, Ross SA, Milner JA. Garlic and onions: their cancer prevention properties. *Cancer Prev Res* (Phila). 2015 Mar;8(3):181-9.

Owen RW, Giacosa A, et al. The antioxidant/anticancer potential of phenolic compounds isolated from olive oil. *Eur J Cancer*. 2000 Jun; 36(10):1235-47.

Park EM, Chelvanambi M, Bhutiani N, et al. Targeting the gut and tumor microbiota in cancer. *Nat Med*. 2022 Apr;28(4):690-703.

Petrovic V, Nepal A, Olaisen C, Bachke S, et al. Anti-Cancer Potential of Homemade Fresh Garlic Extract Is Related to Increased Endoplasmic Reticulum Stress. *Nutrients*. 2018 Apr 5;10(4):450.

Peyrot des Gachons C, Breslin PAS. Salivary amylase: digestion and metabolic syndrome. *Curr Diab Rep*. 2016;16(10):102.

Phan TT, See P, Lee ST, et al. Protective effects of curcumin against oxidative damage on skin cells in vitro: its implication for wound healing. *J Trauma*. 2001;51:927-931.

Poff AM, Ari C, et al. Ketone supplementation decreases tumor cell viability and prolongs survival of mice with metastatic cancer. *Int J Cancer*. 2014 Feb 26;135(7):1722-20.

Poutahidis T, Cappelle K, Levkovich T, et al. Pathogenic intestinal bacteria enhance prostate cancer development via systemic activation of immune cells in mice. *PLoS One*. 2013 Aug 26;8(8):e73933.

Proctor LM. The Human Microbiome Project in 2011 and beyond. *Cell Host Microbe*. 2011 Oct 20;10(4):287-91.

Psaltopoulou T, Kosti RI, Haidopoulos D, Dimopoulos M, Panagiotakos DB. Olive oil intake is inversely related to cancer prevalence: a systematic review and a meta-analysis of 13,800 patients and 23,340 controls in 19 observational studies. *Lipids Health Dis*. 2011 Jul 30;10:127.

Rebersek M. Gut microbiome and its role in colorectal cancer. *BMC Cancer*. 2021 Dec 11;21(1):1325.

Romer M, Dorfler J, Huebner J. The use of ketogenic diets in cancer patients: a systematic review. *Clin Exp Med*. 2021 Nov;21(4):501-536.

Schwingshackl L, Schwedhelm C, Galbete C, Hoffmann G. Adherence to Mediterranean Diet and Risk of Cancer: An Updated Systematic Review and Meta-Analysis. *Nutrients*. 2017 Sep 26;9(10):1063.

Selvam R, Subramanian L, Gayathri R, Angayarkanni N. The anti-oxidant activity of turmeric (*Curcuma longa*). *J Ethnopharmacol*. 1995;47: 59-67.

Sfanos KS, Isaacs WB, De Marzo AM. Infections and inflammation in prostate cancer. *Am J Clin Exp Urol*. 2013 Dec 25;1(1):3-11.

Ursell LK, et al. Defining the Human Microbiome. *Nutr Rev*. 2012 Aug;70(Suppl 1):S38–S44.

Visioli F, Grande S, Bogani P, Galli C. The role of antioxidants in the Mediterranean diets: focus on cancer. *Eur J Cancer Prev*. 2004 Aug;13(4):337-43.

Weber DD, Aminzadeh-Gohari S, et al. Ketogenic diet in the treatment of cancer - Where do we stand? *Mol Metab*. 2020 Mar;33:102-121.

Chapter 9

Abiri B, Vafa M. Vitamin C and Cancer: The Role of Vitamin C in Disease Progression and Quality of Life in Cancer Patients. *Nutr Cancer*. 2021;73(8):1282-1292.

Andreeva VA, Touvier M, Kesse-Guyot E, Julia C, Galan P, Hercberg S. B vitamin and/or ω-3 fatty acid supplementation and cancer: ancillary findings from the supplementation with folate, vitamins B6 and B12, and/or omega-3 fatty acids (SU.FOL.OM3) randomized trial. *Arch Intern Med*. 2012;172:540-7.

Azemar M, Hildenbrand B, et al. Clinical benefit in patients with advanced solid tumors treated with modified citrus pectin: a prospective pilot study. *Clin Med: Oncology* 2007;1:73-80.

Balk JL. Indole-3-carbinol for cancer prevention. *Altern Med Alert* 2000; 3:105-7.

Bemis DL, Capodice JL, Gorroochurn P, Katz AE, Buttyan R. Anti-prostate cancer activity of a Beta-carboline alkaloid enriched extract from Rauwolfia vomitoria. *J. Oncol.* 2006;29:1065–1073.

Bemis DL, Capodice JL, Desai M, Katz AE, Buttyan R. Beta-carboline alkaloid-enriched extract from the Amazonian rain forest tree Pao pereira suppresses prostate cancer cells. *J Soc Integr Oncol.* Spring 2009;7:59–65.

Bencze, G., Bencze, S., Rivera, K.D. et al. Mito-oncology agent: fermented extract suppresses the Warburg effect, restores oxidative mitochondrial activity, and inhibits in vivo tumor growth. *Sci Rep.* 2020 Aug 25;10:14174.

Bettuzzi S, Brausi M, Rizzi F, Castagnetti G, Peracchia G, Corti A. Chemoprevention of human prostate cancer by oral administration of green tea catechins in volunteers with high-grade prostate intraepithelial neoplasia: a preliminary report from a one-year proof-of-principle study. *Cancer Res.* 2006 Jan 15;66(2):1234-40.

Block K, Koch A, et al. Impact of antioxidant supplementation on chemotherapeutic efficacy: a systematic review of the evidence from randomized controlled trials. *Cancer Treatment Reviews.* 2007. 33(5):407-18.

Bradlow HL, Sepkovic DW, et al. Multifunctional aspects of the action of indole-3-carbinol as an antitumor agent. *Ann NY Acad Sci* 1999;889:204-13.

Byar D, Blackard C. Comparisons of placebo, pyridoxine, and topical thiotepa in preventing recurrence of stage I bladder cancer. *Urology.* 1977;10:556-61.

Carlberg C, Velleuer E. Vitamin D and the risk for cancer: A molecular analysis. *Biochem Pharmacol.* 2022 Feb;196:114735.

Ceci C, Lacal PM, Tentori L, et al. Experimental Evidence of the Antitumor, Antimetastatic and Antiangiogenic Activity of Ellagic Acid. *Nutrients*. 2018 Nov 14;10(11):1756.

Chai W, Cooney RV, Franke AA, et al. Plasma coenzyme Q10 levels and prostate cancer risk: the multiethnic cohort study. *Cancer Epidemiol Biomarkers Prev*. 2011 Apr;20(4):708-10.

Chang YC, et al. 1999. Cytostatic and antiestrogenic effects of 2-(indole-3-ylmethyl)-3,3'-diindolylmethane, a major in vivo product of dietary indole-3-carbinol. *Biochem Pharm* 58:825-34.

Chang C, Zhao W, Xie B, Deng Y, et al. Pao pereira Extract Suppresses Castration-Resistant Prostate Cancer Cell Growth, Survival and Invasion Through Inhibition of NFkB Signaling. *Integrative Cancer Therapies*. 2013;(11)13:3.

Chen, BH., Hsieh, CH., Tsai, SY. et al. Anticancer effects of epigallocatechin-3-gallate nanoemulsion on lung cancer cells through the activation of AMP-activated protein kinase signaling pathway. *Sci Rep*. 2020 Mar 20;10:5163.

Chen I, et al. Aryl hydrocarbon receptor-mediated antiestrogenic and antitumorigenic activity of diindolylmethane. *Carcinogenesis* 19:1631-9.

Cheshomi H, Bahrami AR, Matin MM. Ellagic acid and human cancers: a systems pharmacology and docking study to identify principal hub genes and main mechanisms of action. *Mol Divers*. 2021 Feb;25(1):333-349.

Cho JH, Bhutani S, Kim CH, Irwin MR. Anti-inflammatory effects of melatonin: A systematic review and meta-analysis of clinical trials. *Brain Behav Immun*. 2021 Mar;93:245-253.

Corrie PG, Bulusu R, Wilson CB, et al. A randomised study evaluating the use of pyridoxine to avoid capecitabine dose modifications. *Br J Cancer*. 2012;107:585-7.

Cover CM, et al. 1998. Indole-3-carbinol inhibits the expression of cyclin-dependent kinase-6 and induces a G1 cell cycle arrest of human breast cancer cells independent of estrogen receptor signaling. *J Biol Chem* 273:3838-47.

Crane FL, Sun IL, Sun EE. The essential functions of coenzyme Q. *Clin Investig.* 1993;71(8 Suppl):S55-9.

de La Puente-Yagüe M, Cuadrado-Cenzual MA, et al. Vitamin D: And its role in breast cancer. *Kaohsiung J Med Sci.* 2018 Aug;34(8):423-427.

den Besten G, van Eunen K, Groen AK, Venema K, Reijngoud DJ, Bakker BM. The role of short-chain fatty acids in the interplay between diet, gut microbiota, and host energy metabolism. *J Lipid Res.* 2013 Sep;54(9):2325-40.

Denner G, Horneber M. Selenium for relieving the side effects of chemotherapy, radiotherapy, and surgery in cancer patients. *Cochrane Library.* Updated 02/16/09.

Doskey CM, Visarut Buranasudja V, et al. Tumor cells have decreased ability to metabolize H2O2: Implications for pharmacological ascorbate in cancer therapy. *Redox Biology*, 2016;10:274.

Dresler, H. et al. Long term effect of PectaSol-C modified citrus pectin treatment in non-metastatic biochemically relapsed prostate cancer patients: Results of a prospective phase II study. *Eur Urology Supplements*, 2019 Nov; 18(11):e3467.

Du GJ, Zhang Z, Wen XD, et al. Epigallocatechin Gallate (EGCG) is the most effective cancer chemopreventive polyphenol in green tea. *Nutrients.* 2012 Nov 8;4(11):1679-91.

Egnell M, Fassier P, Lécuyer L, et al. B-vitamin intake from diet and supplements and breast cancer risk in middle-aged women: results from the prospective NutriNet-Santé cohort. *Nutrients.* 2017;9:488-504.

Fabian CJ, Kimler BF, Hursting SD Omega-3 fatty acids for breast cancer prevention and survivorship. *Breast Cancer Res.* 2015 May 4;17:article number 62.

Figueiredo JC, Levine AJ, Grau MV, et al. Vitamins B2, B6, and B12 and risk of new colorectal adenomas in a randomized trial of aspirin use and folic acid supplementation. *Cancer Epidemiol Biomarkers Prev.* 2008;17:2136-45.

Folkers K. The potential of coenzyme Q 10 (NSC-140865) in cancer treatment. *Cancer Chemother Rep 2.* 1974 Dec;4(4):19-22.

Folkers K, Morita M, McRee J Jr. The activities of coenzyme Q10 and vitamin B6 for immune responses. *Biochem Biophys Res Commun.* 1993 May 28;193(1):88-92.

Folkers K, Osterborg A, Nylander M, Morita M, Mellstedt H. Activities of vitamin Q10 in animal models and a serious deficiency in patients with cancer. *Biochem Biophys Res Commun.* 1997 May 19;234(2):296-9.

Folkers K, Porter TH, Bertino JR, Moroson B. Inhibition of two human tumor cell lines by antimetabolites of coenzyme Q10. *Res Commun Chem Pathol Pharmacol.* 1978 Mar;19(3):485-90.

Fried LE, Arbiser JL. Honokiol, a multifunctional antiangiogenic and antitumor agent. *Antioxid Redox Signal.* 2009 May;11(5):1139-48.

Fujiki H, Watanabe T, Sueoka E, Rawangkan A, Suganuma M. Cancer Prevention with Green Tea and Its Principal Constituent, EGCG: from Early Investigations to Current Focus on Human Cancer Stem Cells. *Mol Cells.* 2018 Feb 28;41(2):73-82.

Gillner M, et al. Interactions of indoles with specific binding sites for 2,3,7,8-tetrachlorodibenzo-p-dioxin in rat liver. *Mol Pharm* 28: 357-63.

Gruber BM. B-group vitamins: chemoprevention? *Adv Clin Exp Med.* 2016;25:561-8.

Gu JJ, Qiao KS, Sun P, Chen P, Li Q. Study of EGCG induced apoptosis in lung cancer cells by inhibiting PI3K/Akt signaling pathway. *Eur Rev Med Pharmacol Sci.* 2018 Jul;22(14):4557-4563.

Gu JW, Makey KL, Tucker KB, et al. EGCG, a major green tea catechin suppresses breast tumor angiogenesis and growth via inhibiting the activation of HIF-1α and NFκB, and VEGF expression. *Vasc Cell.* 2013 May 2;5(1):9.

Guess BW, Scholz MC, Strum SB, et al. Modified citrus pectin (MCP) increases the prostate-specific antigen doubling time in men with prostate cancer: a phase II pilot study. *Prostate Cancer Prostatic Dis.* 2003;6(4):301-4.

Guillermo-Lagae R, Santha S, et al. Antineoplastic Effects of Honokiol on Melanoma. *Biomed Res Int.* 2017;2017:5496398.

Guo S, Xu JJ, Wei N, et al. Honokiol Attenuates the Memory Impairments, Oxidative Stress, Neuroinflammation, and GSK-3β Activation in Vascular Dementia Rats. *J Alzheimers Dis.* 2019;71(1):97-108.

Halgamuge MN. Pineal melatonin level disruption in humans due to electromagnetic fields and ICNIRP limits. *Radiat Prot Dosimetry.* 2013 May;154(4):405-16.

Hartman TJ, Woodson K, Stolzenberg-Solomon R, et al. Association of the B-vitamins pyridoxal 5′-phosphate (B(6)), B(12), and folate with lung cancer risk in older men. *Am J Epidemiol.* 2001;153:688-94.

Hertz N, Lister R. Improved Survival in Patients with Endstage Cancer Treated with Coenzyme Q10 and Other Antioxidants: a Pilot Study. *Intl J Med Research.* 2009;37:1961-7 1.

Honjo Y, Nangia-Makker P, Inohara H, Raz A. Down-regulation of galectin-3 suppresses tumorigenicity of human breast carcinoma cells. *Clin Cancer Res*. 2001 Mar;7(3):661-8.

Imran M, Aslam Gondal T, Atif M, et al. Apigenin as an anticancer agent. *Phytother Res*. 2020 Aug;34(8):1812-1828.

Jatoi A, Ellison N, Burch PA, et al. A phase II trial of green tea in the treatment of patients with androgen independent metastatic prostate carcinoma. *Cancer*. 2003 Mar 15;97(6):1442-6.

Jellinck PH, et al. 1993. Ah receptor binding properties of indole carbinols and induction of hepatic estradiol hydroxylation. *Biochem Pharmacol* 45:1129-36.

Jellinck PH, et al. 1994. Distinct forms of hepatic androgen 6 beta-hydroxylase induced in the rat by indole-3-carbinol and pregnenolone carbonitrile. *J Steroid Biochem Mol Biol* 51:219-25.

Jolliet P, Simon N, Barré J, Pons JY, Boukef M, Paniel BJ, Tillement JP. Plasma coenzyme Q10 concentrations in breast cancer: prognosis and therapeutic consequences. *Int J Clin Pharmacol Ther*. 1998 Sep;36(9):506-9.

Kim YS, Milner JA. Targets for indole-3-carbinol in cancer prevention. *J Nutr Biochem*. 2005 Feb;16(2):65-73.

Kouakanou L, Peters C, Brown CE, Kabelitz D, Wang LD. Vitamin C, From Supplement to Treatment: A Re-Emerging Adjunct for Cancer Immunotherapy? *Front Immunol*. 2021 Nov 12;12:765906.

Lai H, Sasaki T, Singh NP. Targeted treatment of cancer with artemisinin and artemisinin-tagged iron-carrying compounds. *Expert Opin Ther Targets*. 2005 Oct;9(5):995-1007.

Lamson DW, Plaza SM. The anticancer effects of vitamin K. *Altern Med Rev*. 2003 Aug;8(3):303-18.

Lardone PJ, Alvarez-Sanchez SN, Guerrero JM, Carrillo-Vico A. Melatonin and glucose metabolism: clinical relevance. *Curr Pharm Des*. 2014;20(30):4841-53.

Lee J, Im YH, Jung HH, et al. Curcumin inhibits interferon-alpha-induced NF-kappaB and COX-2 in human A549 non-small cell lung cancer cells. *Biochem Biophys Res Commun*. 2005;334:313-318.

Li D, Zhang J, Zhao X. Mechanisms and Molecular Targets of Artemisinin in Cancer Treatment. *Cancer Invest*. 2021 Sep;39(8):675-684.

Li H, Jia J, Wang W, et al. Honokiol Alleviates Cognitive Deficits of Alzheimer's Disease (PS1V97L) Transgenic Mice by Activating Mitochondrial SIRT3. *J Alzheimers Dis*. 2018;64(1):291-302.

Li Y, Li S, Zhou Y, et al. Melatonin for the prevention and treatment of cancer. *Oncotarget*. 2017 Jun 13;8(24):39896-39921.

Lin JK, Shih CA. Inhibitory effect of curcumin on xanthine dehydrogenase/oxidase induced by phorbol-12-myristate-13-acetate in NIH3T3 cells. *Carcinogenesis*. 1994;15:1717-2171.

Liontas A, Yeger H. Curcumin and resveratrol induce apoptosis and nuclear translocation and activation of p53 in human neuroblastoma. *Anticancer Res*. 2004;24:987-988.

Liu T, Liu H, Wang P, et al. Honokiol Inhibits Melanoma Growth by Targeting Keratin 18 *in vitro* and *in vivo*. *Front Cell Dev Biol*. 2020 Nov 24;8:603472.

Lockwood K, Moesgaard S, Hanioka T, Folkers K. Apparent partial remission of breast cancer in 'high risk' patients supplemented with nutritional antioxidants, essential fatty acids and coenzyme Q10. *Mol Aspects Med*. 1994;15 Suppl:s231-40.

Luo H, Tang L, Tang M, Billam M, et al. Phase IIa chemoprevention trial of green tea polyphenols in high-risk individuals of liver cancer: modulation of urinary excretion of green tea polyphenols and 8-hydroxydeoxyguanosine. *Carcinogenesis.* 2006 Feb;27(2):262-8.

Magrì A, Germano G, Lorenzato A, et al. High-dose vitamin C enhances cancer immunotherapy. *Sci Transl Med.* 2020 Feb 26;12(532):eaay8707.

Malik A, Afaq S, Shahid M, Akhtar K, Assiri A. Influence of ellagic acid on prostate cancer cell proliferation: a caspase-dependent pathway. *Asian Pac J Trop Med.* 2011 Jul;4(7):550-5.

Meng Q, et al. 2000. Indole-3-carbinol is a negative regulator of estrogen receptor- signaling in human tumor cells. *J Nutr* 130:2927-31.

Milacic V, Banerjee S, Landis-Piwowar KR, et al. Curcumin inhibits the proteasome activity in human colon cancer cells in vitro and in vivo. *Cancer Res.* 2008;68(18):7283-7292.

Mohammadinejad A, Mohajeri T, Aleyaghoob G, Heidarian F, Kazemi Oskuee R. Ellagic acid as a potent anticancer drug: A comprehensive review on in vitro, in vivo, in silico, and drug delivery studies. *Biotechnol Appl Biochem.* 2022 Dec;69(6):2323-2356.

Muñoz A, Grant WB. Vitamin D and Cancer: An Historical Overview of the Epidemiology and Mechanisms. *Nutrients.* 2022 Mar 30;14(7):1448.

Nagai S, Kurimoto M, Washiyama K, et al., Inhibition of cellular proliferation and induction of apoptosis by curcumin in human malignant astrocytoma cell lines. *J Neurooncol.* 2005;74(2):105-11.

Nakamura Y, Ohto Y, Murakami A, et al. Inhibitory effects of curcumin and tetrahydrocurcuminoids on the tumor promoter-induced reactive oxygen species in leukocytes in vitro and invivo. *Jpn J Cancer Res.* 1998;89:-361-370.

Newling DW, Robinson MR, Smith PH, et al. Tryptophan metabolites, pyridoxine (vitamin B6) and their influence on the recurrence rate of superficial bladder cancer. Results of a prospective, randomised phase III study performed by the EORTC GU Group. EORTC Genito-Urinary Tract Cancer Cooperative Group. *Eur Urol.* 1995;27:110-6.

Ong CP, Lee WL, Tang YQ, Yap WH. Honokiol: A Review of Its Anticancer Potential and Mechanisms. *Cancers (Basel).* 2019 Dec 22;12(1):48.

Ota M, Tatsumi K, Suwa H, et al. The effect of pyridoxine for prevention of hand-foot syndrome in colorectal cancer patients with adjuvant chemotherapy using capecitabine: a randomized study. *Hepatogastroenterology.* 2014;61:1008-13.

Overvad K, Diamant B, Holm L, Holmer G, Mortensen SA, Stender S. Coenzyme Q10 in health and disease. *Eur J Clin Nutr.* 1999 Oct;53(10):764-70.

Pan J, Lee Y, Wang Y, You M. Honokiol targets mitochondria to halt cancer progression and metastasis. *Mol Nutr Food Res.* 2016 Jun;60(6):1383-95.

Patel D, Shukla S, Gupta S. Apigenin and cancer chemoprevention: progress, potential and promise (review). *Int J Oncol.* 2007 Jan;30(1):233-45.

Phan TT, See P, Lee ST, et al. Protective effects of curcumin against oxidative damage on skin cells in vitro: its implication for wound healing. *J Trauma.* 2001;51:927-931.

Prasad R, Katiyar SK. Honokiol, an Active Compound of Magnolia Plant, Inhibits Growth, and Progression of Cancers of Different Organs. *Adv Exp Med Biol.* 2016;928:245-265.

Ramachandran C, Wilk BJ, et al. Activation of human T-helper/inducer cell, T-cytotoxic cell, B-cell, and natural killer (NK)-cells and induction of natural killer cell activity against K562 chronic myeloid leukemia cells with modified citrus pectin. *BMC Complement Altern Med*. 2011 Aug 4;11:59.

Ramachandran L, Krishnan CV, Nair CK. Radioprotection by alpha-lipoic acid palladium complex formulation (POLY-MVA) in mice. *Cancer Biother Radiopharm*. 2010 Aug;25(4):395-9.

Ramesh S, Govindarajulu M, Lynd T, et al. SIRT3 activator Honokiol attenuates β-Amyloid by modulating amyloidogenic pathway. *PLoS One*. 2018 Jan 11;13(1):e0190350.

Rauf A, Patel S, Imran M, et al. Honokiol: An anticancer lignan. *Biomed Pharmacother*. 2018 Nov;107:555-562.

Riby JE, et al. 2000. Ligand-independent activation of estrogen receptor function by 3,3'-diindolylmethane in human breast cancer cells. *Biochem Pharm* 60:167-77.

Rickert U, Cossais F, Heimke M, et al. Anti-inflammatory properties of Honokiol in activated primary microglia and astrocytes. *J Neuroimmunol*. 2018 Oct 15;323:78-86.

Romano A, Martel F. The Role of EGCG in Breast Cancer Prevention and Therapy. *Mini Rev Med Chem*. 2021;21(7):883-898.

Sahu Rp, Batra S, Srivastava SK. Activation of ATM/Chk1 by curcumin causes cell cycle arrest and apoptosis in human pancreatic cancer cells. *Br J Cancer*. 2009;100(9):1425-1433.

Shamsuddin AM, Vucenik I, Cole KE. IP6: a novel anti-cancer agent. *Life Sci*. 1997;61(4):343-54.

Shamsuddin AM. Inositol phosphates have novel anticancer function. *J Nutr*. 1995 Mar;125(3 Suppl):725S-732S.

Shamsuddin AM. Metabolism and cellular functions of IP6: a review. *Anticancer Res.* 1999 Sep-Oct;19(5A):3733-6.

Shukla S, Gupta S. Apigenin: a promising molecule for cancer prevention. *Pharm Res.* 2010 Jun;27(6):962-78.

Singh S. Aggarwal BB. Activation of transcription factor NF-kappa B is suppressed by curcumin (diferuloylmethane) [corrected]. *J Biol Chem.* 1995;270:24,995-25,000.

Song Y, Manson JE, Lee IM, et al. Effect of combined folic acid, vitamin B(6), and vitamin B(12) on colorectal adenoma. *J Natl Cancer Inst.* 2012;104:1562-75.

Sudarshana P, Berliner A, Suraj SF, et al. Curcumin blocks brain tumor formation. Brain Research. 2009;1266:130-138.

Sun C, Liu X, Chen Y, et al., Anticancer effect of curcumin on human B cell non-Hodgkin's lymphoma. *J Huazhong Univ Sci Technolog Med Sci.* 2005;25(4):404-7.

Talarek S, Listos J, Barreca D, et al. Neuroprotective effects of honokiol: from chemistry to medicine. Biofactors. 2017 Nov;43(6):760-769.

Talib WH. Melatonin and Cancer Hallmarks. *Molecules.* 2018 Feb 26;23(3):518.

Talib WH, Alsayed AR, Abuawad A, Daoud S, Mahmod AI. Melatonin in Cancer Treatment: Current Knowledge and Future Opportunities. *Molecules.* 2021 Apr 25;26(9):2506.

Tsao AS, Liu D, Martin J, Tang XM, et al. Phase II randomized, placebo-controlled trial of green tea extract in patients with high-risk oral premalignant lesions. *Cancer Prev Res* (Phila). 2009 Nov;2(11): 931-41.

Veena RK, Ajith TA, Janardhanan KK, Antonawich F. Antitumor Effects of Palladium-α-Lipoic Acid Complex Formulation as an Adjunct in Radiotherapy. *J Environ Pathol Toxicol Oncol.* 2016;35(4):333-342.

Verma SP, Salamone E, Goldin BR. Curcumin and genistein, plant natural products, show synergistic inhibitory effects on the growth of human breast cancer MCF-7 cells induced by estrogenic pesticides. *Biochem Biophys Res Commun.* 1997;233(3):692-696.

Vitamin D and cancer prevention.(2013). www.cancer.gov/about-cancer/causes-prevention/risk/diet/vitamin-d-fact-sheet

von Gruenigen V, Frasure H, Fusco N, et al. A double-blind, randomized trial of pyridoxine versus placebo for the prevention of pegylated liposomal doxorubicin-related hand-foot syndrome in gynecologic oncology patients. *Cancer.* 2010;116:4735-43.

Vucenik I, Shamsuddin AM. Cancer inhibition by inositol hexaphosphate (IP6) and inositol: from laboratory to clinic. *J Nutr.* 2003 Nov;133(11 Suppl 1):3778S-3784S.

Vucenik I, Shamsuddin AM. Protection against cancer by dietary IP6 and inositol. *Nutr Cancer.* 2006;55(2):109-25.

Wang LD, Zhou Q, Feng CW, et al. Intervention and follow-up on human esophageal precancerous lesions in Henan, northern China, a high-incidence area for esophageal cancer. *Gan To Kagaku Ryoho.* 2002 Feb;29 Suppl 1:159-72.

Wang YM, Jin BZ, Ai F, et al. The efficacy and safety of melatonin in concurrent chemotherapy or radiotherapy for solid tumors: a meta-analysis of randomized controlled trials. *Cancer Chemother Pharmacol.* 2012 May;69(5):1213-20.

Wang L, Wang C, Choi WS. Use of Melatonin in Cancer Treatment: Where Are We? *Int J Mol Sci.* 2022 Mar 29;23(7):3779.

Wattenberg LW, et al. 1978. Inhibition of polycyclic aromatic hydrocarbon-induced neoplasia by naturally occurring indoles. *Cancer Res* 38:1410-13.

Weitzen R, Epstein N, Oberman B, Shevetz R, Hidvegi M, Berger R. Fermented Wheat Germ Extract (FWGE) as a Treatment Additive for Castration-Resistant Prostate Cancer: A Pilot Clinical Trial. *Nutr Cancer*. 2022;74(4):1338-1346. doi: 10.1080/01635581.2021.

Welsh J, Bak MJ, Narvaez CJ. New insights into vitamin K biology with relevance to cancer. *Trends Mol Med*. 2022 Oct;28(10):864-881.

Wiernik PH, Yeap B, Vogl SE, et al. Hexamethylmelamine and low or moderate dose cisplatin with or without pyridoxine for treatment of advanced ovarian carcinoma: a study of the Eastern cooperative Oncology Group. *Cancer Invest*. 1992;10:1-9.

Wong GY, Bradlow L, Sepkovic D, et al. Dose-ranging study of indole-3-carbinol for breast cancer prevention. *J Cell Biochem Suppl*. 1997;28-29:111-6.

Wong YK, Xu C, Kalesh KA, et al. Artemisinin as an anticancer drug: Recent advances in target profiling and mechanisms of action. *Med Res Rev*. 2017 Nov;37(6):1492-1517.

Yan X, Qi M, Li P, Zhan Y, Shao H. Apigenin in cancer therapy: anti-cancer effects and mechanisms of action. *Cell Biosci*. 2017 Oct 5;7:50.

Yang GY, Shamsuddin AM. IP6-induced growth inhibition and differentiation of HT-29 human colon cancer cells: involvement of intracellular inositol phosphates. *Anticancer Res*. 1995 Nov-Dec;15(6B):2479-87.

Yeend T, Robinson K, Lockwood C, McArthur A. The effectiveness of fermented wheat germ extract as an adjunct therapy in the treatment of cancer: A systematic review. *JBI Libr Syst Rev*. 2012;10(42 Suppl):1-12.

Yu J, Drisko J, Chen Q. Antitumor Activities of Rauwolfia Vomitoria Extract and Potentiation of Carboplatin Effects Against Ovarian Cancer. *Curr Ther Res Clin Exp*. 2013 Dec;75:8-14.

Yu J, Chen Q. Antitumor Activities of Rauwolfia vomitoria Extract and Potentiation of Gemcitabine Effects Against Pancreatic Cancer. *Integrative Cancer Therapy*. 2014 Apr 24;13(3):217-225.

Yu J, Drisko J, Chen Q. Inhibition of Pancreatic Cancer and Potentiation of Gemcitabine Effects by the Extract of Pao Pereira. *Oncology Reports Journal* (doi: 10.3892/or.2013.2461).

Yu J, Drisko J, Chen Q. The Plant Extract of Pao Pereira Potentiates Carboplatin Effects Against Ovarian Cancer. Informa Healthcare USA, Inc.– ISSN 1388-0209 print/ISSN 1744-5116 – *Pharmaceutical Biology*.

Zasowska-Nowak A, Nowak PJ, Ciałkowska-Rysz A. High-Dose Vitamin C in Advanced-Stage Cancer Patients. *Nutrients*. 2021 Feb 26;13(3):735.

Zhang Y, Xu G, Zhang S, Wang D, Saravana Prabha P, Zuo Z. Antitumor Research on Artemisinin and Its Bioactive Derivatives. *Nat Prod Bioprospect*. 2018 Aug;8(4):303-319.

Zhurakivska K, Troiano G, Caponio VCA, et al. The Effects of Adjuvant Fermented Wheat Germ Extract on Cancer Cell Lines: A Systematic Review. *Nutrients*. 2018 Oct 19;10(10):1546.

Chapter 10

Behrens G, Jochem C, Keimling M, et al. The association between physical activity and gastroesophageal cancer: systematic review and meta-analysis. *European Journal of Epidemiology* 2014; 29(3):151-170.

Behrens G, Leitzmann MF. The association between physical activity and renal cancer: systematic review and meta-analysis. *British Journal of Cancer* 2013; 108(4):798-811.

Bernstein H, Bernstein C, Payne CM, Dvorakova K, Garewal H. Bile acids as carcinogens in human gastrointestinal cancers. *Mutation Research* 2005; 589(1):47-65.

Borch KB, Weiderpass E, Braaten T, et al. Physical activity and risk of endometrial cancer in the Norwegian Women and Cancer (NOWAC) study. *International Journal of Cancer* 2017; 140(8):1809-1818.

Chevalier G, Sinatra ST, Oschman JL, Sokal K, Sokal P. Earthing: health implications of reconnecting the human body to the Earth's surface electrons. *J Environ Public Health*. 2012;2012:291541.

Contrepois K, Wu S, Moneghetti KJ, et al. Molecular Choreography of Acute Exercise. *Cell*. 2020 May 28;181(5):1112-1130.e16.

Cook AL. *The shear effect of exercise.* The Physiological Society, Feb 22, 2018. www.physoc.org/blog/the-shear-effect-of-exercise

Dimitrov S, Hulteng E, Hong S. Inflammation and exercise: Inhibition of monocytic intracellular TNF production by acute exercise via β2-adrenergic activation. *Brain Behav Immun*. 2017 March;61:60-68.

Du M, Kraft P, Eliassen AH, et al. Physical activity and risk of endometrial adenocarcinoma in the Nurses' Health Study. *International Journal of Cancer* 2014; 134(11):2707-2716.

Eliassen AH, Hankinson SE, Rosner B, Holmes MD, Willett WC. Physical activity and risk of breast cancer among postmenopausal women. *Archives of Internal Medicine* 2010; 170(19):1758-1764.

Fournier A, Dos Santos G, Guillas G, et al. Recent recreational physical activity and breast cancer risk in postmenopausal women in the E3N cohort. *Cancer Epidemiology, Biomarkers & Prevention* 2014; 23(9):1893-1902.

Friedenreich C, Cust A, Lahmann PH, et al. Physical activity and risk of endometrial cancer: The European prospective investigation into cancer and nutrition. *International Journal of Cancer* 2007; 121(2):347-355.

Hardefeldt PJ, Penninkilampi R, Edirimanne S, Eslick GD. Physical activity and weight loss reduce the risk of breast cancer: A meta-analysis of 139 prospective and retrospective studies. *Clinical Breast Cancer* 2018; 18(4):e601-e612.

Keimling M, Behrens G, Schmid D, Jochem C, Leitzmann MF. The association between physical activity and bladder cancer: systematic review and meta-analysis. *British Journal of Cancer* 2014; 110(7):1862-1870.

Liu L, Shi Y, Li T, et al. Leisure time physical activity and cancer risk: evaluation of the WHO's recommendation based on 126 high-quality epidemiological studies. *British Journal of Sports Medicine* 2016; 50(6):372-378.

Ma S, Fu A, Chiew GG, Luo KQ. Hemodynamic shear stress stimulates migration and extravasation of tumor cells by elevating cellular oxidative level. *Cancer Lett.* 2017 Mar 1;388:239-248.

McTiernan A, Friedenreich CM, Katzmarzyk PT, et al. Physical activity in cancer prevention and survival: A systematic review. *Medicine and Science in Sports and Exercise* 2019; 51(6):1252-1261.

Metsios GS, Moe RH, Kitas GD. Exercise and inflammation. *Best Pract Res Clin Rheumatol.* 2020 Apr;34(2):101504.

Minihan AK.; Patel AV; et al. Proportion of Cancer Cases Attributable to Physical Inactivity by US State, 2013–2016. *Medicine & Science in Sports & Exercise.* Mar 2022; 54(3): 417-423.

Moore SC, Lee IM, Weiderpass E, et al. Association of leisure-time physical activity with risk of 26 types of cancer in 1.44 million adults. *JAMA Intern Med* 2016; 176(6):816-825.

Patel AV, Friedenreich CM, Moore SC, et al. American College of Sports Medicine Roundtable Report on physical activity, sedentary behavior, and cancer prevention and control. *Medicine and Science in Sports and Exercise* 2019; 51(11):2391-2402.

Pedersen BK. Anti-inflammatory effects of exercise: role in diabetes and cardiovascular disease. Eur J. Clin Investigation. 2017 Jul17;47(8):600-11.

Pizot C, Boniol M, Mullie P, et al. Physical activity, hormone replacement therapy and breast cancer risk: A meta-analysis of prospective studies. *European Journal of Cancer* 2016; 52:138-154.

Psaltopoulou T, Ntanasis-Stathopoulos I, Tzanninis IG, et al. Physical activity and gastric cancer risk: A systematic review and meta-analysis. *Clinical Journal of Sports Medicine* 2016; 26(6):445-464.

Rezende LFM, Sá TH, Markozannes G, et al. Physical activity and cancer: an umbrella review of the literature including 22 major anatomical sites and 770 000 cancer cases. *British Journal of Sports Medicine* 2018; 52(13):826-833.

Rundqvist H, et al. Cytotoxic T-cells mediate exercise-induced reductions in tumor growth. *eLife.* 2020;9:e59996.

Schmid D, Behrens G, Keimling M, et al. A systematic review and meta-analysis of physical activity and endometrial cancer risk. *European Journal of Epidemiology* 2015; 30(5):397-412.

Wertheim BC, Martinez ME, Ashbeck EL, et al. Physical activity as a determinant of fecal bile acid levels. *Cancer Epidemiology, Biomarkers & Prevention* 2009; 18(5):1591-1598.

Winzer BM, Whiteman DC, Reeves MM, Paratz JD. Physical activity and cancer prevention: a systematic review of clinical trials. *Cancer Causes and Control* 2011; 22(6):811-826.

Chapter 11

Allen BG, et al. Ketogenic diets as an adjuvant cancer therapy: History and potential mechanism. *Redox Biol.* 2014; 2: 963–970.

Barabás J, Németh Z. The opinion of Hungarian Association of Oral and Maxillofacial Surgeons (Magyar Arc-, Állcsont- és Szájsebészeti Társaság) on the justification of supportive treatment of patients with tumorous diseases of the oral cavity. *Hung Med J.* 2006;147(35):1709–1711.

Barisone GA, O'Donnell RT, Ma Y, et al. A purified, fermented, extract of Triticum aestivum has lymphomacidal activity mediated via natural killer cell activation. *PLoS One.* 2018 Jan 5;13(1):e0190860.

Barton DL, Liu H, Dakhil SR, et al. Wisconsin Ginseng (Panax quinquefolius) to improve cancer-related fatigue: a randomized, double-blind trial, N07C2. *J Natl Cancer Inst.* 2013 Aug 21;105(16):1230-8.

Block KI, Mead MN. Immune system effects of echinacea, ginseng, and astragalus: a review. *Integr Cancer Ther.* 2003 Sep;2(3):247-67.

Calder PC. Omega-3 polyunsaturated fatty acids and inflammatory processes: nutrition or pharmacology? *Br J Clin Pharmacol.* 2013 Mar;75(3):645-62.

Canto C, Jiang LQ, Deshmukh AS, et al. Interdependence of AMPK and SIRT1 for metabolic adaptation to fasting and exercise in skeletal muscle. *Cell Metab.* 2010 Mar 3;11(3):213-9.

Canto C, Houtkooper RH, Pirinen E, et al. The NAD(+) precursor nicotinamide riboside enhances oxidative metabolism and protects against high-fat diet-induced obesity. *Cell Metab.* 2012 Jun 6;15(6):838-47.

Chen D, Bruno J, Easlon E, et al. Tissue-specific regulation of SIRT1 by calorie restriction. *Genes Dev.* 2008 Jul 1;22(13):1753-7.

Davis JM, Murphy EA, Carmichael MD, Davis B. Quercetin increases brain and muscle mitochondrial biogenesis and exercise tolerance. *Am J Physiol Regul Integr Comp Physiol.* 2009 Apr;296(4):R1071-7.

Demidov LV, Manziuk LV, Kharkevitch GY, et al. Adjuvant fermented wheat germ extract (Avemar) nutraceutical improves survival of high-risk skin melanoma patients: a randomized, pilot, phase II clinical study with a 7-year follow-up. *Cancer Biother Radiopharm.* 2008;23(4):477–482.

Goodsell DS. The Molecular Perspective: Cytochrome c and Apoptosis. *The Oncologist.* 2004;9(2):226-227.

Guarente L. Mitochondria--a nexus for aging, calorie restriction, and sirtuins? *Cell.* 2008 Jan 25;132(2):171-6.

Hanahan D, Weinberg RA. Hallmarks of cancer: the next generation. *Cell.* 2011 Mar 4;144(5):646-74.

Hanselmann RG, Welter C. Origin of cancer: An information, energy, and matter disease. *Front Cell Develop Biol.* 2016;4:121.

Holmström KM, Kostov RV, Dinkova-Kostova AT. The multifaceted role of Nrf2 in mitochondrial function. *Curr Opin Toxicol.* 2016 Dec;1:80-91.

Hood DA. Mechanisms of exercise-induced mitochondrial biogenesis in skeletal muscle. *Appl Physiol Nutr Metab*. 2009 Jun;34(3):465-72.

Hsu CC, Tseng LM, Lee HC. Role of mitochondrial dysfunction in cancer progression. *Exp Biol Med (Maywood)*. 2016 Jun; 241(12): 1281–1295.

Jakab F, Shoenfeld Y, Balogh A, et al. A medical nutriment has supportive value in the treatment of colorectal cancer. *Br J Cancer*. 2003;89:465–469.

Jin L, Alesi GN, Kang S. Glutaminolysis as a target for cancer therapy. *Oncogene*. 2016 Jul 14;35(28):3619-25.

Kalyanaraman B, Cheng G, Hardy M, et al. A review of the basics of mitochondrial bioenergetics, metabolism, and related signaling pathways in cancer cells: Therapeutic targeting of tumor mitochondria with lipophilic cationic compounds. *Redox Biol*. 2018 Apr;14:316-327.

Khodadadi S, Sobhani N, Mirshekar S, et al. Tumor Cells Growth and Survival Time with the Ketogenic Diet in Animal Models: A Systematic Review. *Int J Prev Med*. 2017 May 25;8:35.

Kienle GS, Kiene H. Review article: Influence of Viscum album L (European mistletoe) extracts on quality of life in cancer patients: a systematic review of controlled clinical studies. *Integr Cancer Ther*. 2010 Jun;9(2):142-57.

Kunnumakkara AB, Bordoloi D, Harsha C, et al. Curcumin mediates anticancer effects by modulating multiple cell signaling pathways. *Clin Sci (Lond)*. 2017 Jul 5;131(15):1781-1799.

Ladas EJ, Kroll DJ, Oberlies NH, et al. A randomized, controlled, double-blind, pilot study of milk thistle for the treatment of hepatotoxicity in childhood acute lymphoblastic leukemia (ALL). *Cancer*. 2010 Jan 15;116(2):506-13.

Lee KM, Hwang MK, Lee DE, Lee KW, Lee HJ. Protective effect of quercetin against arsenite-induced COX-2 expression by targeting PI3K in rat liver epithelial cells. *J Agric Food Chem*. 2010 May 12;58(9):5815-20.

Li Y, Yao J, Han C, et al. Quercetin, Inflammation and Immunity. *Nutrients*. 2016 Mar 15;8(3):167.

Lunby C, Jacobs RA. Adaptations of skeletal mitochondria to exercise training. *Exper Physiol*. 2016 Jan 1;101(1):17-22.

Marcsek Z, et al. The Efficacy of Tamoxifen in Estrogen Receptor–Positive Breast Cancer Cells Is Enhanced by a Medical Nutriment. *Cancer Biother Radiopharm*. 2004;19(6):746-753.

Marie SKN, Oba-Shinjo M. Metabolism and Brain Cancer. *Clinics (Brazil)* 2011;66(S1):33-43.

Menshikova EV, Ritov VB, Fairfull L, et al. Effects of exercise on mitochondrial content and function in aging human skeletal muscle. *J Gerontol A Biol Sci Med Sci*. 2006 Jun;61(6):534-40.

Miriam Valera-Alberni et al. Mitochondrial stress management: a dynamic journey. *Cell Stress*. 2018 Oct 8;2(10): 253 – 274.

McCulloch M, See C, Shu XJ, et al. Astragalus-based Chinese herbs and platinum-based chemotherapy for advanced non-small-cell lung cancer: meta-analysis of randomized trials. *J Clin Oncol*. 2006 Jan 20;24(3):419-30.

Muller AWJ. Cancer is an adaptation that selects in animals against energy dissipation. *Med Hypotheses*. 2017 Jul;104:104-115.

Nigh G. Cancer as Adaptation: Rethinking the Cause and Treatment of Malignancy. *Townsend Letter*. Aug/Sept 2016:37-40.

Ooi VE, Liu F. Immunomodulation and anti-cancer activity of polysaccharide-protein complexes. *Curr Med Chem*. 2000 Jul;7(7):715-29.

Otto C, et al. Antiproliferative and antimetabolic effects behind the anticancer property of fermented wheat germ extract. *BMC Complement Altern Med*. 2016;1:16-160.

Pizzorno J. Mitochondria-Fundamental to Life and Health. *Integr Med (Encinitas)*. 2014 Apr;13(2):8-15.

Potter M, Newport E, Morten KJ. The Warburg effect: 80 years on. *Biochem Soc Trans*. 2016 Oct 15; 44(5): 1499–1505.

Ricca C, Aillon A, Bergandi L, et al. Vitamin D Receptor Is Necessary for Mitochondrial Function and Cell Health. *Int J Mol Sci*. 2018 Jun 5;19(6):1672.

Schmidt M, Pfetzer N, Schwab M, Strauss I, Kämmerer U. Effects of a ketogenic diet on the quality of life in 16 patients with advanced cancer: A pilot trial. *Nutr Metab (Lond)*. 2011 Jul 27;8(1):54.

Seely D, Wu P, Fritz H, et al. Melatonin as adjuvant cancer care with and without chemotherapy: a systematic review and meta-analysis of randomized trials. *Integr Cancer Ther*. 2012 Dec;11(4):293-303.

Seyfried TN, et al. Cancer as a metabolic disease: implications for novel therapeutics. *Carcinogenesis*. 2014 Mar; 35(3): 515–527.

Seyfried TN. Cancer as a mitochondrial metabolic disease. *Front Cell Dev Biol*. 2015;3:43.

Sheng Y, Pero RW, Amiri A, Bryngelsson C. Induction of apoptosis and inhibition of proliferation in human tumor cells treated with extracts of Uncaria tomentosa. *Anticancer Res*. 1998 Sep-Oct;18(5A):3363-8.

Singh BN, Shankar S, Srivastava RK. Green tea catechin, epigallocatechin-3-gallate (EGCG): mechanisms, perspectives and clinical applications. *Biochem Pharmacol*. 2011 Dec 15;82(12):1807-21.

Sinha A, Hollingsworth KG, Ball S, Cheetham T, Improving the Vitamin D Status of Vitamin D Deficient Adults Is Associated With Improved Mitochondrial Oxidative Function in Skeletal muscle. *J Clin Endocrin & Metab. 2012 Mar* 1:98(3):E509–E513.

Tait SW, Green DR. Mitochondrial regulation of cell death. *Cold Spring Harb Perspect Biol*. 2013 Sep 1;5(9):a008706.

Tran B, Jailwala P, Cam M, et al. ONC201 kills breast cancer cells *in vitro* by targeting mitochondria. *Oncotarget*. 2018 Apr 6;9(26):18454-18479.

United Mitochondrial Disease Foundation. What is mitochondrial disease. http://www.umdf.org/what-is-mitochondrial-disease.

Vander Heiden MG. Exploiting tumor metabolism: challenges for clinical translation. *J Clin Invest*. 2013 Sep;123(9):3648-51.

Vander Heiden MG, Cantley LC, Thompson CB. Understanding the Warburg effect: The metabolic requirements of cell proliferation. *Science*. 2009. 324(5930):1029–1033.

Wallace DC. Mitochondria and cancer. *Nat Rev Cancer*. 2012 Oct; 12(10): 685–698.

Wen S, Zhu D, Huang P. Targeting cancer cell mitochondria as a therapeutic approach. *Future Med Chem*. 2013 Jan; 5(1): 53–67.

Wang CW, et al. Preclinical Evaluation on the Tumor Suppression Efficiency and Combination Drug Effects of Fermented Wheat Germ Extract in Human Ovarian Carcinoma Cells. *Evid Based Complement Alternat Med*. 2015: 570-785.

Yang L, Venneti S, Nagrath D. Glutaminolysis: A Hallmark of Cancer Metabolism. *Annu Rev Biomed Eng*. 2017 Jun 21;19:163-194.

Ziello J, Jovin IS, Huanga Y. Hypoxia-Inducible Factor (HIF)-1 Regulatory Pathway and its Potential for Therapeutic Intervention in Malignancy and Ischemia. *Yale J Biol Med*. 2007 Jun; 80(2): 51–60.

Zong WX, Rabinowitz JD, White E. Mitochondria and Cancer. *Molecular Cel*. 2016;61:667-673.

Chapter 12

Abid SH, Malhotra V, Perry MC. Radiation-induced and chemotherapy-induced pulmonary injury.*CurrOpinOncol*. 2001 Jul;13(4): 242-8.

Adnan A, Munoz NM, Prakash P, et al. Hyperthermia and Tumor Immunity.*Cancers (Basel)*. 2021 May 21;13(11):2507. An TT, Liu XY, et al. Primary assessment of treatment effect of thymosin alpha 1 on chemotherapy-induced neurotoxicity. [Article in Chinese].*Ai Zheng 23*.2004 Nov (Suppl 11):1428-30.

Awadalla M, Hassan MZO, Alvi RM, Neilan TG. Advanced imaging modalities to detect cardiotoxicity.*CurrProbl Cancer*. 2018 Jul;42(4): 386-396.

Block KI, Gyllenhaal C, Lowe L, et al. Designing a broad-spectrum integrative approach for cancer prevention and treatment. *Semin Cancer Biol*. 2015 Dec;35 Suppl(Suppl):S276-S304.

Bonuccelli G, De Francesco E, de Boer R, Tanowitz HB, Lisanti MP. NADH autofluorescence, a new metabolic biomarker for cancer stem cells: Identification of Vitamin C and CAPE as natural products targeting "stemness". *Oncotarget*. 2017;8:20667-20678.

Broder H, Gottlieb RA, Lepor NE. Chemotherapy and cardiotoxicity. *Rev Cardiovasc Med*. 2008 Spring;9(2):75-83.

Burnet FM. The concept of immunological surveillance. *Prog Exp Tumor Res*. 1970;13:1-27.

Cancer and Nanotechnology. National Cancer Institute (NCI). www.cancer.gov/nano/cancer-nanotechnology

Champiat S, Lambotte O, Barreau E, et al. Management of immune checkpoint blockade dysimmune toxicities: a collaborative position paper. *Ann Oncol*. 2016 Apr;27(4):559-74.

Chatterjee K, Zhang J, Honbo N, Karliner JS. Doxorubicin cardiomyopathy. *Cardiology*. 2010;115(2):155-62.

Chen DS, Mellman I. Elements of cancer immunity and the cancer-immune set point. *Nature*. 2017 Jan 18;541(7637):321-330.

Chen MY, Li J, Zhang N, et al. In Vitro and in Vivo Study of the Effect of Osteogenic Pulsed Electromagnetic Fields on Breast and Lung Cancer Cells. *Technol Cancer Res Treat*. 2022 Jan-Dec;21: 15330338221124658.

Datta NR, Jain BM, Mathi Z, et al. Hyperthermia: A Potential Game-Changer in the Management of Cancers in Low-Middle-Income Group Countries. Cancers (Basel). 2022 Jan 9;14(2):315.

De Francesco E, Bonuccelli G, Maggiolini M, Sotgia F, Lisanti MP. Vitamin C and Doxycycline: A synthetic lethal combination therapy targeting metabolic flexibility in cancer stem cells (CSCs). *Oncotarget*. 2017;8:67269-67286.

Ding X, Yue W, Chen H. Effect of artesunate on apoptosis and autophagy in tamoxifen resistant breast cancer cells (TAM-R). *Transl Cancer Res*. 2019 Sep;8(5):1863-1872.

Finn OJ. Cancer vaccines: between the idea and the reality. *Nat Rev Immunol.* 2003 Aug;3(8):630-41.

Gettinger SN, Horn L, Gandhi L, et al. Overall Survival and Long-Term Safety of Nivolumab (Anti-Programmed Death 1 Antibody, BMS-936558, ONO-4538) in Patients With Previously Treated Advanced Non-Small-Cell Lung Cancer. *J Clin Oncol.* 2015 Jun 20;33(18):2004-12.

Hodi FS, O'Day SJ, McDermott DF, et al. Improved survival with ipilimumab in patients with metastatic melanoma. *N Engl J Med.* 2010 Aug 19;363(8):711-23.

Integrative Oncology Study Draws Attention for Promising Results. Bastyr University Dec 4, 2013. https://bastyr.edu/about/news/integrative-oncology-study-draws-attention-promising-results

James MO, Jahn SC, Zhong G, et al. Therapeutic applications of dichloroacetate and the role of glutathione transferase zeta-1. *PharmacolTher.* 2017 Feb;170:166-180.

Jiang W, Hu JW, He XR, Jin WL, He XY. Statins: a repurposed drug to fight cancer. *J ExpClin Cancer Res.* 2021 Jul 24;40(1):241.

Jordon MA. Anti-cancer agents. Cur Med Chem. 2002;2:1–17.

Late Effects of Cancer Treatment. National Cancer Institute (NCI). www.cancer.gov/about-cancer/coping/survivorship/late-effects

June CH, Sadelain M. Chimeric Antigen Receptor Therapy. *N Engl J Med.* 2018 Jul 5;379(1):64-73.

Kankotia S, Stacpoole PW. Dichloroacetate and cancer: new home for an orphan drug? *BiochimBiophysActa.* 2014 Dec;1846(2):617-29.

Kato M, Li J, Chuang JL, Chuang DT. Distinct structural mechanisms for inhibition of pyruvate dehydrogenase kinase isoforms by AZD7545, dichloroacetate, and radicicol. *Structure*. 2007 Aug;15(8):992-1004.

Konig M, von Hagens C, Hoth S, et al. Investigation of ototoxicity of artesunate as add-on therapy in patients with metastatic or locally advanced breast cancer: new audiological results from a prospective, open, uncontrolled, monocentric phase I study. *Cancer Chemother-Pharmacol* 77(2): 413-427, 2016.

Lamb R, Ozsvari B, LisantiCL et al. Antibiotics that target mitochondria effectively eradicate cancer stem cells, across multiple tumor types: treating cancer like an infectious disease. *Oncotarget*. 2015 Mar 10;6(7):4569-84.

Lefrak EA, Pitha J, Rosenheim S, Gottlieb JA. A clinicopathologic analysis of adriamycin cardiotoxicity. *Cancer*. 1973 Aug;32(2):302-14.

Li J, Luo Y, Zeng Z, et al. Precision cancer sono-immunotherapy using deep-tissue activatablesemiconducting polymer immunomodulatory nanoparticles. *Nat Commun*. 2022 Jul 12;13(1):4032.

Liu WM, Dalgleish AG. Naltrexone at low doses (LDN) and its relevance to cancer therapy. *Expert Rev Anticancer Ther*. 2022 Mar;22(3): 269-274.

Liubchenko K, Kordbacheh K, Khajehdehi N, et al. Naltrexone's Impact on Cancer Progression and Mortality: A Systematic Review of Studies in Humans, Animal Models, and Cell Cultures. *Adv Ther*. 2021 Feb;38(2):904-924.

Longo J, vanLeeuwen JE, Elbaz M, et al. Statins as Anticancer Agents in the Era of Precision Medicine. *Clin Cancer Res*. 2020 Nov 15; 26 (22): 5791–5800.

Mack MG, Straub R, Eichler K, et al. Breast Cancer Metastases in Liver: Laser-induced Interstitial Thermotherapy—Local Tumor Control Rate and Survival Data. *Radiology* Nov 1, 2004;233(2):400-9.

Miller KD, Nogueira L, et al. Cancer treatment and survivorship statistics, 2022. *CA: A Cancer Journal for Clinicians* Sept/Oct 2022;72(5):409-36.

Mistletoe Extracts (PDQ®), Patient Version. PDQ Integrative, Alternative, and Complementary Therapies Editorial Board. Created: Oct 24, 2005; Published online Feb 28, 2022. https://www.ncbi.nlm.nih.gov/books/NBK65978

Mohammadi S, Soratijahromi E, et al. Phototherapy and Sonotherapy of Melanoma Cancer Cells Using Nanoparticles of Selenium-Polyethylene Glycol-Curcumin as a Dual-Mode Sensitizer. *J Biomed Phys Eng.* 2020 Oct 1;10(5):597-606.

Mudd TW, Guddati AK. Management of hepatotoxicity of chemotherapy and targeted agents. *Am J Cancer Res.* 2021 Jul 15;11(7):3461-3474.

Muñoz NM, Dupuis C, Williams M, et al. Molecularly targeted photothermal ablation improves tumor specificity and immune modulation in a rat model of hepatocellular carcinoma. *Commun Biol.* 2020 Dec 17;3(1):783.

Nanda N, Dhawan DK, Bhatia A, Mahmood A, Mahmood S. Doxycycline Promotes Carcinogenesis & Metastasis via Chronic Inflammatory Pathway: An In Vivo Approach. *PLoS One.* 2016 Mar 21;11(3):e0151539.

Nowak KM, Schwartz MR, Breza VR, Price RJ. Sonodynamic therapy: Rapid progress and new opportunities for non-invasive tumor cell killing with sound. *Cancer Lett.* 2022 Apr 28;532:215592.

Pardoll DM. The blockade of immune checkpoints in cancer immunotherapy. *Nat Rev Cancer.* 2012 Mar 22;12(4):252-64.

Piccolo S, Cordenonsi M, Dupont S. Molecular pathways: YAP and TAZ take center stage in organ growth and tumorigenesis. *Clin Cancer Res*. 2013 Sep 15;19(18):4925-30.

Pirali M, Taheri M, Zarei S, Majidi M, Ghafouri H. Artesunate, as a HSP70 ATPase activity inhibitor, induces apoptosis in breast cancer cells. *Int J BiolMacromol*. 2020 Dec 1;164:3369-3375.

Postow MA, Sidlow R, Hellmann MD. Immune-Related Adverse Events Associated with Immune Checkpoint Blockade. *N Engl J Med*. 2018 Jan 11;378(2):158-168.

Radiation Therapy Side Effects. National Cancer Institute (NCI). www.cancer.gov/about-cancer/treatment/types/radiation-therapy/side-effects

Radiation Therapy To Treat Cancer. National Cancer Institute (NCI). www.cancer.gov/about-cancer/treatment/types/radiation-therapy

Ramadori G, Cameron S. Effects of systemic chemotherapy on the liver. *Ann Hepatol*. 2010 Apr-Jun;9(2):133-43.

Ribas A, Wolchok JD. Cancer immunotherapy using checkpoint blockade. *Science*. 2018 Mar 23;359(6382):1350-1355.

Rosenberg SA, Yang JC, Restifo NP. Cancer immunotherapy: moving beyond current vaccines. *Nat Med*. 2004 Sep;10(9):909-15.

Sanchez W, McGee S, Connor T. et al. Dichloroacetate inhibits aerobic glycolysis in multiple myeloma cells and increases sensitivity to bortezomib. *Br J Cancer*. 2013 Mar 26;108:1624–1633.

Saraei P, Asadi I, Kakar MA, Moradi-Kor N. The beneficial effects of metformin on cancer prevention and therapy: a comprehensive review of recent advances. *Cancer Manag Res*. 2019 Apr 17;11:3295-3313.

Scatena C, Roncella M, Di Paolo A, et al. Doxycycline, an Inhibitor of Mitochondrial Biogenesis, Effectively Reduces Cancer Stem Cells (CSCs) in Early Breast Cancer Patients: A Clinical Pilot Study. *Front Oncol.* 2018 Oct 12;8:452.

Schuster SJ, Bishop MR, Tam CS, et al; JULIET Investigators. Tisagenlecleucel in Adult Relapsed or Refractory Diffuse Large B-Cell Lymphoma. *N Engl J Med.* 2019 Jan 3;380(1):45-56.

Seeds, William A. *Peptide Protocols, Vol. 1.* Geneva, Ohio: Spire Institute, 2020.

Sharma P, Allison JP. The future of immune checkpoint therapy. *Science.* 2015 Apr 3;348(6230):56-61.

Sharma A, Houshyar R, Bhosale P, et al. Chemotherapy induced liver abnormalities: an imaging perspective. *ClinMolHepatol.* 2014 Sep;20(3):317-26.

Singal PK, Deally CM, Weinberg LE. Subcellular effects of adriamycin in the heart: a concise review. *J Mol Cell Cardiol.* 1987 Aug;19(8):817-28.

Slezakova S, Ruda-Kucerova J. Anticancer Activity of Artemisinin and its Derivatives.*Anticancer Res.* 2017 Nov;37(11):5995-6003.

Sorrentino G, Ruggeri N, Specchia V, et al. Metabolic control of YAP and TAZ by the mevalonate pathway. *Nat Cell Biol.* 2014 Apr;16(4):357-66.

Soucek L, Whitfield J, Martins CP, et al. Modelling Myc inhibition as a cancer therapy. *Nature.* 2008 Oct 2;455(7213):679-83.

Su K, Tan L, Liu X, et al. Rapid Photo-Sonotherapy for Clinical Treatment of Bacterial Infected Bone Implants by Creating Oxygen Deficiency Using Sulfur Doping. *ACS Nano.* 2020 Feb 25;14(2):2077-2089.

Sugarman J. Are Mistletoe Extract Injections the Next Big Thing In Cancer Therapy? *John Hopkins Magazine*, Spring 2014. https://hub.jhu.edu/magazine/2014/spring/mistletoe-therapy-cancer

Surgery to Treat Cancer. National Cancer Institute (NCI). www.cancer.gov/about-cancer/treatment/types/surgery

Survival Rates for Colorectal Cancer. American Cancer Society (ACS). www.cancer.org/cancer/types/colon-rectal-cancer/detection-diagnosis-staging/survival-rates.html

Sutendra G, Dromparis P, Kinnaird A, et al. Mitochondrial activation by inhibition of PDKII suppresses HIF1a signaling and angiogenesis in cancer. *Oncogene*. 2013 Mar 28;32(13):1638-50.

Swain SM, Whaley FS, Ewer MS. Congestive heart failure in patients treated with doxorubicin: a retrospective analysis of three trials. *Cancer*. 2003 Jun 1;97(11):2869-79.

Takemura G, Fujiwara H. Doxorubicin-induced cardiomyopathy from the cardiotoxic mechanisms to management. *ProgCardiovasc Dis*. 2007 Mar-Apr;49(5):330-52.

The Pollution in People: Cancer-Causing Chemicals in Americans' Bodies. Environmental Working Group. Jun 14, 2016. https://www.ewg.org/research/pollution-people

Tataranni T, Piccoli C. Dichloroacetate (DCA) and Cancer: An Overview towards Clinical Applications. *Oxid Med Cell Longev*. 2019 Nov 14;2019:8201079.

Toraya-Brown S, Fiering S. Local tumour hyperthermia as immunotherapy for metastatic cancer. *Int J Hyperthermia*. 2014 Dec;30(8):531-9.

Vadala M, Morales-Medina JC, et al. Mechanisms and therapeutic effectiveness of pulsed electromagnetic field therapy in oncology. *Cancer Med*. 2016 Nov;5(11):3128-3139.

Vander Els NJ, Stover D. Chemotherapy-Induced Lung Disease. *Clin Pulmonary Med.* 2004 Mar;11(2):84-91.

Vento S, Cainelli F, Temesgan Z. Lung infections after cancer chemotherapy. *The Lancet Oncology.* 2008 Oct;9(10):982-992.

Von Hoff DD, Layard MW, Basa P, et al. Risk factors for doxorubicin-induced congestive heart failure. *Ann Intern Med.* 1979 Nov;91(5):710-7.

Wang Q, Wu W, Chen X, He C, Liu X. [Effect of pulsed electromagnetic field with different frequencies on the proliferation, apoptosis and migration of human ovarian cancer cells]. Sheng Wu Yi Xue Gong Cheng XueZaZhi. 2012 Apr;29(2):291-5. Chinese. PMID: 22616177.

Weiner LM, Surana R, Wang S. Monoclonal antibodies: versatile platforms for cancer immunotherapy. *Nat Rev Immunol.* 2010 May;10(5):317-27.

Wolchok JD, Chiarion-Sileni V, Gonzalez R, et al. Overall Survival with Combined Nivolumab and Ipilimumab in Advanced Melanoma. *N Engl J Med.* 2017 Oct 5;377(14):1345-1356.

Xu Z, Liu X, Zhuang D. Artesunate inhibits proliferation, migration, and invasion of thyroid cancer cells by regulating the PI3K/AKT/FKHR pathway. *Biochem Cell Biol.* 2022 Feb;100(1):85-92.

Yun J, Mullarky E, Lu C, et al Vitamin C selectively kills KRAS and BRAF mutant colorectal cancer cells by targeting GAPDH. Science 2015 Nov 5;350(6266):1391-1396.

Zhao D, Plotnikoff N, Griffin N, Song T, Shan F. Methionine enkephalin, its role in immunoregulation and cancer therapy. *IntImmunopharmacol.* 2016 Aug;37:59-64.

Zolochevska O, Figueiredo ML. Advances in sonoporation strategies for cancer. Front Biosci (Schol Ed). 2012 Jan 1;4(3):988-1006.

Acknowledgements

This book has grown out of a passion and commitment that would not have taken form without the indispensable individuals who have imparted wisdom, sparked inspiration, and supported me on my journey.

At the outset, my profound gratitude goes to Naturopathic Doctor Ingemar Wiberg. His mentorship in 1987 was instrumental in introducing me to the realm of naturopathy and setting me on the path to this remarkable field of medicine. The foundation of my professional life and my profound respect for this discipline was formed during those seven years of apprenticeship.

Dr. Paul Anderson, whom I consider the godfather of modern integrative oncology, has been an invaluable touchstone. His exhaustive and impartial research serves as a constant reference for my understanding of cancer.

I owe a debt of gratitude to Dr. Neil McKinney for equipping me with invaluable tools. His lifelong commitment to identifying specific cancer drivers and uncovering natural strategies to impact these targets through rigorous scientific research has been truly enlightening.

To Dr. Michael Hamblin and Dr. Michael Weber, I extend my sincere appreciation. Their extensive efforts have advanced our comprehension of light's power in supporting cellular function and inducing cancer cell death through oxidative stress.

Jane McLelland deserves special recognition for her significant contributions in bringing attention to the use of safe, repurposed drugs in the fight against cancer. Her dedicated efforts have paved the way for novel therapeutic interventions.

Nasha Winters, with her infectious enthusiasm, has underscored the importance of addressing the terrain of cancer, fundamentally changing our approach to this formidable disease.

Following Nasha, I must express my admiration for Dr. Dietrich Klinghardt. His pioneering work in developing the techniques of Autonomic Response Testing (ART) and Applied Psychoneurobiology (APN) has been nothing short of transformative. These techniques have been invaluable in refining my diagnostic and treatment approach, enabling me to offer more personalized and specific therapies to my patients.

My heartfelt gratitude goes out to the revered herbalists who shaped my training - Edward Shook, John Christophers, Jethro Kloss, Bernard Jensen, Henry Lindlahr, Alfred Vogel, and Birger Ledin. Their profound wisdom has illuminated my practice.

To my patients, who have continually pushed me to delve deeper for answers, thank you. Your journeys have fuelled my growth and inspiration.

After acknowledging my patients, it is essential to express my deepest gratitude to Larry Trivieri Jr. His tireless contributions have been instrumental to this project, and without him, this book would not have materialized.

Last, but by no means least, I acknowledge the enduring support and love of my wife, Miste, and my mother. Your unwavering belief in my work has been the bedrock of this endeavor.

My deep gratitude extends to all those named and unnamed here. This book stands as a tribute to your influence and support.

About the Author

Michael Karlfeldt, ND, PhD, has been in clinical practice since 1987 and runs a busy integrative medicine center, The Karlfeldt Center, in Boise, Idaho. Dr. Karlfeldt and his staff pride themselves on being compassionate cancer warriors focusing on cutting edge integrative cancer therapies working with international leaders to provide metabolic, genetic, and nutritional solutions to cancer while triggering cancer cell death through targeted oxidation. His drive to investigate and implement effective, restorative and safe cancer therapies was fueled by losing his father to colon cancer in his twenties.

Dr. Karlfeldt's passion to promote Natural Health publicly has lead him to be a sought after lecturer, writer, and educator. He was the host of the Dr. Michael Show, which aired 100 episodes discussing important health-related topics, reaching approximately a million viewers. Currently, he hosts the TV show True Health: Body, Mind, Spirit, which has been available on Amazon Prime for many years. He was also the host of the radio show Health Made Radio where he connects with international leaders in the integrative health arena, and the host of his internationally recognized podcast Integrative Cancer Solutions with Dr. Karlfeldt, where he features cancer survivors sharing how they beat cancer. He also hosts the podcast Integrative Lyme Solutions with Dr. Karlfeldt. where he features people who have successfully conquered Lyme disease.

Dr. Karlfeldt believes in the innate intelligence and healing power of the body and that if it is properly supported spiritually, emotionally and nutritionally it can find its way back to health. Learn more at thekarlfeldt-center.com.

www.ingramcontent.com/pod-product-compliance
Lightning Source LLC
Chambersburg PA
CBHW080538030426
42337CB00024B/4794